METHODS IN MOLECULAR BIOLOGY

Series Editor
John M. Walker
School of Life and Medical Sciences
University of Hertfordshire
Hatfield, Hertfordshire, AL10 9AB, UK

For further volumes:
http://www.springer.com/series/7651

The Wilms' Tumor (WT1) Gene

Methods and Protocols

Edited by

Nicholas Hastie

MRC Human Genetics Unit, University of Edinburgh, Edinburgh, UK

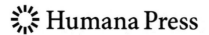

Editor
Nicholas Hastie
MRC Human Genetics Unit
University of Edinburgh
Edinburgh, UK

ISSN 1064-3745   ISSN 1940-6029   (electronic)
Methods in Molecular Biology
ISBN 978-1-4939-8156-4   ISBN 978-1-4939-4023-3   (eBook)
DOI 10.1007/978-1-4939-4023-3

Cover illustration: Section of the kidney of an adult Wt1-GFP knock-in mouse (Hosen et al., Leukemia 21:1783–1791, 2007) showing green fluorescence in the Wt1-expressing podocytes of the glomeruli. Label was enhanced with an anti-GFP antibody and an Alexa480-conjugated secondary antibody. Endothelial cells are labelled in red with an anti-Pecam1 antibody and a Cy5-conjugated secondary antibody. Nuclei are counterstained with DAPI. Author: Dr. Rita Carmona, University of Málaga (Spain).

Printed on acid-free paper

This Humana Press imprint is published by Springer Nature
The registered company is Springer Science+Business Media LLC New York

Preface

I was delighted when asked by John Walker whether I would be interested in editing a volume on the Wilms' tumor gene (WT1), for the distinguished Methods in Molecular Biology Series. However my first thought was to question whether a single gene would cover sufficient ground for a complete volume. I was heartened by the fact that similar successful volumes in the series had been compiled on other genes, notably p53. Also on further consideration I realized WT1 would be ideal. It is a multifunctional protein, mutations in which may lead to a variety of disorders in humans, including the eponymous pediatric kidney cancer, leukemia, gonadal dysgenesis, and occasionally diaphragmatic hernia and heart disease. WT1 is a key regulator of the development of a number of tissues, particularly those involving switches between mesenchymal-epithelial switches; in addition to the kidney, gonads, and heart it has been shown to mark and regulate stem/progenitors for visceral fat. Beyond its role in development, WT1 has been shown to be required for the homeostasis of a number of adult tissues and to be activated in tissue repair. WT1 is a zinc finger protein that clearly in part regulates all these cellular processes by functioning as a transcription factor. However an increasing body of evidence suggests that WT1 also regulates post-transcriptional processes by binding to RNA. What is more, two major WT1 splice isoforms differing by only three amino acids appear to have different relative roles in transcription and post-transcriptional processes. Finally, as WT1 is expressed in a number of adult epithelial tumors but not the healthy tissue counterparts immune cancer therapies against the protein are being trialed. All these facets ensure that WT1 is a rich source for methods chapters. The volume starts with three review chapters to set the scene. These cover the involvement of WT1 in pediatric cancer, kidney disease, and tissue development and homeostasis. These are followed by methods chapters, firstly on tools for studying developmental and cellular processes. These include chapters on cell marking and lineage tracing, epicardial cell methodology, colony forming assays for bone marrow stem cells, isolation of adipocyte progenitors using Fluorescence Activated Cell Sorting, methods for studying angiogenesis, and multiphoton imaging of lipids. All these chapters deal exclusively with mice and mouse tissues/cells. Zebrafish provide another valuable organism for studying Wt1 biology and function, so there is an overview of Wt1 in zebrafish followed by two valuable methods chapters on immunohistochemistry in zebrafish and isolation of kidney podocytes. The remaining methods chapters cover some of the latest tools in Genomics, Molecular Biology, and Biochemistry. These begin with methods for dissecting transcription factor function in cell-free systems and for measuring the binding constants of protein-nucleic acid interaction. These are followed by chapters on ChIP-Seq to identify transcriptional targets and methods for identifying WT1-interacting RNA and proteins. The final methods chapter describes bioinformatic approaches for analyzing Next Generation Sequence data. To round the volume off there is a chapter on Cancer Immune Therapy based on antibodies to WT1. This is a combination of overview and some methodological detail. All the chapters are by experts in the field and I was delighted when everyone approached agreed to write a chapter. I thank the authors and editors and do hope the readers find this volume helpful.

Edinburgh, UK   *Nicholas Hastie*

Contents

Contributors

STUART AITKEN • *Medical Research Council—Human Genetics Unit, Institute of Genetics and Molecular Medicine, Western General Hospital, University of Edinburgh, Edinburgh, Scotland, UK*

THOMAS J.D. BATES • *Leibniz Institute for Age—Fritz Lipmann Institute, Jena, Germany*

RUTHROTHASELVI BHARATHAVIKRU • *Medical Research Council-Human Genetics Unit, Institute of Genetics and Molecular Medicine, Western General Hospital, University of Edinburgh, Edinburgh, Scotland, UK*

JOCELYN CHARLTON • *UCL Institute of Child Health, London, UK*

YOU-YING CHAU • *MRC Human Genetics Unit, MRC Institute of Genetics and Molecular Medicine, University of Edinburgh, Edinburgh, UK; British Heart Foundation Centre for Cardiovascular Science, The Queen's Medical Research Institute, University of Edinburgh, Edinburgh, UK*

LOUISE CLEAL • *MRC Human Genetics Unit, MRC Institute of Genetics and Molecular Medicine, University of Edinburgh, Edinburgh, UK*

TATIANA DUDNAKOVA • *Wellcome Trust Centre for Cell Biology, The University of Edinburgh, Edinburgh, UK*

CHRISTOPH ENGLERT • *Leibniz Institute for Age—Fritz Lipmann Institute, Jena, Germany; Friedrich Schiller University, Jena, Germany*

JANAT FAZAL-SALOM • *CELLTEC-UB, Cellular Biology Department, University of Barcelona, Barcelona, Spain*

PWF HADOKE • *University/BHF Centre for Cardiovascular Science, The Queen's Medical Research Institute, University of Edinburgh, Edinburgh, Scotland, UK*

NICHOLAS HASTIE • *MRC Human Genetics Unit, Institute of Genetics and Molecular Medicine, Western General Hospital, University of Edinburgh, Edinburgh, Scotland, UK*

ALEX VON KRIEGSHEIM • *Systems Biology Ireland, Conway Institute, Belfield, Ireland*

MARTIN LEE • *Institute of Genetics and Molecular Medicine, University of Edinburgh, Edinburgh, Scotland, UK*

OFELIA M. MARTÍNEZ-ESTRADA • *CELLTEC-UB, Cellular Biology Department, University of Barcelona, Barcelona, Spain*

FILIPPO MASSA • *Institute of Biology Valrose, Université de Nice-Sophia, Nice, Cedex 2, France; Inserm, UMR1091, Nice, France; CNRS, UMR7277, Nice, France*

RICHARD J. MCGREGOR • *University/BHF Centre for Cardiovascular Science, The Queen's Medical Research Institute, University of Edinburgh, Edinburgh, Scotland, UK; MRC Human Genetics Unit, Institute of Genetics and Molecular Medicine, Western General Hospital, University of Edinburgh, Edinburgh, Scotland, UK*

SOPHIE MCHAFFIE • *MRC Human Genetics Unit, MRC Institute of Genetics and Molecular Medicine, University of Edinburgh, Edinburgh, Scotland, UK*

EVE MILLER-HODGES • *ECAT Clinical Lecturer—Nephrology, IGMM Human Genetics Unit, Western General Hospital, University of Edinburgh, Edinburgh, Scotland, UK*

RAMON MUÑOZ-CHAPULI • *Department of Animal Biology, University of Malaga, Malaga, Spain*

UTA NAUMANN • *Leibniz Institute for Age—Fritz Lipmann Institute, Jena, Germany*

SUMIYUKI NISHIDA • *Department of Respiratory Medicine, Allergy and Rheumatic Disease, Graduate School of Medicine, Osaka University, Suita-City, Osaka, Japan*

R. OGLEY • *University/BHF Centre for Cardiovascular Science, The Queen's Medical Research Institute, University of Edinburgh, Edinburgh, Scotland, UK*

BIRGIT PERNER • *Leibniz Institute for Age—Fritz Lipmann Institute, Jena, Germany*

KATHY PRITCHARD-JONES • *Hugh and Catherine Stevenson Professor of Paediatric Oncology, UCL Institute of Child Health, London, UK*

STEFAN G.E. ROBERTS • *School of Cellular and Molecular Medicine, University of Bristol, Office G50, Biomedical Sciences Building, University Walk, Bristol, UK*

PAUL J. ROMANIUK • *Department of Biochemistry and Microbiology, University of Victoria, Victoria, BC, Canada*

ANDREAS SCHEDL • *Institute of Biology Valrose, Université de Nice-Sophia, Nice, Cedex 2, France; Inserm, UMR1091, Nice, France; CNRS, UMR7277, Nice, France*

ALAN SERRELS • *Institute of Genetics and Molecular Medicine, University of Edinburgh, Edinburgh, Scotland, UK*

FABIO DA SILVA • *Institute of Biology Valrose, Université de Nice-Sophia, Nice, Cedex 2, France; Inserm, UMR1091, Nice, France; CNRS, UMR7277, Nice, France*

HARUO SUGIYAMA • *Department of Functional Diagnostic Science, Graduate School of Medicine, Osaka University, Osaka, Japan*

VÍCTOR VELECELA • *MRC Human Genetics Unit, Institute of Genetics and Molecular Medicine, University of Edinburgh, Edinburgh, UK; CELLTEC-UB, Cellular Biology Department, University of Barcelona, Barcelona, Spain*

BETTINA WILM • *Department of Cellular and Molecular Physiology, Institute of Translational Medicine, University of Liverpool, Liverpool, UK*

Chapter 1

WT1 Mutation in Childhood Cancer

Jocelyn Charlton and Kathy Pritchard-Jones

Abstract

In this chapter, the role of *WT1* in childhood cancer is discussed, using the key examples Wilms' tumor, desmoplastic small round cell of childhood, and leukemia. The role of *WT1* in each disease is described and mirrored to the role of *WT1* in normal development.

Key words Childhood cancer, Development, Desmoplastic small round cell tumor of childhood, Leukemia, Minimal residual disease, Wilms' tumor

1 Introduction

Since the first description of its tissue-specific expression pattern in 1990, it has been evident that *WT1* is essential for the development of several organs [1–3]. Hence, it is not surprising that genetic aberrations involving the gene are identified in various childhood cancers, including Wilms' tumor, desmoplastic small round cell tumor of childhood, and some leukemias. In this chapter, the role of *WT1* in each of these cancers will be discussed and similarities drawn between tumorigenesis and the role of *WT1* in development.

2 WT1 in Wilms' Tumor

2.1 WT1, Kidney Development and Wilms' Tumor

The gene *WT1* (Wilms' tumor 1) was first characterized in the context of the childhood kidney cancer, Wilms' tumor, also known as nephroblastoma, and was rapidly shown to play a role in normal renal development [1, 3, 4]. Wilms' tumor affects 1 in 10,000 children, generally before their 15th birthday. It is the most common childhood renal tumor, comprising ~85 % of all renal tumors in childhood. The median age at diagnosis is only just over 3 years of age, and it occurs at much higher frequencies in children with specific malformation syndromes that confer a greatly increased risk of genetic predisposition, some of which are due to heritable

Nicholas Hastie (ed.), *The Wilms' Tumor (WT1) Gene: Methods and Protocols*, Methods in Molecular Biology, vol. 1467, DOI 10.1007/978-1-4939-4023-3_1, © Springer Science+Business Media New York 2016

WT1 mutation. Based on the earlier age of onset in patients with bilateral Wilms' tumor or family history, the two-hit model of cancer generation was proposed by Knudson for the role of the *WT1* gene in Wilms' tumor [5]. Further research showed that this model does not fit the majority of Wilms' tumor cases and somatic *WT1* mutation or deletion is observed in only 5–25 % of sporadic Wilms' tumors, depending on the ethnicity of the population [6]. Although this may seem low, it is actually one of the most frequently mutated genes in Wilms' tumor.

The majority of Wilms' tumors consist of a triphasic mixed composition of blastemal, epithelial, and stromal cells, often showing remarkable resemblance to embryonic kidney, albeit with a disrupted architecture. These tumors are often associated with presumed precursor lesions of undifferentiated embryonic tissue retained in the post-natal kidney, termed nephrogenic rests (NRs). Wilms' tumors associated with *WT1* aberration, both germline and sporadic, often show a stromal predominant composition and are associated with intralobar NRs (ILNRs) [7].

ILNRs are thought to rise earlier in development in comparison to their counterpart, the perilobar NR (PLNR). This deduction is based on their presence towards the renal medulla where early nephrogenesis is initiated, and their histological composition, with so-called "heterologous" elements, suggesting that their precursor cells retain the full differentiation capacity of uncommitted metanephric mesenchyme [5]. *WT1* mutation has been observed frequently in ILNRs but not PLNRs, suggesting a timing dependence for *WT1* aberration and tumor formation in renal development.

The driving role of aberrant *WT1* in Wilms' tumor stems from its essential function in kidney development (reviewed in refs. 8 and 9). During renal development, the ureteric bud, extending from the Wolffian duct, invades the metanephric mesenchyme and reciprocal signaling between these components induces both ureteric bud branching and condensation of the mesenchyme. The mesenchyme then undergoes mesenchymal to epithelial transition (MET) before forming the epithelial nephron. During this process, Wt1 has been shown to be essential for MET [10]. Various lines of evidence indicate that the pre-MET mesenchymal renal progenitor is the Wilms' tumor cell of origin [11], thereby confirming the significance of *WT1* in both renal development and Wilms' tumorigenesis. Despite the clear relationship between *WT1* aberration during development and Wilms' tumor, there is clear evidence that the timing is extremely significant, as *WT1* mutations occurring very early or very late in renal development do not necessarily result in tumor formation. Although *WT1* is a bone fide Wilms' tumor gene, the first knock out mouse model (deletion of exon 1) showed embryonic lethality due to failure of kidney and gonad development, instead of Wilms' tumor [4]. This lack of tumors in mice homozygous for the *Wt1* mutation is due to complete apoptosis of the metanephric blastema, with no mesenchymal cells detectable by gestational day E12. These mice also showed abnormal growth of the mesothelium, heart, and lungs. Mutations in late renal development result in glomerular sclerosis rather than cancer, demonstrating further roles of *WT1* in late nephrogenesis [12].

Despite many efforts to generate a *WT1* mutant mouse model that developed Wilms' tumor, this was not achieved until 21 years after *WT1* was originally characterized in humans and required combined *Wt1* mutation with activation of *Igf2* [13]. This showed that, at least in murine embryonic kidney, *Wt1* mutation alone was insufficient to induce tumor formation, with 0/23 *Wt1* mutant mice with normal *Igf2* developing tumors compared to 7/11 with *Wt1* mutation and loss of imprinting of *Igf2*, causing overexpression. This study demonstrates that disruption of two different cellular processes is required for Wilms' tumor formation, likely dysregulation of normal renal differentiation (i.e., *Wt1* mutation) combined with cellular proliferation (i.e., *Igf2* overexpression).

3 Constitutional WT1 Loss and Wilms' Tumor

It was the discovery of large, cytogenetically visible deletions encompassing the short arm of chromosome 11, cytoband p13 in children with Wilms' tumor, aniridia, genitourinary abnormalities, and mental retardation (WAGR) syndrome that pointed the way to the positional cloning of *WT1* [14]. Here, aniridia and genitourinary malformation are dominant phenotypes whereas Wilms' tumor occurs in only 45–57% of cases [15, 16]. Patients with WAGR syndrome were shown to harbor genetic deletion of contiguous genes on chromosome 11, including the *WT1* gene whose impact on genitourinary malformation and Wilms' tumor predisposition is inseparable. The related phenotype of aniridia is associated with loss of the nearby *PAX6* gene whilst only children with large deletions that presumably affect hundreds of genes have mental retardation.

Denys-Drash syndrome (DDS), recognized as a triad of gonadal dysgenesis, early onset nephropathy, and Wilms' tumor predisposition, was also shown to be due to constitutional mutation of the *WT1* gene, but this time with intragenic mutation rather than gene deletion [17]. As originally defined, around 74% of children born with DDS develop Wilms' tumor [18]. However, a wide range of mutations have been associated with the syndrome, with the majority affecting the *WT1* DNA-binding domain, specifically within exon 9 [18]. Subsequently, it has been recognized that children with a partial DDS phenotype may carry *WT1* mutation, and these may be at atypical sites causing a truncated protein rather than a missense mutation [19]. In these cases, the renal nephropathy phenotype may be less severe than those cases originally described, as indeed may the risk of developing Wilms' tumor [19].

Frasier syndrome is caused by *WT1* mutation, however not within the DNA-binding domain but within the intronic region affecting splicing of the gene. These mutations prevent formation of one of two potential isoforms affecting inclusion of three amino acids (KTS) between the third and fourth zinc fingers of WT1. The +KTS and −KTS isoforms have different DNA-binding capabilities and the +KTS isoform, which is hemizygous in Frasier syndrome, is believed to be more important in WT1's RNA binding properties. It is therefore intriguing that the typical tumor found in Frasier syndrome is gonadoblastoma rather than Wilms' tumor. Also, the progressive glomerulopathy results in end-stage renal failure in adolescence rather than the very early childhood years typical of DDS. Both syndromes are associated with a similar spectrum of genitourinary abnormalities that can include complete pseudohermaphroditism.

Germline *WT1* aberrations significantly increase the likelihood of developing bilateral Wilms' tumor. Overall, 5 % Wilms' tumors are bilateral; however 20% patients with DDS [18] and 17% patients with WAGR [20] get bilateral Wilms' tumors or Wilms' tumor in one kidney with nephroblastomatosis in the other.

Several studies of constitutional predisposition syndromes and Wilms' tumor [21–24] clearly demonstrate that tumors due to *WT1* mutation can follow the two-hit tumor suppressor model as proposed by Knudson; however, the genetic pathways are often more complex and may involve WT1 acting in a dominant (onco-genic) or dominant-negative fashion or requiring additional events for full malignant conversion. Demonstrating this, a different clinical phenotype is observed for patients with *WT1* loss and *WT1* mutation, where a more severe genitourinary phenotype is observed in patients whose tissues should express a mutant WT1 protein compared to those with complete loss and therefore a "simple" difference in dosage of the wild-type protein. Furthermore, the selection pressure to lose the second allele may differ between genotypes as the risk of WT is lower in WAGR than DDS cases. This may be due to a lower frequency of loss of the second allele when the first hit is a large deletion that encompasses neighboring genes, some of which may be required for cell survival. Wilms' tumor is very infrequently observed in patients with Frasier syndrome, who have only altered splicing of *WT1*.

4   WT1 and Other Mutations in Wilms' Tumor

Compared to other mutations commonly found in sporadic Wilms' tumor, *WT1* is considered an early event, as the presence of *WT1* mutations have also been observed in NRs [25]. Conversely, activating mutations in *CTNNB1* have been described as late events due to their absence in NRs. *CTNNB1* and *WT1* mutations often occur in the same tumor [26], indicating a strong selection for β-catenin activation and an increase in Wnt signaling in *WT1* mutant cases.

Other mutations commonly found in sporadic WTs include *WTX* (also known as *AMER1*) (18%), *TP53* (5%), and *MYCN* (3.8%). *WTX* has been associated with *WT1* transcriptional control [27], *TP53* directly interacts with WT1 [28, 29], and in the developing kidney, WT1 and MYCN are co-expressed and WT1 mediates MYCN expression. Upon mutation of the *WT1* DNA-binding domain, MYCN has shown to be upregulated [30, 31]. This evidence demonstrates the dependent role of WT1 in Wilms' tumorigenesis. WT1 also interacts with the epigenome, both at a chromatin level where Wt1 has been shown to mediate Wnt4 expression in a tissue-dependent manner [32] and at the level of DNA methylation where WT1 has been shown to regulate DNMT3A expression [33]. Epigenetic alterations are common in cancer and may be driven by initial WT1 aberration in these cases.

5   WT1 and Desmoplastic Small Round Cell Tumor of Childhood

Desmoplastic small round cell tumor (DSRCT) of childhood and adolescence is also associated with aberration of *WT1*; however in this instance, *WT1* is involved in a reciprocal chromosomal translocation that results in overexpression of an aberrant fusion protein. DSRCT is most commonly found in the abdomen and shows a male predominance of 90%. The tumor shows a characteristic histology, not dissimilar to Wilms' tumor, with extensive stromal tissue surrounding islands of undifferentiated desmoplastic cells displaying epithelial, neural, myogenic, and mesenchymal markers [34]. Due to this observed histology, DSRCTs are thought to originate from mesothelial or submesothelial progenitor cells maintaining their potential for multilineage differentiation. Of note, the mesothelium is a tissue that shows strong *WT1* expression in embryogenesis [1] that continues into adult life where the WT1 expressing cells are thought to indicate adult "stem cells" for maintenance of tissues of mesodermal origin [35].

The chromosomal translocation responsible for DSRCTs involves fusion of 11p13 and 22q12, bringing together the N-terminal domains of *EWS* and the C-terminal DNA-binding domain (zinc fingers 2–4) of *WT1* [36]. *EWS*, originally identified as the gene involved in translocations causing Ewing's sarcoma, encodes a putative RNA binding protein, which is a member of the TET family of proteins. The chimeric protein functions as an aberrant transcription factor, resulting in a difference in target gene specificity. Several downstream events have been associated with an upregulation of EWS-WT1 including upregulation of endogenous platelet-derived growth factor A (PDGFA) [37], induction of IL2 receptor β [38], induction of the exocytosis regulator BAIAP3 [39], and induction of TALLA-1 [40], reviewed in ref. 41. However, none of these have been able to recapitulate the transforming potential attributed to EWS-WT1 and the chimera itself is difficult to characterize due to uncertainty of the cell of origin as well as challenging cell culture conditions and the heterologous nature of the primary tumor. Interestingly, the fusion protein is not oncogenic in other cell lines, again showing a cell specificity and timing dependence during development [37].

6   WT1 and Leukemia

6.1   Leukemia and WT1 Expression

Leukemia is a cancer of the hematopoietic system. There are four main types of leukemia including acute myeloid leukemia (AML), acute lymphoblastic leukemia (ALL), chronic myeloid leukemia (CML), and chronic lymphocytic leukemia (CLL). The initial indication that *WT1* abnormalities may be involved in leukemia came from two observations. First, *WT1* mRNA "overexpression" was found in acute leukemia cell lines when these were assessed as part of a panel of cell types that showed its tight tissue-specific expression [1]. Second, an independent somatic *WT1* mutation was found in a case of AML that developed many years later in a survivor of Wilms' tumor who had WAGR syndrome. The different "second hits" in the initial Wilms' tumor and the subsequent AML showed that the two cancers were more likely to be the result of the underlying genetic predisposition due to constitutional deletion of one copy of *WT1* rather than due to any mutagenic consequence of the chemotherapy for Wilms' tumor which had consisted only of vincristine and actinomycin D [42]. Subsequently it has been found that the frequency of *WT1* mutations in leukemia is relatively low and the more commonly observed aberration is a high level of WT1 expression. *WT1* is expressed at very low levels in normal human bone marrow, specifically in CD34+ cells [43]; conversely, *WT1* is highly expressed in around 80 % leukemias with immature leukemia cells showing higher levels of WT1 expression than more mature cells [44].

So what is the role of WT1 overexpression in leukemia? As previously mentioned, Wt1 knockout in mice is embryonic lethal, although no hematopoietic defect was noted. Furthermore, fetal liver cells from WT1 deficient mice can reconstitute the hematopoietic system of irradiated adult mice, showing no defect in differentiation potential or proliferation [45]. Despite this evidence suggesting that WT1 is not required for normal hematopoiesis, further evidence demonstrated a role for Wt1 in self-renewal of early murine hematopoietic cells [46, 47]. In one of these studies, forced overexpression of Wt1 resulted in increased bone marrow cellularity. However production of mature cells was normal and these mice did not develop leukemia without the presence of "second-hit" AML-ETO (a common gene fusion in

AML) transfection [47]. In this case, Wt1 maintained self-renewal capacity while AML-ETO blocked differentiation resulting in leukemia onset. Forced expression of *WT1* in human hematopoietic progenitor cells resulted in strong anti-proliferative effects due to induced maturation [48]. However in leukemia cells, WT1 is a surrogate marker of proliferation [49] and has been shown to confer oncogenic properties in AML cell lines [50]. Overall, WT1 is considered to be a marker of early progenitor cells that becomes aberrantly overexpressed in leukemia and is associated with leukemia cell proliferation.

6.2 WT1 Mutation in Leukemia

For both childhood and adult AML with normal karyotype, *WT1* mutations occurred at a frequency of 10–12% [51–53]. In the latter study, 54% patients with mutations had at least one *WT1* aberration (i.e., two mutations or mutation and deletion) suggesting a dominant-negative role for *WT1* in AML. For each of these studies, significantly inferior overall survival was observed in cases carrying *WT1* mutation. In a separate study, *WT1* mutation frequency was 5% in childhood AML with mutations occurring in younger patients ($P=0.02$); however, in this study, the mutations were not observed in cases with normal karyotype but a similar inferior overall survival was observed [54]. The largest study to date investigated 3157 AML patients for *WT1* mutation in exons 7 and 9, finding a frequency of 5.5%, but an absence of mutations in cases with complex karyotypes and the mutations occurring, generally, in samples with no other common genetic mutations in AML [55]. These mutations were not stable as, from analysis of 35 relapsed patients, one-third lost their *WT1* mutation at relapse. Across the whole cohort, mutation of *WT1* had no clinical impact. However for normal karyotype AML, *WT1* mutation was associated with shorter event-free survival (10.8 vs. 17.9 m, $P=0.008$). Furthermore, a multivariate analysis showed that *WT1* mutation had an independent inverse impact on event-free survival. Overall, *WT1* mutation occurs at a low frequency in AML, in cases with favorable cytogenetics, and is associated with poor prognosis.

WT1 mutation is less common in ALL (found in 1 of 23) [56] and not common in CML blast crisis (found in 0 of 39) [57]. Acute T-lymphoblastic leukemia showed *WT1* exon 7 mutations in 20/238 cases and showed higher WT1 expression as well as immature histological features [58]. For those patients with *WT1* mutation, patients showed similar inferior relapse-free survival as seen in AML.

The mechanisms by which point mutations in *WT1* may drive poor prognosis are poorly characterized. However, leukemia cells with deletions of the entire zinc-finger binding domain (delZ), a leukemia-associated phenotype was identified; inducing delZ in vitro caused increased proliferation of human hematopoietic CD34+ cells and upregulation of genes involved in cell division and maturation, promoting cell proliferation and expansion of progenitor cells [59].

In contrast to *WT1* mutations, a SNP (rs16754) in exon 7 of *WT1* has been shown to correlate with favorable outcome for patients with childhood AML [60], and a follow-up study showed that stratification based on the presence of the SNP may aid prognosis [61].

6.3 WT1 and Prognosis in Leukemia

WT1 overexpression is an independent negative indicator for predicting complete remission rate, disease-free survival, and overall survival of cytogenetically normal AML patients [62], and correlates with progression of clinical phase in acute leukemia [63]. In particular, the level of WT1 in the bone marrow present at the first complete remission was shown to be an independent prognostic factor for disease-free and overall survival in 89 patients with AML followed from diagnosis through treatment [64]. For accurate measurement of WT1 levels, the authors suggest that bone marrow is superior to peripheral blood for relapse prediction [64]. For both acute promyelocytic leukemia (APL) and T-lymphoblastic leukemia, either very low or very high expression of WT1 at diagnosis showed inferior overall survival in comparison to intermediate expression levels [58, 65]. Conversely, WT1 expression at diagnosis did not correlate with relapse, disease-free or overall survival for childhood ALL [66].

6.4 Minimal Residual Disease

Minimal residual disease (MRD) is a term used to describe the very low, microscopically invisible levels of leukemia cells that must still be present in the bone marrow when morphological remission is achieved. According to the molecular method used, a threshold level of residual leukemia can be defined which can be monitored during treatment. MRD status is used for risk stratification and if MRD remains "positive," this is predictive of relapse. Therefore, early detection of MRD can save lives as further treatment can be given prior to major relapse. In the mid-1990s it became apparent that levels of WT1 mRNA could be used as a marker of MRD, and could predict clinical relapse. In some cases, levels of WT1 mRNA were detected 2–8 months prior to clinical relapse becoming apparent [63, 67]. Another study showed detectable WT1 levels by reverse transcriptase (rt)-PCR 1–18 months (mean 7 months) before clinical relapse became apparent [68]. The same study compared the use of bone marrow and peripheral blood to detect MRD and concluded that peripheral blood was superior for WT1 quantitation for the detection of MRD. In general, levels of WT1 are assayed for using rt-PCR; however it was recently shown that flow cytometry to detect MRD in combination with analysis of WT1 gene expression improved the reliability of MRD-based prognostic stratification [69].

Despite some controversial evidence [70], in general, using WT1 as a marker for MRD in adult AML seems promising [71, 72]. For childhood AML, WT1 quantification was deemed an informative molecular marker for MRD and was studied in a prospective study as part of the French ELAM02 protocol [73].

An increase of WT1 levels was detected in 16/44 cases, which subsequently relapsed within a median of 38 days (range 8–180 days). This study concluded that quantification of WT1 may be used for MRD studies and for prognostication in AML [74]. Similarly, despite the absence of WT1 mutation as discussed previously, CML patients in accelerate phase or blast crisis showed much higher WT1 expression levels than normal blood or CML patients in chronic phase [75]. Therefore, WT1 could be a useful marker for MRD and therapeutic efficacy in CML. Conversely, for childhood ALL, WT1 appears to be expressed variably and at much lower levels than AML and is thought to be an unattractive marker for MRD; however it does represent an independent risk factor with very low or very high levels associated with increased likelihood of relapse [76]. This was confirmed for adult ALL whereby WT1 expression did not correlate with MRD detection or relapse [77].

Overall, analysis of WT1 in AML seems to show the most promising results. A panel of genes including WT1 simplified into a small TacMan Low Density array has been proposed for this purpose and shows strong prognostic impact independent of previously defined AML risk factors [78].

6.5 Using Antibodies Against WT1 to Target Leukemia

As a therapy to treat patients with leukemia, targeting cells that express WT1 is a good approach as WT1 shows such low expression in other normal tissues. Current post-remission treatment aims to make the immune system sensitized to WT1 antigen so that upon relapse, the immune system responds by destroying the WT1 expressing tumor cells. For this purpose the use of antigen-loaded dendritic cells to activate immune response against WT1 in patients with AML in a phase I/II trial showed positive immune responses; however further studies are needed [79].

Another, more widely used approach uses *WT1* peptides to stimulate cytotoxic T cells to target WT1-expressing leukemia cells and has shown encouraging early results [80–85] and was shown to not inhibit colony formation of normal hematopoietic cells that express WT1 at physiological levels. This approach was shown to be successful in the mouse [86, 87], and promising human clinical trials for WT1 peptide-based cancer immunotherapy have been described [88, 89]. Worryingly, some patients enrolled in a WT1 peptide phase II vaccination trial (NCT00153582) relapsed despite forming a WT1-specific T cell response; however it was shown that this was not due to defects in antigen presentation caused by loss or mutation of WT1 [90]. Furthermore, one phase I/II clinical trial of subcutaneous peptide vaccination in AML showed poor secondary expansion [91]. In general, this therapy shows great potential, and combined vaccines for several leukemia antigens are now being tested (phase I/II trials) with promising results (reviewed in ref. 92).

Instead of using a peptide to stimulate a patient's immune system, it is possible to transfect patient's T cells (using retroviral gene transfer) with a specific receptor for WT1 [93]. TCR-transduced T cells kill leukemia cells in vitro and in a mouse model and display WT1-specific cytokine production [94]. Another potential therapy involved targeting WT1 using siRNA therapy. In cell lines, WT1 expression was reduced, proliferation was inhibited, and apoptosis was induced [95]. Finally, monoclonal antibodies (mAbs) could be used to target WT1 expressing leukemia cells. MAbs H2 and HCl7 could readily detect WT1 in newly diagnosed acute leukemia [96]. The mAb ESK1, a fully human "T cell receptor like" mAb specific for WT1, was shown to bind in vitro and in vivo and cleared disseminated leukemia from mice models showing its potential as a therapeutic agent [97]. This mAb was later enhanced to improve antibody-dependent cell-mediated cytotoxicity, improving its efficacy [98].

7   Conclusion

In summary, *WT1* plays a significant role in a variety of cancers occurring mainly in childhood and adolescence, but with involvement in some adult cancers, as described here for leukemia and elsewhere in this book for solid tumors. The consequence of *WT1* aberration depends on the tissue and time point during development at which the aberration occurs (or whether it is constitutional), and the specific mutation or change in expression levels of the protein. Whilst we now have a vast knowledge of the complex structure and potential functions of the WT1 protein and its isoforms, we have much less understanding of how these cancer-associated aberrations drive tumorigenesis. The simple "two-hit" inactivation of its tumor suppressor function may explain a proportion of Wilms' tumors but has not yet led to any targeted therapeutic interventions. WT1 clearly can have oncogenic properties as well, and it may be that overexpression of the wild-type protein provides a meaningful therapeutic target for intervention, as is currently being tested in clinical trials in adult leukemias.

References

1. Pritchard-Jones K, Fleming S, Davidson D et al (1990) The candidate Wilms' tumour gene is involved in genitourinary development. Nature 346(6280):194–197

2. Moore AW, Mcinnes L, Kreidberg J, Hastie ND, Schedl A (1999) Yac complementation shows a requirement for WT1 in the development of epicardium, adrenal gland and throughout nephrogenesis. Development 126(9):1845–1857

3. Call KM, Glaser T, Ito CY et al (1990) Isolation and characterization of a zinc finger polypeptide gene at the human chromosome 11 Wilms' tumor locus. Cell 60(3):509–520

4. Kreidberg JA, Sariola H, Loring JM et al (1993) Wt-1 is required for early kidney development. Cell 74(4):679–691

5. Knudson AG Jr, Strong LC (1972) Mutation and cancer: a model for Wilms' tumor of the kidney. J Natl Cancer Inst 48(2):313–324

6. Kaneko Y, Okita H, Haruta M et al (2015) A high incidence of WT1 abnormality in bilateral Wilms' tumours in Japan, and the penetrance rates in children with WT1 germline mutation. Br J Cancer 112:1121–1133

7. Beckwith JB, Kiviat NB, Bonadio JF (1990) Nephrogenic rests, nephroblastomatosis, and the pathogenesis of Wilms' tumor. Fetal Pediatr Pathol 10(1-2):1–36

8. Ozdemir DD, Hohenstein P (2014) WT1 in the kidney—a tale in mouse models. Pediatr Nephrol 29(4):687–693

9. Hohenstein P, Pritchard-Jones K, Charlton J (2015) The yin and yang of kidney development and Wilms' tumors. Genes Dev 29(5):467–482

10. Davies JA, Ladomery M, Hohenstein P et al (2004) Development of an siRNA-based method for repressing specific genes in renal organ culture and its use to show that the WT1 tumour suppressor is required for nephron differentiation. Hum Mol Genet 13(2):235–246

11. Li CM, Guo M, Borczuk A et al (2002) Gene expression in Wilms' tumor mimics the earliest committed stage in the metanephric mesenchymal-epithelial transition. Am J Pathol 160(6):2181–2190

12. Miller-Hodges E, Hohenstein P (2012) WT1 in disease: shifting the epithelial–mesenchymal balance. J Pathol 226(2):229–240

13. Hu Q, Gao F, Tian W et al (2011) WT1 ablation and Igf2 upregulation in mice result in Wilms' tumors with elevated ERK1/2 phosphorylation. J Clin Invest 121(1):174–183

14. Rose EA, Glaser T, Jones C et al (1990) Complete physical map of the WAGR region of 11p13 localizes a candidate Wilms' tumor gene. Cell 60(3):495–508

15. Fischbach BV, Trout KL, Lewis J, Luis CA, Sika M (2005) WAGR syndrome: a clinical review of 54 cases. Pediatrics 116(4):984–988

16. Muto R, Yamamori S, Ohashi H, Osawa M (2002) Prediction by fish analysis of the occurrence of Wilms' tumor in Aniridia patients. Am J Med Genet 108(4):285–289

17. Pelletier J, Bruening W, Kashtan CE et al (1991) Germline mutations in the Wilms' tumor suppressor gene are associated with abnormal urogenital development in Denys-Drash syndrome. Cell 67(2):437–447

18. Mueller RF (1994) The Denys-Drash syndrome. J Med Genet 31(6):471–477

19. Bardeesy N, Zabel B, Schmitt K, Pelletier J (1994) WT1 mutations associated with incomplete Denys-Drash syndrome define a domain predicted to behave in a dominant-negative fashion. Genomics 21(3):663–664

20. Breslow NE, Norris R, Norkool PA et al (2003) Characteristics and outcomes of children with the Wilms' tumor-Aniridia syndrome: a report from the National Wilms' Tumor Study Group. J Clin Oncol 21(24):4579–4585

21. Shibata R, Takata A, Hashiguchi A, Umezawa A, Yamada T, Hata J (2003) Responsiveness of chemotherapy based on the histological type and Wilms' tumor suppressor gene mutation in bilateral Wilms' tumor. Pathol Int 53(4):214–220

22. Royer-Pokora B, Weirich A, Schumacher V et al (2008) Clinical relevance of mutations in the Wilms' tumor suppressor 1 gene WT1 and the cadherin-associated protein beta1 gene CTNNB1 for patients with Wilms' tumors: results of long-term surveillance of 71 patients from International Society of Pediatric Oncology study 9/Society for Pediatric Oncology. Cancer 113(5):1080–1089

23. Santin S, Fraga G, Ruiz P et al (2011) Wt1 mutations may be a cause of severe renal failure due to nephroblastomatosis in Wilms' tumor patients. Clin Nephrol 76(3):244–248

24. Hu M, Fletcher J, Mccahon E et al (2013) Bilateral Wilms' tumor and early presentation in pediatric patients is associated with the truncation of the Wilms' tumor 1 protein. J Pediatr 163(1):224–229

25. Fukuzawa R, Heathcott RW, More HE, Reeve AE (2007) Sequential WT1 and CTNNB1 mutations and alterations of β-catenin localisation in intralobar nephrogenic rests and associated Wilms' tumours: two case studies. J Clin Pathol 60(9):1013–1016

26. Li CM, Kim CE, Margolin AA et al (2004) CTNNB1 mutations and overexpression of wnt/beta-catenin target genes in WT1-mutant Wilms' tumors. Am J Pathol 165(6):1943–1953

27. Rivera MN, Kim WJ, Wells J et al (2009) The tumor suppressor WTX shuttles to the nucleus and modulates WT1 activity. Proc Natl Acad Sci 106(20):8338–8343

28. Maheswaran S, Park S, Bernard A et al (1993) Physical and functional interaction between WT1 and p53 proteins. Proc Natl Acad Sci U S A 90(11):5100–5104

29. Maheswaran S, Englert C, Bennett P, Heinrich G, Haber DA (1995) The WT1 gene product stabilizes p53 and inhibits p53-mediated apoptosis. Genes Dev 9(17):2143–2156

30. Zhang X, Xing G, Saunders GF (1999) Proto-oncogene n-myc promoter is down regulated by the Wilms' tumor suppressor gene WT1. Anticancer Res 19(3A):1641–1648

31. Udtha M, Lee SJ, Alam R, Coombes K, Huff V (2003) Upregulation of c-MYC in WT1-

mutant tumors: assessment of WT1 putative transcriptional targets using cDNA microarray expression profiling of genetically defined Wilms' tumors. Oncogene 22(24):3821–3826

32. Essafi A, Webb A, Rachel B et al (2011) A wt1-controlled chromatin switching mechanism underpins tissue-specific wnt4 activation and repression. Dev Cell 21(3):559–574

33. Szemes M, Dallosso AR, Melegh Z et al (2013) Control of epigenetic states by WT1 via regulation of de novo DNA methyltransferase 3A. Hum Mol Genet 22(1):74–83

34. Chang F (2006) Desmoplastic small round cell tumors: cytologic, histologic, and immunohistochemical features. Arch Pathol Lab Med 130(5):728–732

35. Chau YY, Brownstein D, Mjoseng H et al (2011) Acute multiple organ failure in adult mice deleted for the developmental regulator wt1. PLoS Genet 7(12):e1002404

36. Ladanyi M, Gerald W (1994) Fusion of the EWS and WT1 genes in the desmoplastic small round cell tumor. Cancer Res 54(11):2837–2840

37. Lee SB, Kolquist KA, Nichols K et al (1997) The EWS-WT1 translocation product induces PDGFA in desmoplastic small round-cell tumour. Nat Genet 17(3):309–313

38. Wong JC, Lee SB, Bell MD et al (2002) Induction of the interleukin-2/15 receptor beta-chain by the EWS-WT1 translocation product. Oncogene 21(13):2009–2019

39. Palmer RE, Lee SB, Wong JC et al (2002) Induction of BAIAP3 by the EWS-WT1 chimeric fusion implicates regulated exocytosis in tumorigenesis. Cancer Cell 2(6):497–505

40. Ito E, Honma R, Imai J et al (2003) A tetraspanin-family protein, T-cell acute lymphoblastic leukemia-associated antigen 1, is induced by the Ewing's sarcoma-Wilms' tumor 1 fusion protein of desmoplastic small round-cell tumor. Am J Pathol 163(6):2165–2172

41. Gerald WL, Haber DA (2005) The EWS-WT1 gene fusion in desmoplastic small round cell tumor. Semin Cancer Biol 15(3):197–205

42. Pritchard-Jones K, Renshaw J, King-Underwood L (1994) The Wilms' tumour (WT1) gene is mutated in a secondary leukaemia in a WAGR patient. Hum Mol Genet 3(9):1633–1637

43. Hosen N, Sonoda Y, Oji Y et al (2002) Very low frequencies of human normal CD34+ haematopoietic progenitor cells express the Wilms' tumour gene WT1 at levels similar to those in leukaemia cells. Br J Haematol 116(2):409–420

44. Inoue K, Ogawa H, Sonoda Y et al (1997) Aberrant overexpression of the Wilms' tumor gene (WT1) in human leukemia. Blood 89(4):1405–1412

45. King-Underwood L, Little S, Baker M et al (2005) Wt1 is not essential for hematopoiesis in the mouse. Leuk Res 29(7):803–812

46. Alberta JA, Springett GM, Rayburn H et al (2003) Role of the WT1 tumor suppressor in murine hematopoiesis. Blood 101(7):2570–2574

47. Nishida S, Hosen N, Shirakata T et al (2006) AML1-ETO rapidly induces acute myeloblastic leukemia in cooperation with the Wilms' tumor gene, WT1. Blood 107(8):3303–3312

48. Svedberg H, Richter J, Gullberg U (2001) Forced expression of the Wilms' tumor 1 (WT1) gene inhibits proliferation of human hematopoietic CD34(+) progenitor cells. Leukemia 15(12):1914–1922

49. Olszewski M, Huang W, Chou PM, Duerst R, Kletzel M (2005) Wilms' tumor 1 (WT1) gene in hematopoiesis: a surrogate marker of cell proliferation as a possible mechanism of action? Cytotherapy 7(1):57–61

50. Li Y, Wang J, Li X et al (2014) Role of the Wilms' tumor 1 gene in the aberrant biological behavior of leukemic cells and the related mechanisms. Oncol Rep 32(6):2680–2686

51. Paschka P, Marcucci G, Ruppert AS et al (2008) Wilms' tumor 1 gene mutations independently predict poor outcome in adults with cytogenetically normal acute myeloid leukemia: A cancer and leukemia group b study. J Clin Oncol 26(28):4595–4602

52. Bowen D, Groves MJ, Burnett AK et al (2009) TP53 gene mutation is frequent in patients with acute myeloid leukemia and complex karyotype, and is associated with very poor prognosis. Leukemia 23(1):203–206

53. Hollink IH, Van Den Heuvel-Eibrink MM, Zimmermann M et al (2009) Clinical relevance of Wilms' tumor 1 gene mutations in childhood acute myeloid leukemia. Blood 113(23):5951–5960

54. Renneville A, Boissel N, Zurawski V et al (2009) Wilms' tumor 1 gene mutations are associated with a higher risk of recurrence in young adults with acute myeloid leukemia: a study from the Acute Leukemia French Association. Cancer 115(16):3719–3727

55. Krauth MT, Alpermann T, Bacher U et al (2014) WT1 mutations are secondary events in AML, show varying frequencies and impact on prognosis between genetic subgroups. Leukemia 29(3):660–667

56. King-Underwood L, Pritchard-Jones K (1998) Wilms' tumor (WT1) gene mutations occur mainly in acute myeloid leukemia and may confer drug resistance. Blood 91(8):2961–2968

57. Carapeti M, Goldman JM, Cross NC (1997) Dominant-negative mutations of the Wilms' tumour predisposing gene (WT1) are infrequent in CML blast crisis and de novo acute leukaemia. Eur J Haematol 58(5):346–349

58. Heesch S, Goekbuget N, Stroux A et al (2010) Prognostic implications of mutations and expression of the Wilms' tumor 1 (WT1) gene in adult acute T-lymphoblastic leukemia. Haematologica 95(6):942–949

59. Vidovic K, Ullmark T, Rosberg B et al (2013) Leukemia associated mutant Wilms' tumor gene 1 protein promotes expansion of human hematopoietic progenitor cells. Leuk Res 37(10):1341–1349

60. Ho PA, Kuhn J, Gerbing RB et al (2011) WT1 synonymous single nucleotide polymorphism rs16754 correlates with higher mRNA expression and predicts significantly improved outcome in favorable-risk pediatric acute myeloid leukemia: a report from the children's oncology group. J Clin Oncol 29(6):704–711

61. Ho PA, Alonzo TA, Gerbing RB et al (2014) The prognostic effect of high diagnostic WT1 gene expression in pediatric AML depends on WT1 SNP rs16754 status: report from the children's oncology group. Pediatr Blood Cancer 61(1):81–88

62. Lyu X, Xin Y, Mi R et al (2014) Overexpression of Wilms' tumor 1 gene as a negative prognostic indicator in acute myeloid leukemia. PLoS One 9(3):e92470

63. Inoue K, Sugiyama H, Ogawa H et al (1994) Wt1 as a new prognostic factor and a new marker for the detection of minimal residual disease in acute leukemia. Blood 84(9):3071–3079

64. Ommen HB, Nyvold CG, Braendstrup K et al (2008) Relapse prediction in acute myeloid leukaemia patients in complete remission using WT1 as a molecular marker: development of a mathematical model to predict time from molecular to clinical relapse and define optimal sampling intervals. Br J Haematol 141(6):782–791

65. Hecht A, Nolte F, Nowak D et al (2015) Prognostic importance of expression of the Wilms' tumor 1 gene in newly diagnosed acute promyelocytic leukemia. Leuk Lymphoma 56(8):1–7

66. Gaiger A, Linnerth B, Mann G et al (1999) Wilms' tumour gene (WT1) expression at diagnosis has no prognostic relevance in childhood acute lymphoblastic leukaemia treated by an intensive chemotherapy protocol. Eur J Haematol 63(2):86–93

67. Brieger J, Weidmann E, Maurer U, Hoelzer D, Mitrou PS, Bergmann L (1995) The Wilms' tumor gene is frequently expressed in acute myeloblastic leukemias and may provide a marker for residual blast cells detectable by PCR. Ann Oncol 6(8):811–816

68. Inoue K, Ogawa H, Yamagami T et al (1996) Long-term follow-up of minimal residual disease in leukemia patients by monitoring WT1 (Wilms' tumor gene) expression levels. Blood 88(6):2267–2278

69. Marani C, Clavio M, Grasso R et al (2013) Integrating post induction WT1 quantification and flow-cytometry results improves minimal residual disease stratification in acute myeloid leukemia. Leuk Res 37(12):1606–1611

70. Elmaagacli AH, Beelen DW, Trenschel R, Schaefer UW (2000) The detection of wt-1 transcripts is not associated with an increased leukemic relapse rate in patients with acute leukemia after allogeneic bone marrow or peripheral blood stem cell transplantation. Bone Marrow Transplant 25(1):91–96

71. Nowakowska-Kopera A, Sacha T, Florek I, Zawada M, Czekalska S, Skotnicki AB (2009) Wilms' tumor gene 1 expression analysis by real-time quantitative polymerase chain reaction for monitoring of minimal residual disease in acute leukemia. Leuk Lymphoma 50(8):1326–1332

72. Bergmann L, Miething C, Maurer U et al (1997) High levels of Wilms' tumor gene (wt1) mRNA in acute myeloid leukemias are associated with a worse long-term outcome. Blood 90(3):1217–1225

73. Lapillonne H, Renneville A, Auvrignon A et al (2006) High WT1 expression after induction therapy predicts high risk of relapse and death in pediatric acute myeloid leukemia. J Clin Oncol 24(10):1507–1515

74. Weisser M, Kern W, Rauhut S et al (2005) Prognostic impact of RT-PCR-based quantification of WT1 gene expression during MRD monitoring of acute myeloid leukemia. Leukemia 19(8):1416–1423

75. Cao XS, Gu WY, Chen ZX, Hu SY, He J, Cen JN (2007) Bone marrow WT1 gene expression and clinical significance in chronic myelogenous leukemia. Zhonghua Nei Ke Za Zhi 46(4):277–279

76. Boublikova L, Kalinova M, Ryan J et al (2006) Wilms' tumor gene 1 (WT1) expression in childhood acute lymphoblastic leukemia: a

wide range of WT1 expression levels, its impact on prognosis and minimal residual disease monitoring. Leukemia 20(2):254–263

77. Imashuku S, Terui K, Matsuyama T et al (2003) Lack of clinical utility of minimal residual disease detection in allogeneic stem cell recipients with childhood acute lymphoblastic leukemia: Multi-institutional collaborative study in Japan. Bone Marrow Transplant 31(12):1127–1135

78. Osumi K, Fukui T, Kiyoi H et al (2002) Rapid screening of leukemia fusion transcripts in acute leukemia by real-time PCR. Leuk Lymphoma 43(12):2291–2299

79. Van Tendeloo VF, Van De Velde A, Van Driessche A et al (2010) Induction of complete and molecular remissions in acute myeloid leukemia by Wilms' tumor 1 antigen-targeted dendritic cell vaccination. Proc Natl Acad Sci U S A 107(31):13824–13829

80. Oka Y, Elisseeva OA, Tsuboi A et al (2000) Human cytotoxic T-lymphocyte responses specific for peptides of the wild-type Wilms' tumor gene (WT1) product. Immunogenetics 51(2):99–107

81. Ohminami H, Yasukawa M, Fujita S (2000) HLA class I-restricted lysis of leukemia cells by a CD8(+) cytotoxic T-lymphocyte clone specific for WT1 peptide. Blood 95(1):286–293

82. Azuma T, Makita M, Ninomiya K, Fujita S, Harada M, Yasukawa M (2002) Identification of a novel WT1-derived peptide which induces human leucocyte antigen-A24-restricted anti-leukaemia cytotoxic t lymphocytes. Br J Haematol 116(3):601–603

83. Yasukawa M (2001) Immunotherapy for leukemia targeting the Wilms' tumor gene. Leuk Lymphoma 42(3):267–273

84. Tsuboi A, Oka Y, Udaka K et al (2002) Enhanced induction of human WT1-specific cytotoxic T lymphocytes with a 9-mer WT1 peptide modified at HLA-A*2402-binding residues. Cancer Immunol Immunother 51(11-12):614–620

85. Guo Y, Niiya H, Azuma T et al (2005) Direct recognition and lysis of leukemia cells by WT1-specific CD4+ T lymphocytes in an HLA class II-restricted manner. Blood 106(4):1415–1418

86. Oka Y, Tsuboi A, Elisseeva OA, Udaka K, Sugiyama H (2002) Wt1 as a novel target antigen for cancer immunotherapy. Curr Cancer Drug Targets 2(1):45–54

87. Nakajima H, Kawasaki K, Oka Y et al (2004) WT1 peptide vaccination combined with BCG-CWS is more efficient for tumor eradication than WT1 peptide vaccination alone. Cancer Immunol Immunother 53(7):617–624

88. Oka Y, Tsuboi A, Murakami M et al (2003) Wilms' tumor gene peptide-based immunotherapy for patients with overt leukemia from myelodysplastic syndrome (MDS) or MDS with myelofibrosis. Int J Hematol 78(1):56–61

89. Oka Y, Tsuboi A, Taguchi T et al (2004) Induction of WT1 (Wilms' tumor gene)-specific cytotoxic T lymphocytes by WT1 peptide vaccine and the resultant cancer regression. Proc Natl Acad Sci U S A 101(38):13885–13890

90. Busse A, Letsch A, Scheibenbogen C et al (2010) Mutation or loss of Wilms' tumor gene 1 (WT1) are not major reasons for immune escape in patients with AML receiving WT1 peptide vaccination. J Transl Med 8:5

91. Uttenthal B, Martinez-Davila I, Ivey A et al (2014) Wilms' tumour 1 (WT1) peptide vaccination in patients with acute myeloid leukaemia induces short-lived WT1-specific immune responses. Br J Haematol 164(3):366–375

92. Casalegno-Garduno R, Schmitt A, Schmitt M (2011) Clinical peptide vaccination trials for leukemia patients. Expert Rev Vaccines 10(6):785–799

93. Xue SA, Gao L, Hart D et al (2005) Elimination of human leukemia cells in NOD/SCID mice by WT1-TCR gene-transduced human T cells. Blood 106(9):3062–3067

94. Xue SA, Gao L, Thomas S et al (2010) Development of a Wilms' tumor antigen-specific T-cell receptor for clinical trials: engineered patient's T cells can eliminate autologous leukemia blasts in NOD/SCID mice. Haematologica 95(1):126–134

95. Elmaagacli AH, Koldehoff M, Peceny R et al (2005) WT1 and BCR-ABL specific small interfering RNA have additive effects in the induction of apoptosis in leukemic cells. Haematologica 90(3):326–334

96. Menssen HD, Renkl HJ, Rodeck U, Kari C, Schwartz S, Thiel E (1997) Detection by monoclonal antibodies of the Wilms' tumor (WT1) nuclear protein in patients with acute leukemia. Int J Cancer 70(5):518–523

97. Dao T, Yan S, Veomett N et al (2013) Targeting the intracellular WT1 oncogene product with a therapeutic human antibody. Sci Transl Med 5(176):176ra133

98. Veomett N, Dao T, Liu H et al (2014) Therapeutic efficacy of an Fc-enhanced TCR-like antibody to the intracellular WT1 oncoprotein. Clin Cancer Res 20(15):4036–4046

Chapter 2

Clinical Aspects of *WT1* and the Kidney

Eve Miller-Hodges

Abstract

For more than 30 years, *WT1* mutations have been associated with complex developmental syndromes involving the kidney. Acting as a transcription factor, *WT1* is expressed throughout the nephron and controls the reciprocal interactions and phenotypic changes required for normal renal development. In the adult, WT1 expression remains extremely high in the renal podocyte, and at a lower level in the parietal epithelial cells. Wt1-null mice are unable to form kidneys [1]. Unsurprisingly, *WT1* mutations lead to significant abnormalities of the renal and genitourinary tract, causing a number of human diseases including syndromes such as Denys–Drash syndrome, Frasier syndrome, and WAGR syndrome. Recent methodological advances have improved the identification of *WT1* mutations, highlighting its importance even in nonsyndromic renal disease, particularly in steroid-resistant nephrotic syndrome. This vast spectrum of *WT1*-related disease typifies the varied and complex activity of WT1 in development, disease, and tissue maintenance.

Key words Renal podocyte, Nephrotic syndrome, Glomerular sclerosis, Mesangial cells, Genitourinary syndromes, Genetic testing, Transplantation

1   WAGR Syndrome

The first *WT1*-associated disease to be identified was WAGR syndrome (Wilms' tumor, Aniridia, Genitourinary malformation, and mental Retardation), caused by deletions of 11p13, and the loss of both *WT1* and *Pax6* [2]. Approximately 50 % of WAGR patients develop Wilms' tumor [2, 3] and the renal prognosis for patients both with and without Wilms' tumor is poor, with a cumulative risk of renal failure ranging from 40 to 60 % by the age of 20 [4]. The most common pathological finding is focal segmental sclerosis (FSGS), originally attributed to glomerular hyperfiltration, as a consequence of reduced nephron mass following nephrectomy. However, proteinuria and nephrotic syndrome, with FSGS on renal biopsy, have been identified in WAGR patients without Wilms' tumor, indicating complete loss of one *WT1* allele alone may induce FSGS [5]. Animal models of the renal phenotype, such as the *Wt1*-heterozygous mouse, support this conclusion, as glomerular sclerosis develops in this model with aging [6, 7].

Nicholas Hastie (ed.), *The Wilms' Tumor (WT1) Gene: Methods and Protocols*, Methods in Molecular Biology, vol. 1467, DOI 10.1007/978-1-4939-4023-3_2, © Springer Science+Business Media New York 2016

2   Denys–Drash Syndrome

Denys–Drash syndrome (DDS) is the best characterized *WT1*-related disorder. The classic syndrome consists of Wilms' tumor, rapidly progressive glomerular disease, and genitourinary abnormalities, particularly male pseudohermaphroditism. The characteristic renal disease is diffuse mesangial sclerosis, assumed to be a developmental or paracrine effect, as WT1 is not expressed in mature mesangial cells. DDS tends to be associated with mutations in the DNA-binding domains of *WT1*. This is thought to affect transcription factor activity, and the profound phenotype may result from the mutant protein acting in a dominant negative manner, as cell lines expressing DDS mutations abolish binding to known WT1-binding targets [8].

A number of animal models of DDS have been developed, which partially recapitulate the human disease, although only one Wilms' tumor has ever been described [9, 10]. These, in combination with conditionally immortalized DDS podocytes in culture, provide evidence of an abnormal podocyte phenotype in DDS. This is unsurprising given the continued high expression of WT1 in the adult podocyte, and profound podocyte damage following conditional Wt1 loss [11]. Histology and immunohistochemical analysis of DDS kidneys demonstrates podocytes are hypertrophied and effaced, with areas of continued proliferation, especially where WT1 expression is lowest. Overexpression of PDGFa and TGFB in these areas is consistent with a pathological epithelial to mesenchymal transition [12]. More recently, evidence has emerged indicating that podocytes in DDS resemble an earlier developmental stage, having not differentiated fully. DDS podocytes continue to express the stimulatory form of VEGF-A (VEGF165), which is normally only expressed from the S-shaped body stage of nephron development, and stimulates glomerular endothelial cell proliferation, migration, and differentiation [13]. Upon differentiation, mature podocytes begin to express an inhibitory form of VEGF (VEGF165b). Using semiquantitative PCR to analyze human biopsy specimens, this is completely lacking in DDS podocytes [14]. This study also revealed that glomerular basement membrane constituents in DDS patients also resemble those at the S-shaped body developmental stage, with high levels of collagen α1(IV) and laminin β1 and a relative lack of collagen α4(IV) and laminin β2, which are normally found in normal adult glomeruli. The authors interpret this to mean that DDS podocytes are halted in development and do not proceed fully through differentiation. The paracrine influence of abnormal podocytes and an impaired glomerular filtration barrier would explain the profound nephrosis and diffuse mesangial sclerosis in these patients.

3 Frasier Syndrome

Frasier syndrome (FS) describes the combination of male pseudohermaphroditism, predisposition to gonadoblastoma and glomerular disease (usually FSGS), which causes renal failure within the first two decades of life. It is usually caused by point mutations affecting the splice sites in exon 9 of the *WT1* gene. The risk of Wilms' tumor is much lower than in DDS [15, 16]. Splice site mutations lead to an imbalance in the expression of the *WT1*-KTS isoforms, with relative underexpression of the +KTS isoform. This is known to play a role post-transcriptionally as a binding partner for splicing factors and is located in splicing speckles [17–19]. Mouse models unable to express either the +KTS or –KTS isoform have differing renal phenotypes, although neither is as severe as the *Wt1*-null mouse, implying a degree of redundancy is present [17, 18]

4 Meacham Syndrome

Meacham syndrome describes a rare and complex multi-malformation syndrome reminiscent of the *Wt1*-null mouse. The phenotype includes male pseudohermaphroditism, abnormal female internal genitalia, complex congenital heart defects, and diaphragmatic hernia [20]. *WT1* mutations have been found in a number of cases, affecting the DNA-binding zinc finger regions and including mutations previously described in DDS.

Importantly, these genotype-phenotype correlations are not clear-cut. The mutations described are generally associated with their relevant syndromes, but exceptions exist. Intron 9 splice site mutations have been described in patients with clinical DDS but without Wilms' tumor [21], and intron 9 mutations which should not have affected splicing have been found in patients with clinical Frasier syndrome [22]. The influence of other modifying genes or environmental factors remains a subject for further research.

Stronger correlation between genotype and phenotype is found with regard to risk from Wilms' tumor. A recent paper reviewed over 50 patients with nephrotic syndrome. Those with missense or nonsense mutations, as is usually found in DDS, were found to have a high risk of Wilms' tumor, whereas splice mutations, as seen in patients with Frasier Syndrome, had a very low risk [23]. The mechanisms explaining this difference are not clear, but are attributed to the potential dominant negative effect of DDS mutant protein.

5   Nonsyndromic Renal Disease

Advances in genetic technology and sequencing techniques have led to an increased recognition of the role of *WT1* mutations in nonsyndromic renal disease. *WT1* mutations have been found to cause up to 12% of SRNS in children and young adults, particularly in phenotypic females. This is on par with the most common genetic cause of SRNS, *NPHS2* (podocin) mutations, which account for up to 26% of cases [24].

Given its complexity, screening for *WT1* and other genetic mutations in SRNS has been difficult. Traditional Sanger sequencing techniques were time-consuming and expensive, particularly as there exists significant genetic heterogeneity and phenotypic variability amongst the various causes of SRNS. Even limiting genetic analysis to the most frequently mutated causative genes remained expensive, and therefore missed unusual and/or multiple mutations [25].

Next Generation sequencing allows for increased throughput and decreased cost, thus facilitating the cost-effective and simultaneous analysis of multiple genes. This has led to the identification of novel genes associated with SRNS as well as expanding the genetic heterogeneity of the condition. *WT1*-associated renal diseases are no exception, with the identification of a familial form of incomplete DDS due to a classic exon 9 DDS mutation (1180C>T: R394W). An unaffected father passed the mutation to his son and daughter [26]. This family demonstrated a DDS-like phenotype in the son, FS-like phenotype in the daughter, and an unaffected father despite all carrying the same classic DDS mutation. Widespread application of NGS techniques to allow simultaneous analysis of multiple genes may provide answers as to the phenotypic variability demonstrated in *WT1*-related disorders by identifying novel genetic variants and disease-modifying alleles [23].

Nonsyndromic *WT1* mutations have also been identified as a cause of inherited autosomal dominant FSGS. Whole exome and direct sequencing techniques were used to investigate the cause of AD FSGS in two northern-European families. A nonsynonymous heterozygous missense change in exon 9 (1327G>A; R458Q) was identified. Unlike WT mRNA, R458Q mRNA was unable to rescue zebrafish morpholinos unable to express Wt1a (one of the two zebrafish Wt1 orthologs) and expression of WT1R458Q in HEK293 cells reduced the expression of podocyte-specific genes including nephrin, synaptopodin, and CD2AP relative to wild-type WT1, consistent with an abnormal podocyte phenotype leading to FSGS [27].

This is the first paper to demonstrate potentially direct regulation of synaptopodin expression by WT1. However, efficacious treatment of SRNS caused by *WT1* mutations has been demonstrated via the use of cyclosporin. This is not thought to be via its immunosuppressive effect, but via prevention of synaptopodin degradation, and thus stabilization of the podocyte cytoskeleton [28].

Nonsyndromic forms of kidney disease have been caused by splice site mutations in intron 9 in 46,XX females (usually associated with Frasier syndrome). Missense mutations in exons 8 and 9 (usually associated with DDS) have also been found in cases of isolated diffuse mesangial sclerosis without Wilms' tumor [29, 30].

From a methodological point of view, these developments have highlighted the importance of genetic testing in steroid resistant nephrotic syndrome in the clinic. As described above, a few cases of nephrotic syndrome caused by *WT1* mutations have been reported which demonstrated a partial response to cyclosporin treatment. In general, genetic causes of nephrotic syndrome do not respond well to immunosuppression so given the toxic side effect profile and lack of efficacy, expert opinion suggests these agents should be avoided or used cautiously [31]. The ability to rapidly screen for *WT1* mutations, and/or specific WT1 mutations that may confer a more favorable risk/benefit profile could offer important therapeutic options to this subgroup of patients. Given the variability of genotype-phenotype correlations, genetic testing also remains vital for other family members when screening for potential organ donors and for the likelihood of disease recurrence in a transplanted graft, and, in theory, for pre-emptive treatment strategies. Although no evidence yet exists for preventative treatment in affected individuals, it is known in other genetic forms of kidney disease that such strategies can be successful, such as the specific use of Angiotensin Converting Enzyme inhibitors in Alport syndrome [32, 33].

6   Conclusion

The importance of *WT1* mutations in developmental renal disorders has been long recognized. Novel genetic technologies, particularly rapid sequencing techniques, have allowed the identification of far more *WT1* mutations, relevant to clinical practice, and thus highlighting the range of *WT1* disease and variable phenotype-genotype correlation. The cause of these profound differences and the wide range of phenotypes provide a focus for further research into the molecular biology of *WT1* as described in subsequent chapters.

References

1. Kreidberg JA, Sariola H, Loring JM et al (1993) WT-1 is required for early kidney development. Cell 74(4):679–691

2. Fischbach BV, Trout KL, Lewis J et al (2005) WAGR syndrome: a clinical review of 54 cases. Pediatrics 116(4):984–988

3. Muto R, Yamamori S, Ohashi H et al (2002) Prediction by FISH analysis of the occurrence of Wilms' tumor in aniridia patients. Am J Med Genet 108(4):285–289

4. Breslow NE, Takashima JR, Ritchey ML et al (2000) Renal failure in the Denys-Drash and Wilms' tumor-aniridia syndromes. Cancer Res 60(15):4030–4032

5. Iijima K, Someya T, Ito S et al (2012) Focal segmental glomerulosclerosis in patients with complete deletion of one WT1 allele. Pediatrics 129(6):e1621–e1625

6. Guo JK, Menke AL, Gubler MC et al (2002) WT1 is a key regulator of podocyte function:

reduced expression levels cause crescentic glomerulonephritis and mesangial sclerosis. Hum Mol Genet 11(6):651–659

7. Menke AL, IJpenberg A, Fleming S, Ross A et al (2003) The wt1-heterozygous mouse; a model to study the development of glomerular sclerosis. J Pathol 200(5):667–674

8. Little M, Holmes G, Bickmore W et al (1995) DNA binding capacity of the WT1 protein is abolished by Denys-Drash syndrome WT1 point mutations. Hum Mol Genet 4(3):351–358

9. Gao F, Maiti S, Sun G et al (2004) The Wt1+/ R394W mouse displays glomerulosclerosis and early-onset renal failure characteristic of human Denys-Drash syndrome. Mol Cell Biol 24(22):9899–9910

10. Ratelade J, Arrondel C, Hamard G et al (2010) A murine model of Denys-Drash syndrome reveals novel transcriptional targets of WT1 in podocytes. Hum Mol Genet 19(1):1–15

11. Chau YY, Brownstein D, Mjoseng H et al (2011) Acute multiple organ failure in adult mice deleted for the developmental regulator Wt1. PLoS Genet 7(12):e1002404

12. Yang AH, Chen JY, Chen BF (2004) The dysregulated glomerular cell growth in Denys-Drash syndrome. Virchows Arch 445(3):305–314

13. Robert B, Zhao X, Abrahamson DR (2000) Coexpression of neuropilin-1, Flk1, and VEGF(164) in developing and mature mouse kidney glomeruli. Am J Physiol Renal Physiol 279(2):F275–F282

14. Schumacher VA, Jeruschke S, Eitner F, Becker JU, Pitschke G, Ince Y, Miner JH, Leuschner I, Engers R, Everding AS, Bulla M, Royer-Pokora B (2007) Impaired glomerular maturation and lack of VEGF165b in Denys-Drash syndrome. J Am Soc Nephrol 18(3):719–729

15. Auber F, Jeanpierre C, Denamur E et al (2009) Management of Wilms' tumors in Drash and Frasier syndromes. Pediatr Blood Cancer 52(1):55–59

16. Barbosa AS, Hadjiathanasiou CG, Theodoridis C et al (1999) The same mutation affecting the splicing of WT1 gene is present on Frasier syndrome patients with or without Wilms' tumor. Hum Mutat 13(2):146–153

17. Hammes A, Guo JK, Lutsch G et al (2001) Two splice variants of the Wilms' tumor 1 gene have distinct functions during sex determination and nephron formation. Cell 106(3):319–329

18. Hastie ND (2001) Life, sex, and WT1 isoforms—three amino acids can make all the difference. Cell 106(4):391–394

19. Larsson SH, Charlieu JP, Miyagawa K et al (1995) Subnuclear localization of WT1 in splicing or transcription factor domains is regulated by alternative splicing. Cell 81(3):391–401

20. Suri M, Kelehan P, O'Neill D et al (2007) WT1 mutations in Meacham syndrome suggest a coelomic mesothelial origin of the cardiac and diaphragmatic malformations. Am J Med Genet A 143A(19):2312–2320

21. Little M, Wells C (1997) A clinical overview of WT1 gene mutations. Hum Mutat 9(3):209–225

22. Kohsaka T, Tagawa M, Takekoshi Y et al (1999) Exon 9 mutations in the WT1 gene, without influencing KTS splice isoforms, are also responsible for Frasier syndrome. Hum Mutat 14(6):466–470

23. Chernin G, Vega-Warner V, Schoeb DS et al (2010) Genotype/phenotype correlation in nephrotic syndrome caused by WT1 mutations. Clin J Am Soc Nephrol 5(9):1655–1662

24. Ruf RG, Lichtenberger A, Karle SM et al (2004) Patients with mutations in NPHS2 (podocin) do not respond to standard steroid treatment of nephrotic syndrome. J Am Soc Nephrol 15(3):722–732

25. Bullich G, Trujillano D, Santin S et al (2015) Targeted next-generation sequencing in steroid-resistant nephrotic syndrome: mutations in multiple glomerular genes may influence disease severity. Eur J Hum Genet 23(9):1192–1199

26. Zhu C, Zhao F, Zhang W et al (2013) A familial WT1 mutation associated with incomplete Denys-Drash syndrome. Eur J Pediatr 172(10):1357–1362

27. Hall G, Gbadegesin RA, Lavin P et al (2015) A novel missense mutation of Wilms' tumor 1 causes autosomal dominant FSGS. J Am Soc Nephrol 26(4):831–843

28. Faul C, Donnelly M, Merscher-Gomez S et al (2008) The actin cytoskeleton of kidney podocytes is a direct target of the antiproteinuric effect of cyclosporine A. Nat Med 14(9):931–938

29. Hahn H, Cho YM, Park YS et al (2006) Two cases of isolated diffuse mesangial sclerosis with WT1 mutations. J Korean Med Sci 21(1):160–164

30. Jeanpierre C, Denamur E, Henry I et al (1998) Identification of constitutional WT1 mutations, in patients with isolated diffuse mesangial sclerosis, and analysis of genotype/ phenotype correlations by use of a computerized mutation database. Am J Hum Genet 62(4):824–833

31. Brown EJ, Pollak MR, Barua M (2014) Genetic testing for nephrotic syndrome and FSGS in the era of next-generation sequencing. Kidney Int 85(5):1030–1038

32. Kashtan CE, Ding J, Gregory M, Alport Syndrome Research Collaborative et al (2013) Clinical practice recommendations for the treatment of Alport syndrome: a statement of the Alport Syndrome Research Collaborative. Pediatr Nephrol 28(1):5–11

33. Webb NJ, Lam C, Shahinfar S et al (2011) Efficacy and safety of losartan in children with Alport syndrome—results from a subgroup analysis of a prospective, randomized, placebo- or amlodipine-controlled trial. Nephrol Dial Transplant 26(8):2521–2526

Chapter 3

The Role of WT1 in Embryonic Development and Normal Organ Homeostasis

Bettina Wilm and Ramon Muñoz-Chapuli

Abstract

The Wilms' tumor suppressor gene 1 (*Wt1*) is critically involved in a number of developmental processes in vertebrates, including cell differentiation, control of the epithelial/mesenchymal phenotype, proliferation, and apoptosis. Wt1 proteins act as transcriptional and post-transcriptional regulators, in mRNA splicing and in protein–protein interactions. Furthermore, Wt1 is involved in adult tissue homeostasis, kidney function, and cancer. For these reasons, Wt1 function has been extensively studied in a number of animal models to establish its spatiotemporal expression pattern and the developmental fate of the cells expressing this gene. In this chapter, we review the developmental anatomy of Wt1, collecting information about its dynamic expression in mesothelium, kidney, gonads, cardiovascular system, spleen, nervous system, lung, and liver. We also describe the adult expression of Wt1 in kidney podocytes, gonads, mesothelia, visceral adipose tissue, and a small fraction of bone marrow cells. We have reviewed the available animal models for Wt1-expressing cell lineage analysis, including direct Wt1 expression reporters and systems for permanent Wt1 lineage tracing, based on constitutive or inducible Cre recombinase expression under control of a Wt1 promoter. Finally we provide a number of laboratory protocols to be used with these animal models in order to assess reporter expression.

Key words Wt1, Wilms' tumor suppressor gene, Cell lineage tracing

1 Introduction

1.1 Developmental Anatomy of Wt1

The Wilms' tumor suppressor gene 1 (*Wt1*) is well known for its dynamic expression pattern during embryonic development, both in mouse and human. The gene gives rise to at least 24 protein isoforms in human, which are involved in the regulation of the expression of target genes acting in tissue development, growth, differentiation, and apoptosis. Target gene expression is frequently regulated through binding to co-regulators. Furthermore, Wt1 proteins also act as post-transcriptional regulators in mRNA splicing and in protein–protein interaction [1].

In this chapter, we first give a short overview of the distribution of Wt1 expression at gene and/or protein level during development in mice and other animal models, and describe the adult expression of Wt1. We then review the murine models available for

Nicholas Hastie (ed.), *The Wilms' Tumor (WT1) Gene: Methods and Protocols*, Methods in Molecular Biology, vol. 1467, DOI 10.1007/978-1-4939-4023-3_3, © Springer Science+Business Media New York 2016

the study of Wt1 function and provide protocols that include the use of some of these models, with special emphasis on *Wt1*-expressing cell lineage tracing (in short: Wt1 lineage tracing).

1.2 Mesothelium

The mesothelium is a simple epithelium that lines the coelomic cavities and the organs that develop within these cavities. It forms from the lateral mesoderm at around E9 in the mouse embryo. By this time *Wt1* transcripts start to be detected in the parietal coelomic lining, and over the heart, intestine, and urogenital ridge [2]. Expression of Wt1 protein appears first over the urogenital ridge at E9.5, but between E10.5 and E11.5 Wt1 protein is present in the mesothelial layers of the parietal coelomic linings, over the heart, intestine, lungs, and liver, and also in the septum transversum and developing diaphragm [3–7]. Wt1 is also found in many submesothelial mesenchymal cells in the parietal layers of the coelom at later stages of development [8].

2 Kidney

Expression analysis of the murine *Wt1* gene in the developing kidney by in situ hybridization and immunohistological analysis revealed that *Wt1* mRNA/Wt1 protein is expressed in the urogenital ridge from E9, the pro- and mesonephric tissues from E10, and the metanephric mesenchyme (MM) from E12 [9, 10]. The functional postnatal kidney develops from two tissues that have their origin in the intermediate mesoderm, the metanephric mesenchyme, and the ureteric bud (UB). Reciprocal induction events between MM and UB lead to the formation of the functional kidney. This involves several rounds of induction and branching events, involving MM condensation into the mesenchymal cap around the UB, and a subsequent differentiation of condensed cap mesenchyme via mesenchymal-to-epithelial transition (MET) into epithelial cells forming the nephron. Expression of Wt1 in metanephric structures is highly dynamic with highest levels of expression in the condensing cap mesenchyme, comma- and s-shaped body of the developing nephrons, and finally remaining restricted to the podocytes of the glomeruli [11–13]. This was confirmed in transgenic mice expressing LacZ under control of YAC fragments that harbored the human *WT1* gene locus including flanking regions of 470 or 280 kb [14]. Wt1 expression is not found in the UB.

Specifically, Wt1 is intimately involved in the regulation of the early steps of nephron formation and the maintenance of the glomeruli, through interactions with a range of nephrogenic and renal proteins. Wt1 regulates kidney development from early stages leading to complete renal agenesis in loss of Wt1 mutants through apoptosis of the mesonephric tubules and the metanephric mesenchyme, resulting in failure to induce ureteric bud outgrowth [15].

Apoptosis of renal progenitors in absence of Wt1 has recently been related with downregulation of fibroblast growth factor and induction of BMP/pSMAD signaling, and this apoptosis can be rescued by recombinant FGFs or inhibition of pSMAD signaling [16]. Analysis of subsequent stages of kidney development, which is precluded due to metanephric apoptosis in the Wt1 null mutants, has been performed using kidney organoid culture in combination with siRNA approaches [17], and conditional inactivation of Wt1 in vivo [18]. These studies showed that Wt1 controls MET to allow formation of renal vesicles and subsequent stages towards nephron formation from MM, through control of Wnt4 expression. Wnt4 has been identified as a crucial regulator of MET during nephron formation [19, 20]. Furthermore, a specific role for Wt1 in the control of Wnt4 expression had been described since Wt1 expression precedes that of Wnt4, Wt1 can control Wnt4 expression in vitro, and Wnt4 expression is lost in the embryonic kidney mesenchyme when Wt1 is inactivated [18, 21, 22].

At later stages, Wt1 protein controls the formation of podocytes and their homeostasis through transcriptional regulation of Pax2, Nephrin, and Podocalyxin [13, 23–26].

Wt1 also regulates the expression of Nestin, an intermediate filament protein, in the glomeruli, although the significance of Nestin expression in the kidney is not well understood [27]. Conditional deletion of Wt1 in embryonic kidneys using a Nestin-Cre model leads to a failure in MET and nephron formation [18].

Using ChIP-PCR to identify Wt1 target sites in vivo, a recent systemic study demonstrated that a range of factors important for kidney development are transcriptional targets of Wt1, including Bmp7 and Sall1 [28]. Taken together, recent studies in the developing kidney have shown that Wt1 is a key regulator of a range of molecular pathways that lead to the formation of functional nephrons from the metanephric mesenchyme.

3 Gonads

Gonads develop from the urogenital ridge, initially as indifferent primordia, but later they specify into testis and ovaries. They start to arise at around E11 from the mesonephros, the embryonic kidney that forms only transiently, and the overlying coelomic mesothelium. The coelomic mesothelial cells contribute to gonad formation by migrating into the gonadal ridge, forming the primary sex cords and later giving rise to the Sertoli cells (male) or granulosa cells (female) [29, 30]. In situ hybridization and immunohistochemical studies have shown that Wt1 is expressed in the mesonephros and the overlying coelomic epithelium from around E10, but as the urogenital ridges thicken during gonad formation, Wt1 is strongly expressed in the mesenchymal component [12, 13].

Development into male or female gonads and genital organs is regulated by Sry expression, leading to testes formation and differentiation of the Wolffian ducts into seminal vesicles, epididymis, and vas deferens in the male, or ovary formation and the emergence of the oviducts, Fallopian tubes, uterus, and upper vagina from the Müllerian ducts in the female. However, most components of the testis arise from mesonephric cells migrating into the gonad, including peritubular and vascular endothelial cells, while the Leydig cells are formed in waves from primary mesonephric and mesonephric-derived cells [31–33]. One can speculate that since Wt1 is expressed in the gonadal anlagen from early on, most gonadal cells have their origin in cells originally expressing Wt1.

Testis: A complex hierarchical cascade of transcription and signaling factors controls the formation and maintenance of the male gonads. Wt1 is involved in this cascade at several levels since Wt1 expression is required for the survival of the early gonadal anlagen [34]. A range of studies have shown that Wt1 is an important regulator of sex determination by controlling the expression of the *Sry* gene [34–39]. Loss of function studies have demonstrated that Wt1 regulates the expression of steroidogenic factor 1 (*Sf1*) in the indifferent gonad [40]. In addition, molecular and in vitro data indicate that Wt1 acts in concert with Sf1 to regulate the expression of the Müllerian inhibiting substance (*MIS*, also called anti-Müllerian hormone, AMH) [41], and it probably indirectly activates Dax1 during early gonadal development [42].

Using a mouse model for testis-specific conditional ablation of Wt1, Vicky Huff and collaborators showed that Wt1 is required for the formation and maintenance of the seminiferous tubules, Sertoli cells, and germ cells in the testicular cords [43]. Specifically, proteins expressed in Sertoli cells including Sox8, Sox9, and MIS were lost when Wt1 function was abolished. Importantly, loss of Wt1 in the testes leads to β-catenin accumulation which in turn results in testicular cord disruption [44]. Further evidence for a role of Wt1 in testicular cord and Sertoli cell maintenance and germ cell survival stems from the finding that testicular cord integrity is associated with the expression of *Col4a1* and *Col4a2* as these collagens are downregulated in the testes of mice with testis-specific loss of Wt1 [45]. Using an siRNA approach and transgenic mice expressing dominant negative *Wt1*, similar results were reported, supporting an essential role for Wt1 in Sertoli cell and germ cell integrity and survival [46].

Ovary: During female gonad development, Wt1 is expressed in stromal cells, granulosa cells, and the overlying coelomic mesothelium of the ovary [10]. Specifically, granulosa cells of the primordial, primary, and secondary follicles express Wt1 during ovary development, and expression is maintained throughout adult life [47], suggesting that Wt1 is involved in folliculogenesis.

Germ cells: Wt1 is expressed in germ cells when they start converting from primary germ cells to gonadal germ cells, beginning at embryonic day E11.5. Chimera experimentation has shown that loss of *Wt1* in ES cells leads to their exclusion from the germ cell lineage, suggesting that Wt1 is involved in germ cells proliferation, maturation, or survival [48].

4 Heart and Blood Vessels

Wt1 expression in the heart is predominantly, but not exclusively, associated with epicardial development. The earliest expression of Wt1 during cardiac morphogenesis is detected in mouse embryos at E9.5 in the proepicardium, which is the epicardial primordium; subsequently, Wt1 expression continues during the epicardial covering of the heart [2, 49]. Wt1 expression is maintained in the epicardial-derived mesenchymal cells (EPDC) which delaminate from the epicardium and invade first the subepicardial space, and then the myocardium. This expression is progressively downregulated as EPDC differentiate and contribute to the vascular and connective tissue of the heart.

The role played by Wt1 in the developing epicardium seems to be critical, since conditional Wt1 loss of function in this tissue leads to impaired generation of EPDC, abnormal coronary morphogenesis, and thinning of the myocardium, resulting in embryonic lethality [50]. The mechanism by which Wt1 acts in the epicardium is not completely understood, but results from recent studies suggest that the balance between Snail and E-cadherin activity [50] and the canonical β-catenin pathway [51] serve as main downstream effectors of Wt1 in regulating epicardial to mesenchymal transition. Additionally, recent data indicate that in the epicardium Wt1 regulates the transcriptional activation of Raldh2, which represents the main retinoic acid synthesizing enzyme in mesodermal tissues [52]. It had been previously established that cross-talk between epicardium and myocardium, facilitating development of both components, is dependent on retinoic acid signaling [53, 54].

Other genes activated by Wt1 in the epicardium include the neurotrophin receptor *TrkB* [55] and *α4 integrin*, required to maintain epicardial adhesion to the myocardium [56]. Wt1 regulates the expression of the erythropoietin receptor [57] in hematopoietic cells and its ligand erythropoietin in in vitro assays [58]. Since the erythropoietin signaling system also acts in the epicardium and its failure causes myocardial thinning [59], Wt1 may also be involved through this pathway in epicardial-myocardial interaction, thus supporting development and differentiation of both tissues. Finally, an unsuspected role of Wt1 in the developing epicardium is the regulation of the expression of some chemokines. Specifically, Wt1 downregulates Ccl5 and Cxcl10, two chemokines that inhibit EPDC migration and myocardial proliferation. This role is performed through increasing of the levels of Irf7 [60].

In summary, in the epicardium Wt1 activates a set of genes related with epicardial adhesion, epithelial-mesenchymal transition, and migration. Thus, *Wt1* represents a key gene for epicardial development and function.

Wt1 expression has also been found in non-epicardial-derived, cardiac cells. A few cells expressing Wt1 are already present in the endocardium and possibly in the myocardium of E9.5 embryos [61].

Lineage tracing studies of Wt1-expressing cells using Cre-LoxP technology have shed further light onto the role of Wt1 during cardiovascular development and function. Importantly, these studies have shown that the fate of Wt1-expressing cells in the heart is clearly related to coronary vascularization and the formation of cardiac connective tissue. Specifically, Wt1-lineage studies have confirmed an extensive contribution to coronary smooth muscle and cardiac fibroblasts [62]. EPDC-derived Wt1-expressing cells have also been shown to contribute to the lateral atrioventricular cushions where they differentiate into fibroblastic cells of the valves [63]. However, contribution of Wt1-expressing cells to coronary endothelium has been more controversial. Using different lineage tracing approaches, it was shown that the proportion of coronary endothelial cells originating from Wt1-expressing cells comprises less than 15 % [3, 62]. Recent data demonstrate a large, but not complete, overlap between the Wt1 lineage and a *bona fide* epicardial-derived lineage characterized by the activation of a Gata4 enhancer in the septum transversum and proepicardium [64]. These epicardial-derived cells contribute to a minor, but significant fraction of the coronary endothelium (about 20 % of all the endothelial cells), at least during embryonic life and early postnatal stages. This agrees with recent findings reporting that the endocardium is a major contributor to the coronary endothelium [65, 66]. Wagner and colleagues showed that Wt1 is expressed in the coronary endothelium of late gestation mouse embryos, while Wt1$^{-/-}$ embryos that survive to close to term reveal a dramatic lack in coronary vasculature [55]. In addition, the group could identify the neurotrophin receptor TrkB as a downstream target of Wt1 in the coronary endothelium [55], and argued that loss of the coronary vasculature in Wt1 mutant embryos was directly linked to downregulation of TrkB expression.

Furthermore, using in vitro experiments, Wt1 was shown to bind to the VEGF promoter and regulate its expression [67, 68]. The intermediate filament and progenitor marker Nestin has also been shown to be downstream of Wt1 in the developing coronary vasculature [27], and to be co-expressed in the vasa vasorum of human tissue samples [69]. The finding that Wt1 regulates VE-cadherin expression in vitro and in vivo since VE-cadherin expression is reduced in the liver and hearts of Wt1 mutant embryos [70], corroborates the hypothesis that Wt1 is important for the regulation of blood vessel formation.

Lineage tracing studies have also added to controversy around the contribution of Wt1-expressing cells to the myocardium. Of note, this hypothetical contribution may originate from two sources, (1) the EPDC and (2) migration of myocardial progenitors from the posterior secondary cardiac field, where Wt1 expression is prominent in mesenchymal cells of the transverse septum. Original evidence for Wt1-derived myocardial cells provided by Zhou et al. [62] was questioned by Rudat and Kispert [61] on the basis of the unsuitability of the Cre drivers used. Zhou and Pu [71] responded by providing new validating evidence for the existence of cardiomyocytes derived from Wt1-expressing cells, which they considered as epicardial-derived. On the other hand, the existence of a sinus venosus defect in Wt1-deficient mouse embryos [8] could be interpreted as the lack of a Wt1 lineage population contributing to the inflow tract myocardium. This possibility was ruled out by Norden et al. [8] who, by using two different models (LacZ reporter and Wt1-Cre), found that Wt1-expressing cells did not give rise to myocardial cells. These authors conclude that the involvement of the Wt1 lineage in sinus venosus development seems to be indirect.

5 Developmental Hematopoiesis

Molecular evidence for Wt1 as a regulator of developmental hematopoiesis is based on studies showing that Wt1 regulates the expression of both Epo and its receptor EpoR in the fetal liver as the primary hematopoietic organ during mid-gestation [57, 58]. Furthermore, loss of Wt1 affects in vitro differentiation of fetal liver cells, suggesting that Wt1 regulates possibly in synergy with EpoR the differentiation potential of fetal hematopoietic stem cells [57]. However, transplantation studies into lethally irradiated mice showed that fetal liver-derived Wt1$^{-/-}$ hematopoietic stem cells were as potent in restoring bone marrow and peripheral blood cells as wild-type cells [72].

6 Spleen

Wt1 is expressed in the spleen rudiment of the dorsal mesogastrium of mouse embryos by E10.5, continuing in the spleen capsule and epithelium by E14.5 [12]. Herzer et al. [73] reported expression by E12.5 and described failure of spleen development in Wt1$^{-/-}$ embryos. Koehler et al. [74] found that the expression of *Wt1* in the spleen follows that of *Hox11* (a homeobox gene required for spleen development) with a delay of one day, while Hox11$^{-/-}$ embryos show reduced expression of Wt1 in the spleen rudiment, suggesting that Wt1 is acting downstream of Hox11 in spleen development.

7   Body Muscle

Expression of Wt1 in musculature of the body wall of E12-E13 mice embryos was described by Armstrong et al. [2], but this observation has not been confirmed by further reports. It is possible that the presence of mesenchymal cells migrating from the dorsolateral coelomic epithelium to the lateral body wall is related with this early description.

8   Nervous System and Eye

Besides its extensive expression in mesodermal cells, there are only a few specific domains of Wt1 expression in the neuroectoderm. In mouse embryos, Wt1 is expressed from E11 in a narrow linear domain located between the mantle and the ependymal layers. This expression domain becomes more pronounced by E12 and expands by E13 before turning more diffuse, extending to the ventral part of the marginal area of the medulla and finally disappearing at the end of gestation [2, 12, 14]. This expression is anatomically related to the area where motoneurons differentiate. A second area of expression is found in the roof of the fourth ventricle, in a diverticulum of the ependymal layer, close to the rostral part of the medulla oblongata [2, 12].

Wt1 is also expressed in developing retina, as shown by RT-PCR in E12.5 mice embryos. In humans, retina expression of Wt1 has been detected in day 42 fetuses [2]. Wt1 seems to be required for retinal development since Wt1-deficient mouse embryos show defects in retinal ganglion cells [75]. This effect could be due to the activation of Pou4f2, a transcription factor essential for the survival of retinal ganglion cells.

9   Lung

Wt1 is expressed in mesothelial cells of the murine lungs from the early sprouting of the lung buds onwards [6, 12, 76]. Differently to the heart, Wt1 is rapidly downregulated in cells delaminating from the mesothelium and incorporating into the pulmonary mesenchyme. These mesothelial-derived cells contribute to most pulmonary mesodermal tissues, including vascular and bronchial smooth muscle, tracheal cartilage, and a small fraction of the vascular endothelium [6, 76]. In neonates, about 1.5% of all the dissociated pulmonary cells and about 11% of all the endothelial cells derive from the Wt1-expressing cell lineage [6]. Another difference with the epicardium is that the migration of the mesothelial-derived cells inside the pulmonary stroma is dependent of hedgehog signaling [5].

10   Liver

Wt1 is expressed in the liver mesothelium from the early stages of hepatic development [2, 14]. Liver mesothelial cells continue to express Wt1 when they migrate from the surface and intermingle with the hepatoblasts and the hematopoietic cells to differentiate into sinusoidal endothelium and stellate cells [14]. In contrast to the heart and the lung, in the liver Wt1 is not downregulated with the onset of differentiation of mesothelium-derived cells. In fact, Wt1 expression is still detectable in sinusoidal endothelial cells [14]. This invasion of mesothelial-derived cells is necessary for proper hepatic development [4, 77].

11   Adult Expression of Wt1

Wt1 expression has been reported in a few sites of adult mice, namely kidney podocytes, Sertoli cells of the testes, granulosa cells of the ovary, mesothelia, pancreatic stellate cells, the stromal vascular component of several fat bodies including visceral adipose tissue progenitors, and a small fraction of bone marrow cells [3, 78–80].

The podocytes are the most prominent site of adult Wt1 expression, and in fact podocyte maintenance and function depends on Wt1 [80]. In postnatal stages, Wt1 is involved in the regulation of the maintenance of the glomerular filtration function of the kidney, as shown through a range of studies. Mice with reduced Wt1 expression and subsequent downregulation of nephrin and podocalyxin expression showed increased glomerulosclerosis [26]. The damage to the glomeruli is possibly caused by insufficient levels of podocalyxin and nephrin both of which are required for the functional morphology of the slit diaphragm and foot processes of the glomerular filtration membrane. Furthermore, recent study from the Ai lab has shown that Wt1 is important for maintaining cross-talk between podocytes and glomerular endothelial cells across glomerular filtration membrane. Specifically, Wt1 controls the expression of the 6-O-endosulfatases Sulf1 and Sulf2 which in turn regulate signaling of VEGFA from podocytes to glomerular endothelial cells across the glomerular filtration barrier [81].

Wt1 expression is not maintained in all adult mesothelial tissues: while it is present in the adult intestine [3] and the mesothelium lining the visceral fat [78, 79], there are conflicting findings about Wt1 expression in the lung mesothelium, with Dixit and colleagues reporting downregulation of Wt1 in postnatal and adult mice, while Que and colleagues have shown continued expression in P45 animals [5, 79]. Karki et al. [82] also stated that the expression of Wt1 remains in the adult pulmonary mesothelium, and its loss is correlated with mesenchymalization and fibrosis. Wt1 expression in the liver mesothelium seems to be downregulated after E13.5 [4]. It is possible that a low basal level of Wt1 expression in adult mesothelium is the basis for these discrepancies.

The expression of Wt1 in the visceral fat mesothelium and in the progenitors of the visceral white adipose tissue (WAT) establishes a key difference with other fat bodies such as subcutaneous WAT and brown adipose tissue that do not develop from Wt1-expressing cells [79]. This difference could be significant given the different potential of visceral and subcutaneous WAT as risk factor for a number of diseases.

Expression of Wt1 is maintained into adulthood in the Sertoli and granulosa cells [2, 10]. Wt1 regulates Sertoli cell polarity in the testes, and it is essential for germ cell survival, differentiation, and spermatogenesis [83, 84]. Additionally, the expression of Wt1 in Sertoli cell is essential to maintain steroidogenesis in Leydig cells [85, 86]. In the ovary, Wt1 is also expressed in granulosa cells, controlling their polarity and differentiation [87]. In a mouse model mimicking the Denys-Drash syndrome (DSS), heterozygous mice have reduced ovulation rates, premature differentiation of granulosa cells, leading to disturbed development of follicles [87]. This study supports the notion that Wt1 is required not only for normal spermatogenesis but also for oogenesis.

Besides the ovary, Wt1 expression has also been reported in the embryonic and adult uterus, specifically the myometrium and human endometrium [10, 88, 89].

Wt1 expression was detected in the bone marrow of mice and humans for the first time by Fraizer et al. [90]. A range of studies showed that Wt1 expression in hematopoietic cells is restricted to the phase of expansion of hematopoietic progenitor cells while expression was found to be reduced in mature hematopoietic cells and absent in the mature peripheral blood ([91] and references therein). Furthermore, it was found that Wt1 expression was downregulated in hematopoietic cell lines that underwent differentiation, while high expression of Wt1 was correlated with induced proliferation of cells in culture [92, 93]. Wt1 seems to have conflicting roles in different stages of hematopoiesis since it can induce quiescence in early (CD34+ CD38−) progenitors, while it stimulates differentiative behavior in more committed progenitor cells. Wt1 is present in erythroblastic progenitors, where it transactivates the EPO receptor [56]. Wt1 is also involved in granulocyte differentiation [94]. Single cell qPCR of cells during hematopoiesis revealed a biphasic expression pattern with high activity in quiescent primitive precursor cells and specific myeloid cell populations [95, 96]. Interestingly, using a genetically modified mouse line which expresses GFP under control of the endogenous Wt1 locus, Hosen and colleagues came to a slightly different finding, since in Wt1$^{GFP/+}$ mice, Wt1 expression was absent or very low in hematopoietic stem cells or fully differentiated granulocytes, respectively, while expression was higher in myeloid progenitor cells [97]. Loss of Wt1 in hematopoietic stem cells was shown to affect their differentiation potential [98]. Furthermore, in an independent study using ES cells lacking Wt1 protein that were differentiated towards the hematopoietic lineage, similar observations were made, as the colony forming/differentiation potential of the cells was greatly reduced [99]. The authors could show that Wt1$^{-/-}$ ES cells undergo apoptosis that is dependent of Vegfa, and that Wt1 is responsible for splicing of Vegfa into functional isoforms. The function of Wt1 in blood cell differentiation could be mediated by p21cip1 induction, leading to growth arrest [95]. This would explain the role played by Wt1 mutations in leukemogenesis (see below).

In some pathological conditions, the adult expression of Wt1 becomes more prominent. Wt1 is expressed in coronary arteries (endothelium and smooth muscle) after myocardial infarction [100]. This is probably due to the hypoxia produced by the local ischemia, since the upregulation of the *Wt1* gene, mediated by a hypoxia responsive element in the Wt1 promoter, is mimicked by exposing rats to hypoxic conditions [101]. Thus, low oxygen tension could be a driver for Wt1-regulated angiogenesis [102].

Wt1 was named after its supposed role in the development of Wilms' tumor [103], although only a fraction of these tumors shows alterations in WT1 expression. In contrast, abnormal overexpression of WT1 has been reported in a number of tumor cells [104], and it is particularly prominent in acute myeloid leukemia (AML) [105–107]. WT1 is overexpressed in malignant cells of 90% of patients with AML and appears mutated in approximately 10% of these patients [108]. Importantly, these observations have raised expectations for Wt1 as a target in cancer immunotherapy [109, 110].

12 Wt1 Expression in Non-mammalian Animal Models

The developmental expression of Wt1 in chicken embryos is in principle similar to that described for mammals [111]. Wt1 has been used as a marker of proepicardial, epicardial, and epicardial-derived cells by a number of groups studying chick development [112–116].

In zebrafish, two *Wt1* genes, *wt1a* and *wt1b*, have been reported, both showing +KTS and –KTS isoforms [117]. In early embryos the expression of both genes is dynamic and restricted to intermediate mesoderm. Expression of wt1a in the zebrafish pronephros is regulated by retinoic acid through a highly conserved enhancer [118]. In addition, wt1a has recently been reported to regulate the expression of osr1, thus controlling the differentiation of zebrafish podocytes [119]. The expression domains of wt1a and wt1b in adult fish tissues are more extensive than in mammals, including gonads, kidneys, heart, spleen, and muscle. Both wt1a and wt1b have also been reported in other fish, such as *Oncorhynchus*, *Oryzias*, *Takifugu*, and *Tetraodon* (reviewed in ref. 120). In *Tetraodon*, the highly conserved motif KTS, distinguishing DNA binding to DNA nonbinding isoforms, is changed to KPS [120].

Information on Wt1 expression in amphibians is more limited. Wt1 is expressed in Sertoli cells, spermatogonia, and mature sperm stages in the testes of the newt *Cynops pyrrhogaster* [121]. In *Xenopus*, Wt1 expression is first restricted to the developing nephric system, and later is also detected in the developing heart [121, 123]. Since Wt1 is not detected in developing pronephric tubules and ducts, its function seems to be related with the development of the glomeruli. In fact, when Wt1 was ectopically expressed in *Xenopus* embryos by mRNA injection, it inhibited pronephric tubule development [124].

Regarding invertebrates, a Wt1 ortholog has been found in the cephalochordate *Branchiostoma floridae* [125]. Furthermore, the *Drosophila* gene *Klumpfuss* has been considered as a Wt1 ortholog and is involved in neuronal [126, 127] and hemocyte differentiation [128]. However, despite the similarity between the four zinc-finger domains with those of the vertebrate Wt1, the N-terminal region is clearly different making this orthology very doubtful.

References

1. Toska E, Roberts SJ (2014) Mechanisms of transcriptional regulation by WT1 (Wilms' tumour 1). Biochem J 461:15–32

2. Armstrong JF, Pritchard-Jones K, Bickmore WA et al (1993) The expression of the Wilms' tumour gene, WT1, in the developing mammalian embryo. Mech Dev 40:85–97

3. Wilm B, Ipenberg A, Hastie ND et al (2005) The serosal mesothelium is a major source of smooth muscle cells of the gut vasculature. Development 132:5317–5328

4. Asahina K, Zhou B, Pu WT et al (2011) Septum transversum-derived mesothelium gives rise to hepatic stellate cells and perivascular mesenchymal cells in developing mouse liver. Hepatology 53:983–995

5. Dixit R, Ai X, Fine A (2013) Derivation of lung mesenchymal lineages from the fetal mesothelium requires hedgehog signaling for mesothelial cell entry. Development 140:4398–4406

6. Cano E, Carmona R, Muñoz-Chápuli R (2013) Wt1-expressing progenitors contribute to multiple tissues in the developing lung. Am J Physiol 305:L322–L332

7. Carmona R, Cano E, Mattiotti A et al (2013) Cells derived from the coelomic epithelium contribute to multiple gastrointestinal tissues in mouse embryos. PLoS One 8:e55890

8. Norden J, Grieskamp T, Lausch E et al (2010) Wt1 and retinoic acid signaling in the subcoelomic mesenchyme control the development of the pleuropericardial membranes and the sinus horns. Circ Res 106:1212–1220

9. Buckler AJ, Pelletier J, Haber DA et al (1991) Isolation, characterization, and expression of the murine Wilms' tumor gene (WT1) during kidney development. Mol Cell Biol 11:1707–1712

10. Pelletier J, Bruening W, Li FP et al (1991) WT1 mutations contribute to abnormal genital system development and hereditary Wilms' tumour. Nature 353(6343):431–434

11. Armstrong JF, Kaufman MH, van Heyningen V et al (1993) Embryonic kidney rudiments grown in adult mice fail to mimic the Wilms' phenotype, but show strain-specific morphogenesis. Exp Nephrol 1:168–174

12. Rackley RR, Flenniken AM, Kuriyan NP et al (1993) Expression of the Wilms' tumor suppressor gene WT1 during mouse embryogenesis. Cell Growth Differ 4:1023–1031

13. Ryan G, Steele-Perkins V, Morris JF et al (1995) Repression of Pax-2 by WT1 during normal kidney development. Development 121:867–875

14. Moore AW, Schedl A, McInnes L et al (1998) YAC transgenic analysis reveals Wilms'

tumour 1 gene activity in the proliferating coelomic epithelium, developing diaphragm and limb. Mech Dev 79:169–184

15. Kreidberg JA, Sariola H, Loring JM et al (1993) WT-1 is required for early kidney development. Cell 74:679–691

16. Motamedi FJ, Badro DA, Clarkson M et al (2014) WT1 controls antagonistic FGF and BMP-pSMAD pathways in early renal progenitors. Nat Commun 5:4444

17. Davies JA, Ladomery M, Hohenstein P et al (2004) Development of an siRNA-based method for repressing specific genes in renal organ culture and its use to show that the Wt1 tumour suppressor is required for nephron differentiation. Hum Mol Genet 13:235–246

18. Essafi A, Webb A, Berry RL et al (2011) A wt1-controlled chromatin switching mechanism underpins tissue-specific wnt4 activation and repression. Dev Cell 21:559–574

19. Stark K, Vainio S, Vassileva G et al (1994) Epithelial transformation of metanephric mesenchyme in the developing kidney regulated by Wnt-4. Nature 372(6507):679–683

20. Kispert A, Vainio S, McMahon AP et al (1998) Wnt-4 is a mesenchymal signal for epithelial transformation of metanephric mesenchyme in the developing kidney. Development 125:4225–4234

21. Sim EU, Smith A, Szilagi E et al (2002) Wnt-4 regulation by the Wilms' tumour suppressor gene, WT1. Oncogene 21:2948–2960

22. Murugan S, Shan J, Kühl SJ et al (2012) WT1 and Sox11 regulate synergistically the promoter of the Wnt4 gene that encodes a critical signal for nephrogenesis. Exp Cell Res 318:1134–1145

23. Guo G, Morrison DJ, Licht JD et al (2004) WT1 activates a glomerular-specific enhancer identified from the human nephrin gene. J Am Soc Nephrol 15:2851–2856

24. Wagner N, Wagner KD, Xing Y et al (2004) The major podocyte protein nephrin is transcriptionally activated by the Wilms' tumor suppressor WT1. J Am Soc Nephrol 15:3044–3051

25. Palmer RE, Kotsianti A, Cadman B et al (2001) WT1 regulates the expression of the major glomerular podocyte membrane protein podocalyxin. Curr Biol 11:1805–1809

26. Guo JK, Menke AL, Gubler MC et al (2002) WT1 is a key regulator of podocyte function: reduced expression levels cause crescentic glomerulonephritis and mesangial sclerosis. Hum Mol Genet 11:651–659

27. Wagner N, Wagner KD, Scholz H et al (2006) Intermediate filament protein nestin is expressed in developing kidney and heart and might be regulated by the Wilms' tumor suppressor Wt1. Am J Physiol Regul Integr Comp Physiol 291:R779–R787

28. Hartwig S, Ho J, Pandey P et al (2010) Genomic characterization of Wilms' tumor suppressor 1 targets in nephron progenitor cells during kidney development. Development 137:1189–1203

29. Albrecht KH, Eicher EM (2001) Evidence that Sry is expressed in pre-Sertoli cells and Sertoli and granulosa cells have a common precursor. Dev Biol 240:92–107

30. Karl J, Capel B (1998) Sertoli cells of the mouse testis originate from the coelomic epithelium. Dev Biol 203:323–333

31. Capel B, Albrecht KH, Washburn LL et al (1999) Migration of mesonephric cells into the mammalian gonad depends on Sry. Mech Dev 84:127–131

32. Martineau J, Nordqvist K, Tilmann C et al (1997) Male-specific cell migration into the developing gonad. Curr Biol 7:958–968

33. Tilmann C, Capel B (1999) Mesonephric cell migration induces testis cord formation and Sertoli cell differentiation in the mammalian gonad. Development 126:2883–2890

34. Hammes A, Guo JK, Lutsch G et al (2001) Two splice variants of the Wilms' tumor 1 gene have distinct functions during sex determination and nephron formation. Cell 106:319–329

35. Shimamura R, Fraizer GC, Trapman J et al (1997) The Wilms' tumor gene WT1 can regulate genes involved in sex determination and differentiation: SRY, Müllerian-inhibiting substance, and the androgen receptor. Clin Cancer Res 3:2571–2580

36. Hossain A, Saunders GF (2001) The human sex-determining gene SRY is a direct target of WT1. J Biol Chem 276:16817–16823

37. Matsuzawa-Watanabe Y, Inoue J, Semba K (2003) Transcriptional activity of testis-determining factor SRY is modulated by the Wilms' tumor 1 gene product, WT1. Oncogene 22:7900–7904

38. Miyamoto Y, Taniguchi H, Hamel F et al (2008) A GATA4/WT1 cooperation regulates transcription of genes required for mammalian sex determination and differentiation. BMC Mol Biol 9:44

39. Bradford ST, Wilhelm D, Bandiera R et al (2009) A cell-autonomous role for WT1 in regulating Sry in vivo. Hum Mol Genet 18:3429–3438

40. Wilhelm D, Englert C (2002) The Wilms' tumor suppressor WT1 regulates early gonad development by activation of Sf1. Genes Dev 16:1839–1851

41. Nachtigal MW, Hirokawa Y, Enyeart-VanHouten DL et al (1998) Wilms' tumor 1 and Dax-1 modulate the orphan nuclear receptor SF-1 in sex-specific gene expression. Cell 93:445–454

42. Kim J, Prawitt D, Bardeesy N et al (1999) The Wilms' tumor suppressor gene (wt1) product regulates Dax-1 gene expression during gonadal differentiation. Mol Cell Biol 19:2289–2299

43. Gao F, Maiti S, Alam N et al (2006) The Wilms' tumor gene, Wt1, is required for Sox9 expression and maintenance of tubular architecture in the developing testis. Proc Natl Acad Sci U S A 103:11987–11992

44. Chang H, Gao F, Guillou F et al (2008) Wt1 negatively regulates beta-catenin signaling during testis development. Development 135:1875–1885

45. Chen SR, Chen M, Wang XN et al (2013) The Wilms' tumor gene, Wt1, maintains testicular cord integrity by regulating the expression of Col4a1 and Col4a2. Biol Reprod 88:56

46. Rao MK, Pham J, Imam JS et al (2006) Tissue-specific RNAi reveals that WT1 expression in nurse cells controls germ cell survival and spermatogenesis. Genes Dev 20:147–152

47. Hsu SY, Kubo M, Chun SY et al (1995) Wilms' tumor protein WT1 as an ovarian transcription factor: decreases in expression during follicle development and repression of inhibin-alpha gene promoter. Mol Endocrinol 9:1356–1366

48. Natoli TA, Alberta JA, Bortvin A et al (2004) Wt1 functions in the development of germ cells in addition to somatic cell lineages of the testis. Dev Biol 268:429–440

49. Moore AW, McInnes L, Kreidberg J et al (1999) YAC complementation shows a requirement for Wt1 in the development of epicardium, adrenal gland and throughout nephrogenesis. Development 126:1845–1857

50. Martínez-Estrada OM, Lettice LA, Essafi A et al (2010) Wt1 is required for cardiovascular progenitor cell formation through transcriptional control of Snail and E-cadherin. Nat Genet 42:89–93

51. von Gise A, Zhou B, Honor LB et al (2011) WT1 regulates epicardial epithelial to mesenchymal transition through β-catenin and retinoic acid signaling pathways. Dev Biol 356:421–431

52. Guadix JA, Ruiz-Villalba A, Lettice L et al (2011) Wt1 controls retinoic acid signalling in embryonic epicardium through transcriptional activation of Raldh2. Development 138:1093–1097

53. Chen T, Chang TC, Kang JO et al (2002) Epicardial induction of fetal cardiomyocyte proliferation via a retinoic acid-inducible trophic factor. Dev Biol 250:198–207

54. Stuckmann I, Evans S, Lassar AB (2003) Erythropoietin and retinoic acid, secreted from the epicardium, are required for cardiac myocyte proliferation. Dev Biol 255:334–349

55. Wagner N, Wagner KD, Theres H et al (2005) Coronary vessel development requires activation of the TrkB neurotrophin receptor by the Wilms' tumor transcription factor Wt1. Genes Dev 19:2631–2642

56. Kirschner KM, Wagner N, Wagner KD et al (2006) The Wilms' tumor suppressor Wt1 promotes cell adhesion through transcriptional activation of the alpha4integrin gene. J Biol Chem 281:31930–31939

57. Kirschner KM, Hagen P, Hussels CS et al (2008) The Wilms' tumor suppressor Wt1 activates transcription of the erythropoietin receptor in hematopoietic progenitor cells. FASEB J 22:2690–2701

58. Dame C, Kirschner KM, Bartz KV et al (2006) Wilms' tumor suppressor, Wt1, is a transcriptional activator of the erythropoietin gene. Blood 107:4282–4290

59. Wu H, Lee SH, Gao J et al (1999) Inactivation of erythropoietin leads to defects in cardiac morphogenesis. Development 126:3597–3605

60. Velecela V, Lettice LA, Chau YY et al (2013) WT1 regulates the expression of inhibitory chemokines during heart development. Hum Mol Genet 22:5083–5095

61. Rudat C, Kispert A (2012) Wt1 and epicardial fate mapping. Circ Res 111:165–169

62. Zhou B, Ma Q, Rajagopal S et al (2008) Epicardial progenitors contribute to the cardiomyocyte lineage in the developing heart. Nature 454:109–113

63. Wessels A, van den Hoff MJB, Adamo RF et al (2012) Epicardially derived fibroblasts preferentially contribute to the parietal leaflets of the atrioventricular valves in the murine heart. Dev Biol 366:111–124

64. Cano E, Carmona R, Ruiz-Villalba A et al (2016) Extracardiac septum transversum/proepicardial endothelial cells pattern embryonic

coronary arterio-venous connections. Proc Natl Acad Sci USA 113:656–661

65. Red-Horse K, Ueno H, Weissman IL et al (2010) Coronary arteries form by developmental reprogramming of venous cells. Nature 464:549–553

66. Wu B, Zhang Z, Lui W et al (2012) Endocardial cells form the coronary arteries by angiogenesis through myocardial-endocardial VEGF signaling. Cell 151:1083–1096

67. Hanson J, Gorman J, Reese J et al (2007) Regulation of vascular endothelial growth factor, VEGF, gene promoter by the tumor suppressor, WT1. Front Biosci 12:2279–2290

68. McCarty G, Awad O, Loeb DM (2011) WT1 protein directly regulates expression of vascular endothelial growth factor and is a mediator of tumor response to hypoxia. J Biol Chem 286:43634–43643

69. Vasuri F, Fittipaldi S, Buzzi M et al (2012) Nestin and WT1 expression in small-sized vasa vasorum from human normal arteries. Histol Histopathol 27:1195–1202

70. Kirschner KM, Sciesielski LK, Scholz H et al (2010) Wilms' tumour protein Wt1 stimulates transcription of the gene encoding vascular endothelial cadherin. Pflugers Arch 460:1051–1061

71. Zhou B, Pu WT (2012) Genetic Cre-loxP assessment of epicardial cell fate using Wt1-driven Cre alleles. Circ Res 111:e276–e280

72. King-Underwood L, Little S, Baker M et al (2005) Wt1 is not essential for hematopoiesis in the mouse. Leuk Res 29:803–812

73. Herzer U, Crocoll A, Barton D et al (1999) The Wilms' tumor suppressor gene wt1 is required for development of the spleen. Curr Biol 9:837–840

74. Koehler K, Franz T, Dear TN et al (2000) Hox11 is required to maintain normal Wt1 mRNA levels in the developing spleen. Dev Dyn 218:201–206

75. Wagner KD, Wagner N, Vidal VP et al (2002) The Wilms' tumor gene Wt1 is required for normal development of the retina. EMBO J 21:1398–1405

76. Que J, Wilm B, Hasegawa H et al (2008) Mesothelium contributes to vascular smooth muscle and mesenchyme during lung development. Proc Natl Acad Sci U S A 105:16626–16630

77. IJpenberg A, Pérez-Pomares JM, Guadix JA et al (2007) Wt1 and retinoic acid signaling are essential for stellate cell development and liver morphogenesis. Dev Biol 312:157–170

78. Chau YY, Hastie ND (2012) The role of Wt1 in regulating mesenchyme in cancer, development, and tissue homeostasis. Trends Genet 28:515–524

79. Chau YY, Bandiera R, Serrels A et al (2014) Visceral and subcutaneous fat have different origins and evidence supports a mesothelial source. Nat Cell Biol 16:367–375

80. Chau YY, Brownstein D, Mjoseng H et al (2011) Acute multiple organ failure in adult mice deleted for the developmental regulator Wt1. PLoS Genet 7:e1002404

81. Schumacher VA, Schlötzer-Schrehardt U, Karumanchi SA et al (2011) WT1-dependent sulfatase expression maintains the normal glomerular filtration barrier. J Am Soc Nephrol 22:1286–1296

82. Karki S, Surolia R, Hock TD et al (2014) Wilms' tumor 1 (Wt1) regulates pleural mesothelial cell plasticity and transition into myofibroblasts in idiopathic pulmonary fibrosis. FASEB J 28:1122–1131

83. Wang XN, Li ZS, Ren Y et al (2013) The Wilms' tumor gene, Wt1, is critical for mouse spermatogenesis via regulation of sertoli cell polarity and is associated with non-obstructive azoospermia in humans. PLoS Genet 9:e1003645

84. Zheng QS, Wang XN, Wen Q et al (2014) Wt1 deficiency causes undifferentiated spermatogonia accumulation and meiotic progression disruption in neonatal mice. Reproduction 147:45–52

85. Chen M, Wang X, Wang Y et al (2014) Wt1 is involved in Leydig cell steroid hormone biosynthesis by regulating paracrine factor expression in mice. Biol Reprod 90:71

86. Wen Q, Zheng QS, Li XX et al (2014) Wt1 dictates the fate of fetal and adult Leydig cells during development in the mouse testis. Am J Physiol Endocrinol Metab 307:E1131–E1143

87. Gao F, Zhang J, Wang X et al (2014) Wt1 functions in ovarian follicle development by regulating granulosa cell differentiation. Hum Mol Genet 23:333–341

88. Makrigiannakis A, Amin K, Coukos G et al (2000) Regulated expression and potential roles of p53 and Wilms' tumor suppressor gene (WT1) during follicular development in the human ovary. J Clin Endocrinol Metab 85:449–459

89. Makrigiannakis A, Coukos G, Mantani A et al (2001) Expression of Wilms' tumor suppressor gene (WT1) in human endometrium: regulation through decidual differentiation. J Clin Endocrinol Metab 86:5964–5972

90. Fraizer GC, Patmasiriwat P, Zhang X et al (1995) Expression of the tumor suppressor gene WT1 in both human and mouse bone marrow. Blood 86:4704–4706

91. Ariyaratana S, Loeb DM (2007) The role of the Wilms' tumour gene (WT1) in normal and malignant haematopoiesis. Expert Rev Mol Med 9:1–17

92. Inoue K, Tamaki H, Ogawa H et al (1998) Wilms' tumor gene (WT1) competes with differentiation-inducing signal in hematopoietic progenitor cells. Blood 91:2969–2976

93. Tsuboi A, Oka Y, Ogawa H et al (1999) Constitutive expression of the Wilms' tumor gene WT1 inhibits the differentiation of myeloid progenitor cells but promotes their proliferation in response to granulocyte-colony stimulating factor (G-CSF). Leuk Res 23:499–505

94. Loeb DM, Summers JL, Burwell EA et al (2003) An isoform of the Wilms' tumor suppressor gene potentiates granulocytic differentiation. Leukemia 17:965–971

95. Ellisen LW, Carlesso N, Cheng T et al (2001) The Wilms' tumor suppressor WT1 directs stage-specific quiescence and differentiation of human hematopoietic progenitor cells. EMBO J 20:1897–1909

96. Algar E (2002) A review of the Wilms' tumor 1 gene (WT1) and its role in hematopoiesis and leukemia. J Hematother Stem Cell Res 11:589–599

97. Hosen N, Shirakata T, Nishida S et al (2007) The Wilms' tumor gene WT1-GFP knock-in mouse reveals the dynamic regulation of WT1 expression in normal and leukemic hematopoiesis. Leukemia 21:1783–1791

98. Alberta JA, Springett GM, Rayburn H et al (2003) Role of the WT1 tumor suppressor in murine hematopoiesis. Blood 101:2570–2574

99. Cunningham TJ, Palumbo I, Grosso M et al (2011) WT1 regulates murine hematopoiesis via maintenance of VEGF isoform ratio. Blood 122:188–192

100. Wagner KD, Wagner N, Bondke A et al (2002) The Wilms' tumor suppressor Wt1 is expressed in the coronary vasculature after myocardial infarction. FASEB J 16:1117–1119

101. Wagner KD, Wagner N, Wellmann S et al (2003) Oxygen-regulated expression of the Wilms' tumor suppressor Wt1 involves hypoxia-inducible factor-1 (HIF-1). FASEB J 17:1364–1366

102. Scholz H, Wagner KD, Wagner N (2009) Role of the Wilms' tumour transcription factor, Wt1, in blood vessel formation. Pflugers Arch 458:315–323

103. Lee SB, Haber DA (2001) Wilms' tumor and the WT1 gene. Exp Cell Res 264:74–99

104. Loeb DM, Sukumar S (2002) The role of WT1 in oncogenesis: tumor suppressor or oncogene? Int J Hematol 76:117–126

105. Brieger J, Weidmann E, Fenchel K et al (1994) The expression of the Wilms' tumor gene in acute myelocytic leukemias as a possible marker for leukemic blast cells. Leukemia 8:2138–2143

106. Menssen HD, Renkl HJ, Rodeck U et al (1995) Presence of Wilms' tumor gene (wt1) transcripts and the WT1 nuclear protein in the majority of human acute leukemias. Leukemia 9:1060–1067

107. Yang L, Han Y, Suarez SF et al (2007) A tumor suppressor and oncogene: the WT1 story. Leukemia 21:868–876

108. Rein LA, Chao NJ (2014) WT1 vaccination in acute myeloid leukemia: new methods of implementing adoptive immunotherapy. Expert Opin Investig Drugs 23:417–426

109. Sugiyama H (2010) WT1 (Wilms' tumor gene 1): biology and cancer immunotherapy. Jpn J Clin Oncol 40:377–387

110. Vasu S, Blum W (2013) Emerging immunotherapies in older adults with acute myeloid leukemia. Curr Opin Hematol 20:107–114

111. Carmona R, González-Iriarte M, Pérez-Pomares JM et al (2001) Localization of the Wilm's tumour protein WT1 in avian embryos. Cell Tissue Res 303:173–186

112. Pérez-Pomares JM, Phelps A, Sedmerova M et al (2002) Experimental studies on the spatiotemporal expression of WT1 and RALDH2 in the embryonic avian heart: a model for the regulation of myocardial and valvuloseptal development by epicardially derived cells (EPDCs). Dev Biol 247:307–326

113. Schlueter J, Männer J, Brand T (2006) BMP is an important regulator of proepicardial identity in the chick embryo. Dev Biol 295:546–558

114. Schulte I, Schlueter J, Abu-Issa R et al (2007) Morphological and molecular left-right asymmetries in the development of the proepicardium: a comparative analysis on mouse and chick embryos. Dev Dyn 236:684–695

115. Ishii Y, Garriock RJ, Navetta AM et al (2007) BMP signals promote proepicardial protrusion necessary for recruitment of coronary vessel and epicardial progenitors to the heart. Dev Cell 19:307–316

116. Torlopp A, Schlueter J, Brand T (2010) Role of fibroblast growth factor signaling during proepicardium formation in the chick embryo. Dev Dyn 239:2393–2403

117. Bollig F, Mehringer R, Perner B et al (2006) Identification and comparative expression analysis of a second wt1 gene in zebrafish. Dev Dyn 235:554–561

118. Bollig F, Perner B, Besenbeck B et al (2009) A highly conserved retinoic acid responsive element controls wt1a expression in the zebrafish pronephros. Development 136:2883–2892

119. Tomar R, Mudumana SP, Pathak N et al (2014) Osr1 is required for podocyte development downstream of wt1a. J Am Soc Nephrol 25:2539–2545

120. Miles C, Elgar G, Coles E et al (1998) Complete sequencing of the Fugu WAGR region from WT1 to PAX6: dramatic compaction and conservation of synteny with human chromosome 11p13. Proc Natl Acad Sci U S A 95:13068–13072

121. Nakayama Y, Yamamoto T, Matsuda Y et al (1998) Cloning of cDNA for newt WT1 and the differential expression during spermatogenesis of the Japanese newt, *Cynops pyrrhogaster*. Dev Growth Differ 40:599–608

122. Semba K, Saito-Ueno R, Takayama G et al (1996) cDNA cloning and its pronephrosspecific expression of the Wilms' tumor suppressor gene, WT1, from *Xenopus laevis*. Gene 175:167–172

123. Carroll TJ, Vize PD (1996) Wilms' tumor suppressor gene is involved in the development of disparate kidney forms: evidence from expression in the Xenopus pronephros. Dev Dyn 206:131–138

124. Wallingford JB, Carroll TJ, Vize PD et al (1998) Precocious expression of the Wilms' tumor gene xWT1 inhibits embryonic kidney development in *Xenopus laevis*. Dev Biol 202:103–112

125. Shimeld SM (2008) C2H2 zinc finger genes of the Gli, Zic, KLF, SP, Wilms' tumour, Huckebein, Snail, Ovo, Spalt, Odd, Blimp-1, Fez and related gene families from *Branchiostoma floridae*. Dev Genes Evol 218:639–649

126. Losada-Pérez M, Gabilondo H, Molina I (2013) Klumpfuss controls FMRFamide expression by enabling BMP signaling within the NB5-6 lineage. Development 140:2181–2189

127. Gabilondo H, Losada-Pérez M, Monedero I et al (2014) A new role of Klumpfuss in establishing cell fate during the GMC asymmetric cell division. Cell Tissue Res 358:621–626

128. Terriente-Felix A, Li J, Collins S, Mulligan A et al (2013) Notch cooperates with Lozenge/Runx to lock haemocytes into a differentiation programme. Development 140:926–937

Chapter 4

Tools and Techniques for Wt1-Based Lineage Tracing

Bettina Wilm and Ramon Muñoz-Chapuli

Abstract

The spatiotemporal expression pattern of Wt1 has been extensively studied in a number of animal models to establish its function and the developmental fate of the cells expressing this gene. In this chapter, we review the available animal models for Wt1-expressing cell lineage analysis, including direct Wt1 expression reporters and systems for permanent Wt1 lineage tracing. We describe the presently used constitutive or inducible genetic lineage tracing approaches based on the Cre/loxP system utilizing Cre recombinase expression under control of a Wt1 promoter.

To make these systems accessible, we provide laboratory protocols that include dissection and processing of the tissues for immunofluorescence and histopathological analysis of the lineage-labeled Wt1-derived cells within the embryo/tissue context.

Key words Wt1, Cell lineage tracing, Cre/loxP, Inducible Cre recombinase, Cre-ERT2, Tamoxifen, Rosa26 reporter mice

1 Introduction

A number of murine models are available to study both Wt1-expressing cell lineage and actual Wt1 expression. The first models are based on a Cre/loxP system, inducing constitutive expression of a reporter gene in those cells where the Wt1 promoter controls expression of the Cre-recombinase enzyme. Different levels of recombination can produce different levels of reporter expression, and rigorous controls using Cre$-$/$-$; Flox+/+ embryos must be performed to discard events of spontaneous recombination. On the other hand, direct activation of a reporter gene by the Wt1 promoter allows to directly monitor Wt1 expression in the tissues. The replacement of the exon 1 of the Wt1 gene by a GFP expressing system (Wt1 knock-in system, [1]) also allows for detection of Wt1 expression in heterozygous (Wt1$^{+/GFP}$) embryos using the original Wt1 promoter (see below).

Nicholas Hastie (ed.), *The Wilms' Tumor (WT1) Gene: Methods and Protocols*, Methods in Molecular Biology, vol. 1467, DOI 10.1007/978-1-4939-4023-3_4, © Springer Science+Business Media New York 2016

1.1 Direct Wt1 Expression Reporters

Wt1-expressing cells in tissues can be analyzed using in situ hybridization and immunohistochemical approaches. However, a set of mouse lines that function as direct Wt1-LacZ or-GFP reporters, enable detection of cells that are expressing Wt1 at any given time [2–5]. The Wt1-LacZ reporters were generated initially by yeast recombineering of YAC clones containing the human WT1 locus with a LacZ-containing cassette, before pronuclear injections of the resulting YAC constructs gave rise to a range of transgenic LacZ reporters (Tg(WT1)HNdh, Tg(WT1)WANdh, Tg(WT1)WCNdh, Tg(WT1)WWNdh; refs. 2, 3). Analysis of these transgenic Wt1-LacZ reporter lines revealed a highly faithful recapitulation of endogenous Wt1 expression in a range of embryonic tissues, and some degree of rescue function by combination with Wt1$^{-/-}$ mutants.

By contrast, the Wt1^{tm1Nhsn} reporter mouse line was generated as knockin of a GFP-cassette containing construct by gene targeting, thus replacing exon1 and part of the intronic region in the resulting mouse line Wt1^{tm1Nhsn} [5]. In Wt1^{tm1Nhsn} heterozygous mice, GFP is expressed directly under control of the endogenous Wt1 promoter elements, while Wt1^{tm1Nhsn} homozygous mice are embryonic lethal due to the inactivation of the Wt1 locus at the GFP insertion site. The GFP expression can be observed directly under the dissecting microscope (Fig. 1a) or by confocal microscopy, but the signal can also be much enhanced by GFP immunolocalization (Fig. 1b).

The GFP reporter line Wt1$^{tm1(EGFP/cre)Wtp}$ was generated following a similar gene targeting strategy, and also results in GFP expression under direct control of the endogenous Wt1 promoter. However, in this mouse line, GFP is fused with the Cre recombinase protein, providing these mice with dual function for direct labeling of Wt1 expression, and as tool for lineage tracing studies [6]. Both mouse lines have been proven useful as tools to study Wt1 expression in embryonic tissues, but also in isolated cells in vitro. Two further transgenic mouse lines which carry eGFP in combination with Cre recombinase under control of a Wt1 promoter have been described (Tg(Wt1-cre)#Jbeb, ref. 7; Tg(Wt1-EGFP/cre)1Akis, ref. 8), but their use as direct reporters for Wt1-controlled GFP expression have not been demonstrated. As shown below, GFP expression in Tg(Wt1-cre)#Jbeb animals is below the detection limit.

1.2 Permanent Wt1 Lineage Tracing: Constitutive Cre Recombinase Expressed Under Control of Wt1

Six different mouse lines have been described that utilize constitutive Cre recombinase expression under control of the mouse or the human WT1 gene for permanent lineage tracing (Fig. 2):

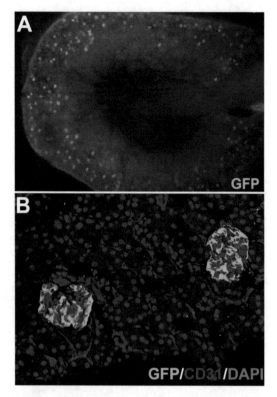

Fig. 1 Direct expression of GFP as a reporter for Wt1, in the Wt1 ^{tm1Nhsn} mouse line, generated by replacing exon1 and part of the intronic region of the Wt1 gene by a GFP-cassette containing construct (98). (**a**) Wt1-GFP expression in glomeruli of an adult kidney bisected shortly after dissection and visualized with a fluorescence dissecting microscope. (**b**) In this section of the kidney of an adult mouse, GFP was immunostained using the chicken polyclonal anti-GFP (Abcam, ab13970). Wt1 (GFP) expression is clearly localized in the glomerular podocytes. Endothelial cells are immunostained in *red*

1. Wt1-Cre, first described by the Bader lab [9] (official nomenclature[1]: Tg(WT1-cre)AG11Dbdr; MGI:3609978).

2. mWt1/IRES/GFP-Cre or $Wt1^{Cre}$, generated by the Burch lab [7] (official nomenclature: Tg(Wt1-cre)#Jbeb; MGI:5308608).

3. Wt1 ^{GFPCre}, generated by the Pu lab [6] (official nomenclature: Wt1 $^{tm1(EGFP/cre)Wtp}$; MGI:3801681).

4. Wt1 $^{BAC-IRES-EGFPCre}$, generated by the Kispert lab [8] (official nomenclature: Tg(Wt1-EGFP/cre)1Akis; MGI:5002800).

5. WT1(RP23-8C14)-Cre, generated by the Burch lab [10] (official nomenclature: Tg(Wt1-cre)1Jbeb; MGI:5562908).

---

[1] Official nomenclature of mouse lines can be found under the Jackson laboratory website: www.informatics.jax.org

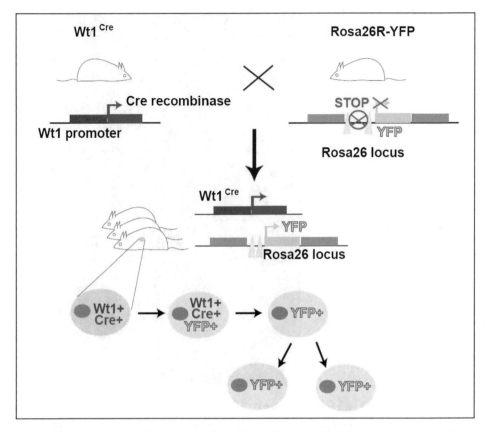

Fig. 2 Schematic diagram delineating the constitutive Cre/loxP-based Wt1 lineage tracing system. The system consists of two genetic components: Transgenic mice generated by inserting a Cre recombinase expressing sequence under control of a Wt1 promoter (Wt1^{Cre}), and gene-targeted mice where a stop sequence flanked by lox sites is placed in front of a YPF cassette in the Rosa26 locus (Rosa26R-YFP reporter). Offspring of crosses between Wt1^{Cre} and Rosa26-YFP reporter mice, result in embryos which carry both genetic modifications, allowing permanent expression of YFP in Wt1-expressing cells and their lineage. Thus, YFP expression remains active even when Wt1 and Cre recombinase expression has been switched off in a particular cell

Similar protocols for permanent lineage tracing of Wt1-expressing cells have been described for all mouse lines of this category. Here, we detail the lineage tracing protocol using the *mWt1/IRES/GFP-Cre* (*Wt1*^{Cre}) mouse line.

The *Wt1*^{Cre} mouse line was developed using a BAC recombineering strategy to insert an IRES/EGFP-CRE cassette 17 bp downstream of the translation stop site of the Wt1 gene in the BAC clone RP23-266M16. The resultant recombinant BAC clone was used to generate several independent transgenic mouse lines that express *Cre* in the epicardial lineage beginning at the proepicardial stage. These *Wt1Cre* transgenic mice have been used in previous studies to trace or delete specific genes in *Wt1*-expressing cells [7, 11–13]. Crossing of homozygote (*Wt1*$^{Cre+/+}$) mice with B6.129X1-Gt(ROSA)26Sortm1(EYFP)Cos/J mice

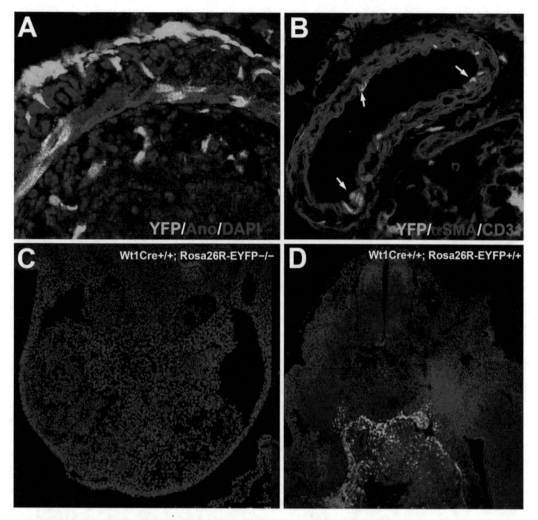

Fig. 3 Permanent lineage tracing with the mWt1/IRES/GFP-Cre;Rosa26R-YFP model. The lineage of the cells that have expressed Wt1, constitutively express YFP which can be directly observed by confocal microscopy. **(a)** Immunostaining of anoctamin (*red*) in the intestine of an E16.5 embryo. The calcium-activated chloride channel anoctamin is expressed in progenitors of the visceral smooth muscle, and some of which express YFP and therefore are part of the Wt1 lineage. **(b)** Double immunofluorescence of an artery in the lungs of an E18.5 embryo. Smooth muscle is shown in *red* and endothelium in *blue*. YFP+ cells can be seen forming part of the endothelium (*arrows*). **(c, d)** Despite the presence of a GFP sequence in the plasmid construct used to generate this model, expression of GFP is too low to be detected (**c**), and does not interfere with the strong expression of YFP (**d**)

(Rosa26R-EYFP in short) allows to generate permanent reporter expression in *Wt1*-expressing cells (Fig. 3a, b).

Of note, the Cre driver used for these studies induces the expression of low levels of GFP, but this expression does not interfere with the YFP expression of the reporter. Control $Wt1^{Cre+/+}$; Rosa26R-EYFP$^{-/-}$ embryos show no detectable GFP levels in the embryonic tissues by confocal microscopy (Fig. 3c, d).

1.3   Temporal Control of Wt1 Lineage Tracing: Inducible Cre Recombinase Expressed Under Control of Wt1

So far, one mouse line has been described that allows temporal induction of Cre recombinase activity under control of *Wt1* transcriptional regulation:

1. Wt1$^{\text{CreERT2}}$, generated in the Pu lab [6] (official nomenclature: Wt1$^{\text{tm2(cre/ERT2)Wtp}}$; MGI:3801682).

The Wt1$^{\text{CreERT2}}$mouse line was generated by gene targeting a construct containing the Cre-ERT2 recombinant expression cassette in alignment with the start codon, thus replacing the first coding exon. In the Wt1$^{\text{CreERT2}}$ mouse line, Cre recombinase activity is induced by administration of tamoxifen to mice. The Cre recombinase in these mice is fused to a modified estrogen receptor (ERT2; ref. 14). The Cre-ERT2 fusion protein can only enter the nucleus when binding of tamoxifen to the ERT2 part of the fusion protein has led to a conformational change; in the absence of tamoxifen, the Cre-ERT2 fusion protein is localized in the cytoplasm. In mice carrying the Wt1$^{\text{CreERT2}}$ allele and a genomic region flanked by loxP recognition sites, the Cre recombinase can remove the loxP-flanked elements after tamoxifen administration.

Because tamoxifen is required for the activation of Cre recombinase activity, it allows for temporal control of reporter gene activity. Thus, the system enables the analysis of the contribution and fate of Wt1-expressing cells at specific, defined time points, either in embryonic development, or in postnatal stages. Tamoxifen as the inducer of Cre recombination acts as a pulse, which results in irreversible activation of the reporter expression only when tamoxifen has led to the Cre-ERT2 conformational change. The time that passes between tamoxifen-induced recombination ("pulse") and time point of analysis represents the "chase" (Fig. 4): cells that change their fate and/or position within the tissue through differentiation and/or migration, may downregulate Wt1 and Cre expression, but will still be detectable for the reporter expression. Assessment of change in fate over time can be performed using immunohistochemistry with differentiation-specific markers.

Wt1$^{\text{CreERT2}}$ mice have been successfully used for lineage tracing studies in combination with Rosa26R-LacZ [15, 16], Rosa26R-EYFP [17] or Rosa26R-mTmG mice ([4, 6, 17, 18] and Wilm et al. in preparation; Fig. 5). For more information on Cre-specific reporter mouse strains, we refer to the Jackson laboratory website (http://cre.jax.org/crereporters.html).

Most applications using the Wt1$^{\text{CreERT2}}$;reporter system involve embryonic lineage tracing studies where tamoxifen is administered once at a specific time point during development [4, 6, 19–22]. However, in studies where adult Wt1-expressing cells are traced, either in unchallenged or injured animals, tamoxifen is usually administered on several occasions within 1–2 weeks, followed by a wash-out period [23, 24], Wilm et al. in preparation).

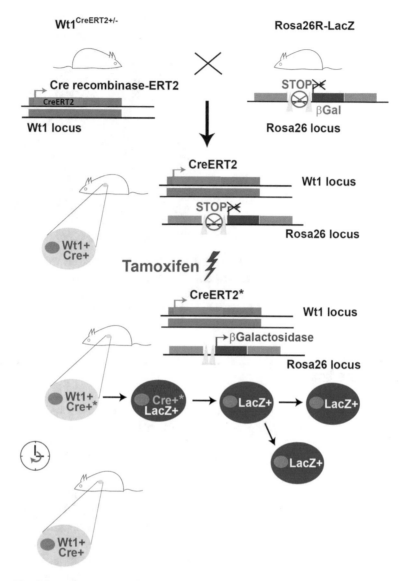

Fig. 4 For temporal control of reporter expression (here: β-galactosidase) in cells of the Wt1 lineage, the system consists of two genetic components similar to the model shown in Fig. 2. However, to allow temporal control of Cre activity in Wt1-expressing cells, the Cre recombinase is fused to a modified estrogen receptor (ERT2; Wt1 CreERT2 mouse line). The Cre-ERT2 fusion protein can only enter the nucleus when binding of tamoxifen to the ERT2 component of the fusion protein has led to a conformational change. In the absence of tamoxifen, the Cre-ERT2 fusion protein is localized in the cytoplasm. In tamoxifen-treated mice carrying both the Wt1 CreERT2 and the Rosa26R-LacZ reporter, the Cre recombinase will remove the loxP-flanked stop cassette after tamoxifen administration leading to permanent reporter expression. However, cells expressing Wt1 in subsequent days will not be labeled through Cre recombination. This means that the lineage of Wt1 expressing cells can be followed from a specific, defined time point, for example during embryonic development

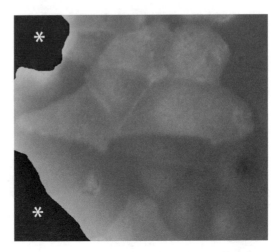

Fig. 5 Endogenous GFP fluorescence of live mesothelial cells grown out of omentum explants in culture, isolated from a Wt1[CreERT2]; Rosa26R-mTmG mouse 15 weeks after tamoxifen-induced recombination. *Indicate artificially blacked out areas of fluorescence of the omentum explant

2   Materials

Solutions for histological analysis are prepared from analytical grade chemicals with autoclaved distilled water. Solutions are autoclaved, where appropriate, and stored at room temperature, 4 °C or –20 °C.

2.1 Tamoxifen Solution and Administration

1. 40 mg/ml tamoxifen solution: weigh 1 g tamoxifen (for example: T5648, Sigma) into a 50 ml universal tube and add 2.5 ml of 100 % ethanol (molecular grade). Mix thoroughly and then add 22.5 ml corn oil (for example: C8267, Sigma). Transfer solution to small bottle wrapped in foil, add a small stir bar and store at 4 °C (*see* **Note 1, 2**).

2. Oral gavage needle (available in a range of sizes from different companies).

2.2 Preparation of Tissue for Frozen Sections

1. 10x PBS stock solution: weigh in 80 g $NaCl_2$, 2 g KCl, 14.4 g Na_2HPO_4, and 2.4 g KH_2PO_4 in a 2 l beaker, and add 800 ml distilled H_2O. Dissolve using a stir bar on a magnetic stirrer, and adjust pH to 7.4 using concentrated HCl. Once pH is adjusted, transfer solution to 1000 ml graduated cylinder and add distilled H_2O to make 1000 ml. Fill into a clean blue-capped bottle, autoclave and store at room temperature.

2. Phosphate Buffered Saline (PBS): either dilute 10× PBS stock solution to 1× working solution, or make up from PBS tablets (for example: P4417, Sigma), using distilled, autoclaved H_2O.

3. 4% Paraformaldehyde (PFA) solution: weigh in 10 g PFA and dissolve in 200 ml distilled H_2O and 25 ml 10× PBS, under constant stirring and by slowly warming up the solution to maximum of 60 °C, in the fume cupboard. Avoid breathing in the toxic fumes! Once solution has cleared, make solution up to 250 ml using distilled H_2O in a measuring cylinder. Transfer 4% PFA solution into a clean bottle, autoclave and store at 4 °C, or aliquot and store at –20 °C.

4. 15% sucrose in PBS: weigh in 15 g Sucrose and dissolve in 80 ml PBS; rotating and warming helps the sucrose to dissolve. Once dissolved, make solution up to 100 ml using PBS in a measuring cylinder, aliquot in 15 ml universal tube and store at –20 °C (*see* **Note 3**).

5. 30% sucrose in PBS: weigh in 30 g Sucrose and dissolve in 60 ml PBS; rotating and warming helps the sucrose to dissolve. Once dissolved, make solution up to 100 ml using PBS in a measuring cylinder, aliquot in 15 ml universal tube and store at –20 °C (*see* **Note 3**).

6. Optimal cutting temperature compound (OCT; Tissue Tek or other suppliers).

7. Cryostat including anti-roll blade, cryoblades.

8. Superfrost Plus glass slides (Thermo Scientific or other suppliers).

9. Isopentane.

2.3 Immuno-fluorescence Analysis

1. Tris-PBS (TPBS): 1× TPBS solution: Weigh 7 g $NaCl_2$, 1.48 g Na_2HPO_4 and 043 g KH_2PO_4 and 5 g of Trizma base (Sigma, T1503) in a 2 l beaker, and add 800 ml distilled H_2O. Dissolve using a stir bar on a magnetic stirrer, and adjust pH to 7.8 using concentrated HCl. Once pH is adjusted, transfer solution to 1000 ml graduated cylinder and add distilled H_2O to make 1000 ml.

2. Serum blocking solution (SB): 16% sheep serum, 1% bovine albumin in TPBS.

3. Serum blocking solution with Triton (SBT): 16% sheep serum, 1% bovine albumin, 0.1% Triton X-100 in TPBS.

4. Avidin-Biotin blocking kit (Vector).

5. Monovalent donkey anti-mouse IgG, Fab fragment (Jackson).

6. Primary antibodies: available from a plethora of companies.

7. Secondary antibodies: take note to match the fluorophore with the filter sets available if using an epifluorescent or confocal microscope.

8. 5 mg/ml DAPI stock solution: dissolve 5 mg DAPI (for example: D9542, Sigma) in 1 ml molecular grade H_2O. Complete dissolution can take some time. Store at –20 °C.

9. 1 μg/ml DAPI working solution: dilute 1 μl DAPI stock solution in 5 ml PBS. This solution can be directly added to the sections.

10. Mounting medium: a 1:1 glycerol–PBS solution can be used for temporal mounting. Alternatively, commercial mounting media are available (e.g., Gel Mount from Biomeda or Sigma).

11. Humid chamber: A closed box containing a horizontal surface covered by filter paper moistened in distilled water.

2.4 X-Gal Staining on Frozen Sections

1. 40 mg/ml X-gal stock solution: Dilute 20 mg of X-gal (for example: Boehringer Mannheim, #745–740) in 0.5 ml of dimethylformamide (for example: 227056, Sigma). Mix well and store at −20 °C in a 1 ml tube protected from light.

2. 100 mM KFerro II solution: Weigh in 2.11 g Potassium hexacyanoferrate(II) trihydrate (for example: P3289, Sigma) into a 50 ml universal container and dissolve in 50 ml distilled, autoclaved H_2O. Wrap in foil to protect from light and store at room temperature.

3. 100 mM KFerro III solution: Weigh in 1.65 g Potassium hexacyanoferrate(III) (for example: 244023, Sigma) into a 50 ml universal container and dissolve in 50 ml distilled, autoclaved H_2O. Wrap in foil to protect from light and store at room temperature.

4. 1 M $MgCl_2$ solution: Weigh in 203.3 g $MgCl_2$ hexahydrate into a 1.5 l glass beaker and dissolve in 800 ml distilled H_2O under stirring. Using a 1000 ml measuring cylinder, fill solution up to 1000 ml with distilled H_2O, fill into blue-capped bottle and autoclave. Store at room temperature.

5. X-gal dilution buffer for frozen sections: In a 50 ml universal container, add 500 μl 100 mM KFerro II solution, 500 μl 100 mM KFerro III solution, 1 ml 10× PBS and 20 μl 1 M $MgCl_2$ to 7730 μl distilled H_2O and mix well.

6. X-gal Working Solution: Warm X-gal dilution buffer to 37 °C and then add 250 μl 40 mg/ml X-gal stock solution. Use immediately and discard any leftover solution.

7. Neutral Red Solution. Weigh 3.3 g neutral red and dissolve in 1000 ml distilled H_2O under stirring. Commercial solutions are available (For example: N2889, Sigma).

8. Eukitt mounting medium (available from different suppliers).

2.5 X-Gal Staining of Tissues

1. 0.2% Glutaraldehyde/2% PFA fixative for whole mount X-gal staining: In a 50 ml universal container, mix 400 μl 25% Glutaraldehyde (grade II, for example G6257 from Sigma) and 25 ml 4% PFA solution with 24.6 ml PBS. Make fresh before each use (see **Note 4**).

2. 20 mg/ml X-gal stock solution: Dilute 20 mg of X-gal (for example: Boehringer Mannheim, #745–740) in 1 ml of

Dimethylformamide (for example: 227056, Sigma). Mix well and store in a 1 ml tube protected from light at −20 °C.

3. 10 % Nonidet P-40 solution: Dilute 1 ml Nonidet P-40 (IGEPAL CA-630, I3021, Sigma) in 9 ml of distilled, autoclaved H_2O in a 15 ml universal container, warm up slightly to aid the detergent to dissolve, and store at room temperature (*see* **Note 5**).

4. 1 % Sodium deoxycholate (NaDOC) solution: Weigh in 500 mg of NaDOC (for example: D6750, Sigma) into a 50 ml universal container and dissolve in 50 ml of distilled, autoclaved H_2O. Store at room temperature.

5. Wash solution: Add 100 μl 10 % Nonidet P-40 to 50 ml PBS to give a final concentration of 0.02 % Nonidet P-40 in PBS.

6. X-gal staining solution: Mix together in a 50 ml universal container 2.5 ml 100 mM KFerro II solution, 2.5 ml 100 mM KFerro III solution, 5 ml 10× PBS, 100 μl 1 M $MgCl_2$, 100 μl 10 % Nonidet P-40 solution and 500 μl 1 % NaDOC solution with 36.8 ml distilled H_2O and mix well. Add 2.5 ml 20 mg/ml X-gal solution and use immediately; discard any leftover solution.

2.6 Eosin-Counterstained Paraffin Sections of X-Gal Stained Tissue

1. Isopropanol/isopropyl alcohol (e.g., W292907, Sigma).

2. Paraffin pellets (various suppliers).

3. Isopropanol–paraffin solution: In a prewarmed 100 ml glass bottle, mix 50 ml isopropanol with 50 ml liquid paraffin, stir and keep in a histology oven at around 58–60 °C until further use.

4. Histology oven, embedding station, microtome, microtome blades, histology water bath, stirrer

5. Embedding cassettes (various suppliers) or Peel-A-Ways embedding molds (for example: 18986 or 18646A, Polysciences).

6. Xylene, histology grade (for example: 534056, Sigma) or Histoclear (for example: HS-200, National Diagnostics).

7. Superfrost Plus glass slides (Thermo Scientific or other suppliers).

8. Glass slide racks with metal handle and staining dish (e.g., 70312-20, EMS).

9. 1 % eosin Y stock solution: Weigh in 10 g eosin Y (e.g., E4009, Sigma), place in a 250 ml bottle, and dissolve in 200 ml distilled, autoclaved H_2O. Add 800 ml 95–100 % ethanol to generate a 1 % eosin Y stock solution. Store at room temperature.

10. 0.25 % eosin Y staining solution: Dilute the eosin Y stock solution further by adding 750 ml of 80 % ethanol to 250 ml eosin Y stock solution. Add 5 ml glacial acetic acid and mix well. Store at room temperature.

11. DPX mountant for histology (06522, Sigma).

12. Coverslip Best No.1, 22 mm×50 mm (12342118, Thermo Scientific).

3 Methods

3.1 Tamoxifen Administration

1. Gently warm the tamoxifen solution on a heated stirrer until completely liquid.

2. Intraperitoneal injection, subcutaneous injection and oral gavage have been reported as successful administration routes [6, 23, 25]. The optimal route of administration depends on a range of factors that need to be considered for each specific experimental design; factors to consider are deposition and leakage of oil after subcutaneous injection; interaction of oil with Wt1-expressing, mesothelial tissues after intraperitoneal injection; and feasibility of oral gavage (25); BW, unpublished observations).

3. Typically, the doses for tamoxifen administration range between 1 and 2 mg tamoxifen per 10 g body weight. Dosing regimens depend on the experimental design and range from once at a specific time point during embryonic development in case of embryonic lineage tracing, to 2–5 times within a week for postnatal or adult lineage tracing (*see* **Note 6**). The pharmacological half-life of tamoxifen after a single dose of tamoxifen has been reported to be about 12 h [26].

3.2 Embryo and Tissue Harvesting

Mouse embryos are staged from the time point when a vaginal plug was observed, which is designated as the stage E0.5. Embryos and neonate/adult mice are sacrificed, dissected and embryos/tissues washed in PBS before further processing. The respective national and local animal experimental guidelines need to be followed for the sacrifice of pregnant dams or newborn/adult animals.

3.3 Immuno-fluorescence Analysis of Reporter Distribution on Frozen Sections

1. Embryos/tissues are fixed at room temperature in 4% freshly prepared paraformaldehyde (PFA) solution in PBS for 2–8 h (depending on the size) in 30–50 ml universal containers. The tissue is washed in PBS and cryoprotected by incubating in 15% sucrose solution at 4 °C until it sinks to the bottom of the container. This is followed by incubation in 30% sucrose solution at 4 °C until the tissue has sunk.

2. Embryos/tissues are placed in Peel-A-Ways or other embedding molds and as much of the sucrose solution is removed as possible using tissue paper before OCT is added to the mold to go at least 1 cm over the embryo/tissue. The embryos/tissues are snap frozen in liquid N_2-cooled isopentane. Plastic tubes with isopentane are kept for a few minutes in liquid N_2 and then the embryos are rapidly submerged in the isopentane. Cooling of isopentane with dry ice is also possible. The frozen embryos are wrapped in foil and stored at –80 °C.

3. Cryosections of 7–10 μm thickness are obtained on a cryostat, collected on glass slides and stored at –20 °C until use. YFP

expression is strong enough to be directly detected by confocal microscopy (Fig. 3a, b).

4. For immunofluorescence detection of reporter and marker proteins, cryosections are air-dried, rehydrated for 5 min in TPBS and blocked during 30 min for nonspecific binding with SB or SBT for membrane-bound and intracellular antigens, respectively. When using biotinylated secondary antibodies, the endogenous biotin must be blocked at this step with the Avidin-Biotin blocking kit, according to the instructions on the supplier. In this case, the sections should be washed for 5 min in TPBS before adding the primary antibody.

5. Single immunofluorescence is performed incubating the sections with the primary antibody overnight at 4 °C. The antibody is dissolved in SB or SBT as indicated in the former point. Then, the sections are washed in TPBS (3×5 min) and incubated with the corresponding fluorochrome-conjugated secondary antibody dissolved in SB or SBT for 1 h at room temperature in the dark. If nuclei are to be counterstained with DAPI, the working solution can be added to the solvent of the secondary antibody to a final concentration of 1 μg/ml of DAPI. Alternatively, the sections can be stained with the working solution described in Subheading 2.3, **item 9** (*see* **Notes 7** and **8**).

6. For double immunofluorescence, two primary antibodies (for example a rabbit polyclonal and a mouse or rat monoclonal) are incubated in combination overnight at 4 °C, in SB or SBT as described in the former section. After a wash step with TPBS, the sections are incubated for 1 h with the corresponding secondary antibodies conjugated to different fluorochromes (e.g., phycoerythrin and Alexa 647) and DAPI (1 μg/mL final concentration), diluted in SB or SBT, allowing for three-color images (Fig. 3a, b).

7. When the primary antibodies are generated in different species (e.g., rat, mouse, and rabbit), it is even possible to perform triple immunofluorescence. In this case, rat and rabbit primary antibodies, and the corresponding secondary antibodies are incubated first as described above. Then, the sections are incubated for 1 h at room temperature with monovalent donkey anti-mouse IgG, Fab fragment (*see* **Note 9**) diluted 1:100 in TPBS, followed by washing in TPBS (3×5 min) and incubation with the mouse primary antibody, washing and the corresponding anti-mouse IgG secondary antibody conjugated to a compatible fluorochrome with those used previously. Counterstaining with DAPI allows for four-color images, but it is important to take in account that confocal images are captured only in three channels (red, green and blue), being any additional color combination of them.

8. After final wash in TPBS (3×5 min), the sections are mounted with glycerol–PBS 1:1 or commercial mounting media and protected from the light.

3.4 X-Gal Staining on Frozen Sections

1. Embryos/tissues can be directly frozen in OCT without prior fixation, and stored at −80 °C until further use. Cryosections obtained from the unfixed tissue are fixed for 10 min in cold 4% PFA and washed three times in PBS.

2. The X-gal dilution buffer is set up, warmed to 37 °C and then 40 mg/ml X-gal stock solution added. The slides are incubated in X-gal working solution in a humidified chamber placed in an incubator at 37 °C for 24 h.

3. The sections are washed in PBS for 2 × 5 min, rinse with distilled water briefly and counterstain with neutral red for 3–5 min. After washing in distilled water the sections can be dehydrated in alcohol and mounted with Eukitt mounting medium.

See **Note 10**.

3.5 X-Gal Whole Mount Staining of Embryos/Tissues

1. Large mouse embryos (over E13.5) or whole organs need to be sectioned with a scalpel (e.g., sagittally) to improve penetration of the staining solution. Embryos/tissues are fixed in 0.2% Glutaraldehyde/2% PFA fixative at 4 °C for 10–15 min (small embryos), 15–30 min (large embryos over E13.5) or 1–2 h (adult tissues) in 20 ml universal containers.

2. The embryos/tissues are washed three times for 30 min in wash solution, followed by incubation in X-gal staining solution in the dark at room temperature (*see* **Note 11**). The stained embryos/tissues are postfixed overnight in 4% PFA at 4 °C, and after a few PBS washes, stored in 70% ethanol.

3.6 Histological Analysis of X-Gal Stained Whole Embryos/Tissues

1. Postfixed X-gal stained embryos/tissues are dehydrated through an ethanol series (25%, 50%, 75%) into 100% ethanol (twice), with each step lasting 15–30 min at room temperature. The ethanol is then replaced by isopropanol for two incubation steps of at least 15 min each.

2. The embryo/tissue is incubated in a pre-warmed, well-mixed 1:1 isopropanol–paraffin solution in a histology incubator at 58–60 °C for 1 h. The isopropanol–paraffin solution is subsequently replaced by fresh paraffin and after a short incubation for 1 h in the incubator, the embryo/tissue is incubated in a fresh change of paraffin in the incubator overnight.

3. The next day, the embryo/tissue is placed inside embedding molds or Peel-A-Ways and covered by paraffin. This step is easiest when done using an embedding station. It is important to consider the desired orientation of the sections and achieving the correct orientation especially for small embryos can be tricky (*see* **Note 12**). The tissue block is allowed to solidify overnight before sectioning. For long-term storage, the blocks are stored at 4 °C.

4. Using a microtome, sections of 5–10 μm are generated as 'ribbons', and collected on glass slides with the help of water

(for example histology water bath at 45–50 °C) to facilitate even spreading of the sections. Sections are subsequently dried for 30 min at RT, followed by baking in an incubator at 45–50 °C overnight. Sections can be stored in slide boxes at room temperature or 4 °C until further use (*see* **Note 13**).

5. For eosin counterstaining, sections are dewaxed by two incubation steps in xylene (or Histoclear as alternative) in a glass rack in a staining dish on a stirrer, where the small stir bar is placed between glass rack and glass trough. Note that xylene steps require work in a fume cupboard.

6. Pass the slides in the glass rack through a series of ethanol changes, starting with two changes of 100 % ethanol, and incubation steps in 95 %, 75 %, and 50 % ethanol for 5 min each. Slides are subsequently placed in PBS. It is important that sections must not be allowed to dry from this step onwards.

7. Slides are incubated for 1 min in eosin staining solution (*see* **Notes 14** and **15**). This is followed by a wash step in tap water for 1 min, and a dehydration series from 50 % to 100 % ethanol for 2–5 min each. Slides are incubated twice for 2 min in xylene (or Histoclear) before embedding with mounting medium using coverslips. A typical result of this procedure is shown in Fig. 8.

4   Notes

1. Note that tamoxifen is an anticancer drug used in cancer patients. Tamoxifen acts as an antagonist of the estrogen receptor through its active metabolite 4-hydroxytamoxifen. It is therefore essential that health and safety aspects of workers exposed to tamoxifen are being considered before work is started.

2. Different concentrations of tamoxifen solutions, using different types of oils (peanut, sunflower), are reported in the literature.

3. Sucrose solutions will be prone to contamination with yeast or fungi. Discard container after 2 weeks.

4. For long term storage, upon opening the bottle, aliquot 25 % glutaraldehyde grade II solution into 10 ml aliquots (15 ml universal containers), and store at –20 °C.

5. Nonidet P-40 is highly viscous, so exact measurement of the 1 ml Nonidet P-40 may not be possible.

6. Tamoxifen can affect the delivery of litters in pregnant females. If lineage tracing is required to last from embryonic to postnatal stages, it is therefore recommended that the pups are recovered by Caesarian section and placed with a foster dam. Lineage tracing in newborn pups can be facilitated via tamoxifen administration to the lactating dam.

7. Cryosections are routinely stained with a panel of antibodies to identify the (developmental) fate of the Wt1-expressing cell lineage. Use of secondary antibodies conjugated to fluorochromes compatible with YFP, such as TRITC, phycoerythrin, Cy5, Alexa 647, or infrared-emitting fluorochromes allows for triple or quadruple staining.

8. Negative controls should always be performed by incubating with non-immune species-matched isotype IgG instead of the primary antibodies.

9. The monovalent antibody blocks potential binding sites on the rat IgG for the anti-mouse IgG secondary antibody.

10. Alternatively, β-galactosidase expression can be detected by immunofluorescence (protocol 3.3) using the rabbit anti-β-galactosidase primary antibody (#559762) from Cappel/MPI (Fig. 6).

11. Depending on the level of β-galactosidase expression, staining may take between a few hours to overnight (Fig. 7).

12. Use fine forceps that are pre-warmed in the histology incubator or the embedding station, to orient the embryo in the paraffin, and place the mold onto the hot spot of the embedding station. This allows the paraffin to stay liquid for a bit longer. One of the problems can be the formation of a solid sheet at the surface, which prevents visualization of the embryo. Removing the solidifying sheet at the surface repeatedly will provide an additional short time window in which to orient the embryo. In general, it is important to work fast, and to know beforehand which way the embryo should be oriented.

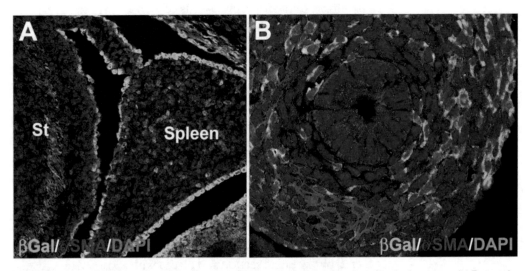

Fig. 6 Detection of the β-Galactosidase reporter by immunofluorescence and confocal microscopy. (**a**) Expression in an E13.5 embryo of the Tg(WT1)HNdh Wt1 reporter line. Putative Wt1 expressing cells can be seen in the mesothelium of the spleen primordium, located in the mesogastrium, and also in cells within the spleen. St, stomach. (**b**) Immunolocalization of β-Galactosidase in the intestine of a E11.5 Wt1[Cre]; Rosa26-LacZ embryo

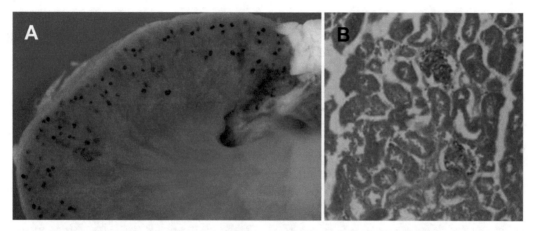

Fig. 7 Detection of the β-Galactosidase reporter by X-gal staining of whole adult tissue. (**a**) X-gal staining of bisected whole kidney of an adult Wt1 ^CreERT2^; Rosa26R-LacZ mouse 5 months after tamoxifen pulse. Only glomeruli show X-gal staining, indicating that they have expressed Wt1 at the time of tamoxifen administration. (**b**) Histological section of the X-gal-stained kidney shown in (**a**), counterstained with eosin. X-gal staining is confined to the glomeruli

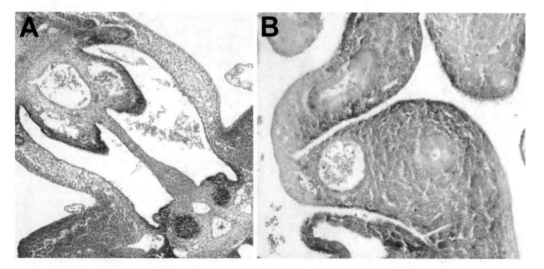

Fig. 8 Detection of the β-Galactosidase reporter by X-gal staining of whole embryos which were stained, paraffin-embedded and sectioned. (**a**) X-gal expression in an E10.5 embryo of the Tg(WT1)HNdh Wt1 reporter line, showing staining in intermediate mesoderm and mesenterium. (**b**) X-gal expression staining cells from the Wt1 lineage in the digestive tract of an E11.5 mWt1/IRES/GFP-Cre; Rosa26LacZ embryo

13. X-gal staining on sections can be detected by eye or under a microscope (depending on the strength of the signal), allowing the selection of relevant sections for eosin counterstaining. It is important to note that the tissue in the paraffin sections does not allow for a proper evaluation unless dewaxed, counterstained (optional), appropriately dehydrated and permanently mounted with coverslips.

14. The eosin counterstaining provides a pink staining to the tissue section. The eosin staining solution is acidic and the staining reaction is based on its binding to basic cells and tissue structures, including the cytoplasm of cells.

15. The optimal time for incubation in the eosin staining solution depends on its strength and needs to be determined individually.

References

1. Algar E (2002) A review of the Wilms' tumor 1 gene (WT1) and its role in hematopoiesis and leukemia. J Hematother Stem Cell Res 11:589–599

2. Moore AW, Schedl A, McInnes L et al (1998) YAC transgenic analysis reveals Wilms' tumour 1 gene activity in the proliferating coelomic epithelium, developing diaphragm and limb. Mech Dev 79:169–184

3. Moore AW, McInnes L, Kreidberg J et al (1999) YAC complementation shows a requirement for Wt1 in the development of epicardium, adrenal gland and throughout nephrogenesis. Development 126:1845–1857

4. Rudat C, Kispert A (2012) Wt1 and epicardial fate mapping. Circ Res 111:165–169

5. Hosen N, Shirakata T, Nishida S et al (2007) The Wilms' tumor gene WT1-GFP knock-in mouse reveals the dynamic regulation of WT1 expression in normal and leukemic hematopoiesis. Leukemia 21:1783–1791

6. Zhou B, Ma Q, Rajagopal S et al (2008) Epicardial progenitors contribute to the cardiomyocyte lineage in the developing heart. Nature 454:109–113

7. del Monte G, Casanova JC, Guadix JA et al (2011) Differential Notch signaling in the epicardium is required for cardiac inflow development and coronary vessel morphogenesis. Circ Res 108:824–836

8. Norden J, Grieskamp T, Lausch E et al (2010) Wt1 and retinoic acid signaling in the subcoelomic mesenchyme control the development of the pleuropericardial membranes and the sinus horns. Circ Res 106:1212–1220

9. Wilm B, IJpenberg A, Hastie ND et al (2005) The serosal mesothelium is a major source of smooth muscle cells of the gut vasculature. Development 132:5317–5328

10. Kolander KD, Holtz ML, Cossette SM et al (2014) Epicardial GATA factors regulate early coronary vascular plexus formation. Dev Biol 386:204–215

11. Cano E, Carmona R, Muñoz-Chápuli R (2013) Wt1-expressing progenitors contribute to multiple tissues in the developing lung. Am J Physiol 305:L322–L332

12. Carmona R, Cano E, Mattiotti A et al (2013) Cells derived from the coelomic epithelium contribute to multiple gastrointestinal tissues in mouse embryos. PLoS One 8:e55890

13. Wessels A, van den Hoff MJB, Adamo RF et al (2012) Epicardially derived fibroblasts preferentially contribute to the parietal leaflets of the atrioventricular valves in the murine heart. Dev Biol 366:111–124

14. Feil R, Wagner J, Metzger D et al (1997) Regulation of Cre recombinase activity by mutated estrogen receptor ligand-binding domains. Biochem Biophys Res Commun 237:752–757

15. Soriano P (1999) Generalized lacZ expression with the ROSA26 Cre reporter strain. Nat Genet 21:70–71

16. Mao X, Fujiwara Y, Orkin SH et al (1999) Improved reporter strain for monitoring Cre recombinase-mediated DNA excisions in mice. Proc Natl Acad Sci U S A 96:5037–5042

17. Srinivas S, Watanabe T, Lin CS et al (2001) Cre reporter strains produced by targeted insertion of EYFP and ECFP into the ROSA26 locus. BMC Dev Biol 1:4

18. Muzumdar MD, Tasic B, Miyamichi K et al (2007) A global double-fluorescent Cre reporter mouse. Genesis 45:593–605

19. Dixit R, Ai X, Fine A (2013) Derivation of lung mesenchymal lineages from the fetal mesothelium requires hedgehog signaling for mesothelial cell entry. Development 140:4398–4406

20. Zhou B, Pu WT (2012) Genetic Cre-loxP assessment of epicardial cell fate using Wt1-driven Cre alleles. Circ Res 111:e276–e280

21. Asahina K, Zhou B, Pu WT et al (2011) Septum transversum-derived mesothelium gives rise to hepatic stellate cells and perivascular mesenchymal cells in developing mouse liver. Hepatology 53:983–995

22. Manuylov NL, Zhou B, Ma Q et al (2011) Conditional ablation of Gata4 and Fog2 genes in mice reveals their distinct roles in mammalian sexual differentiation. Dev Biol 353:229–241

23. Chau YY, Bandiera R, Serrels A et al (2014) Visceral and subcutaneous fat have different origins and evidence supports a mesothelial source. Nat Cell Biol 16:367–375

24. Smart N, Risebro CA, Melville AAD et al (2007) Thymosin beta-4 is essential for coronary vessel development and promotes neovascularization via adult epicardium. Ann N Y Acad Sci 1112:171–188

25. Reinert RB, Kantz J, Misfeldt AA et al (2012) Tamoxifen-Induced Cre-loxP recombination is prolonged in pancreatic islets of adult mice. PLoS One 7:e33529

26. Robinson SP, Langan-Fahey SM, Johnson DA et al (1991) Metabolites, pharmacodynamics, and pharmacokinetics of tamoxifen in rats and mice compared to the breast cancer patient. Drug Metab Dispos 19:36–43

Chapter 5

Biological Systems and Methods for Studying WT1 in the Epicardium

Víctor Velecela, Janat Fazal-Salom, and Ofelia M. Martínez-Estrada

Abstract

The embryonic epicardium is an important source of cardiovascular precursor cells and paracrine factors required for adequate heart formation. During embryonic heart formation, WT1 is mainly expressed in epicardial cells and epicardial derived cells. Its expression has been used to trace epicardial derivatives in embryos and recently it has been used to follow the reactivation of epicardial cells after myocardial infarction. Interestingly, the highest level of expression of WT1 during epicardium development correlates with the highest proliferative state, stem cell properties, and migratory capacity of epicardial cells. Here, we review the various types of tools and strategies used to study WT1 function in the embryonic epicardium and provide examples of their use.

Key words Wt1, Epicardium, Development, Cell culture, In vivo FACS analysis, Migration assay, Transwell assay, Quantitative PCR

1   Introduction

The epicardium originates from a mass of mesothelial cells known as the proepicardium, which is located on the wall of the embryonic pericardial cavity just dorsal and caudal to the developing early heart [1]. Proepicardial cells extend out to reach the surface of the heart around stage E9.5 in mice and spread and cover all the surface of the myocardium by E11.5 [1].

The models in which the epicardium is disrupted are lethal before the onset of normal coronary development and blood flow, suggesting an important role for the epicardium in heart development [2].

The epicardium contributes to the formation of cardiovascular precursor cells that differentiate into various cell types, including coronary smooth muscle and endothelial cells, perivascular and cardiac interstitial fibroblasts, and a low percentage of cardiomyocytes [2]. In addition to cellular contributions to the developing heart, the epicardium and its derivatives provide paracrine signals which influence myocardial maturation and the development of the coronary vasculature [2, 3].

Nicholas Hastie (ed.), *The Wilms' Tumor (WT1) Gene: Methods and Protocols*, Methods in Molecular Biology, vol. 1467, DOI 10.1007/978-1-4939-4023-3_5, © Springer Science+Business Media New York 2016

The understanding of the epicardial potential in development is highly relevant given the crucial role of the epicardium in response to injury [4, 5]. Following myocardial infarction (MI), epicardial cells revert to an embryonic-like phenotype, proliferating at the site of injury and secreting factors to modulate wound healing [4, 5].

During heart development, *Wt1* is mainly expressed in the epicardium and epicardial derived cells, *Wt1* being one of the main hallmarks of the embryonic epicardium signature [6]. Its expression is downregulated during the course of epicardium development and interestingly its expression is reactivated after MI [4, 5].

One of the major challenges in epicardial biology is the identification of novel downstream targets of *Wt1* during heart development. Targeted inactivation of the *Wt1* gene causes embryonic lethality at E13.5 due to defects in heart formation [6]. Histological analyses of hearts from *Wt1* null mice clearly demonstrated severe defects in epicardium formation, with some regions of the heart containing gaps and others with a complete absence of an epicardium [6]. A significant number of apoptotic cells have also been identified in the epicardium and subepicardial region of *Wt1KO* embryos [6]. Thus, these KO mice constitute an important limitation for the study of the function of such an important gene for the epicardium beyond stage E13.5 and which might have a crucial role in heart repair.

Recently, we undertook a conditional gene inactivation strategy using a Cre/loxP system to inactivate *Wt1* in the epicardium from mice containing a floxed *Wt1* allele [3]. *Wt1loxP/loxP* mice were interbred with *Gata5-Cre/Wt1GFP+/−* transgenic mice. The resulting *Wt1KO* mice (*Gata5-Cre+; Wt1loxP/gfp*), henceforth known as epi*Wt1KO*, have its *Wt1* conditional allele located opposite the *Wt1GFPKI* allele (*Wt1loxP/gfp*), allowing us the isolation by FACS of control and *Wt1KO* epicardial cells [3]. The resulting *Wt1* mutants die between embryonic days E16.5 and E18.5 due to cardiovascular failure. The good integrity of epicardial cells covering the surface of the myocardium in these KO mice demonstrated the importance of this *Wt1KO* mouse model in the study of *Wt1* function in the embryonic epicardium [3].

However, the fact that epicardial cells constitute less than 10% of the cells of the developing heart complicates epicardium research and renders the study of the function of *Wt1* in epicardial cells difficult. To bypass this problem and to further study the mechanism of action and role of *Wt1* at a cellular and molecular level, we generated a series of immortalized epicardial cell lines.

Firstly, we generated immortalized epicardial cells from control (*Wt1gfp/+*) and KO embryos (*Wt1gfp/−*), where both are GFP positive and express epicardial cell markers; however their morphology is different [7] (Fig. 1). Interestingly, this change in morphology (size) is also observed in the *Wt1KO* epicardium in vivo

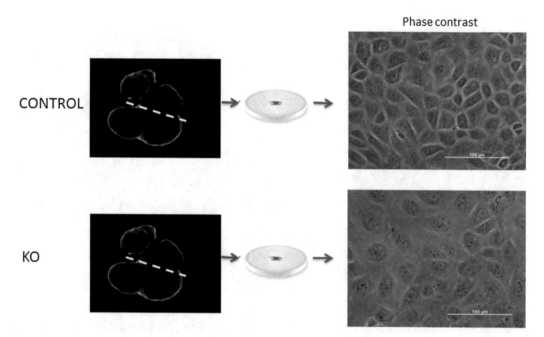

Fig. 1 Generation of immortalized epicardial cells. Schematic representation of the isolation of *Wt1GFP+* E11.5 ventricles (*left panels*) and generation of immortalized epicardial cells from control and *Wt1KO* mice ventricles that were placed on a gelatin coated dish. Phase-contrast micrograph of Control and *Wt1KO* immortalized epicardial cells is shown on the *right hand side panels* where the typical cobblestone morphology of epicardial cells can be observed in both cultures; however KO cells can also be observed to be bigger in size

(data not shown), suggesting that *Wt1KO* immortalized cells and the *Wt1KO* epicardium have acquired some modification during embryonic epicardium development.

We also generated tamoxifen inducible *Wt1KO* epicardial cells [3, 8]. The use of tamoxifen inducible *Wt1KO* cells has helped us in the identification of direct targets of WT1. The genes that are switched on or off shortly after the deletion of *Wt1* are more likely to be directly regulated by WT1.

We generated these immortalized cells using two strategies: the first one involves immortalized epicardial cells that were produced from *Wt1loxP/loxP* mice, and which were transfected with a CAGGs-CreERT2-IRES-puro R expression construct to enable the generation of stable clones using puromycin selection (kind gift from Dr. Lars Grotewold) [3]. The second strategy consisted in the generation of immortalized epicardial cells from CAGG-CreER+; *Wt1loxP/gfp* and CAGG-CreER−; *Wt1loxP/gfp* mice [8].

These strategies allowed us to generate clones and mixed populations of immortalized epicardial cells; thus we are able to produce enough cells and material to enable us to study the epicardium from a cellular and molecular biology point of view (Fig. 2).

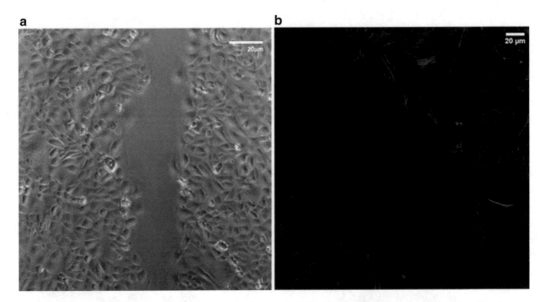

Fig. 2 Migrating epicardial cells in a wound healing assay. (**a**) Phase-contrast micrograph of migrating immortalized epicardial cells in a wound healing assay. (**b**) Actin filament staining (*red*) of migrating epicardial cells

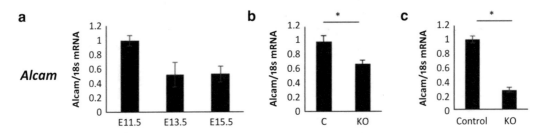

Fig. 3 Gene expression analysis of GFP sorted epicardial cells. (**a**) qRT-PCR analysis of *Alcam* in GFP+ epicardial cells at different days of development. (**b**) qRT-PCR analysis of freshly isolated GFP+ epicardial cells using FACS from *Gata-5 Cre−/Wt1loxP/gfp* (C) and *Gata-5 Cre+/Wt1loxP/gfp* (KO) mice. (**c**) qRT-PCR analysis of GFP+ immortalized control and *Wt1KO* epicardial cells. Arbitrary Units are used

The embryonic epicardium constitutes a heterogeneous population of cells that dynamically changes during heart development; taking into account this fact an accurate characterization of epicardial cells at each embryonic stage will help us understand their nature and composition. The possibility to generate immortalized epicardial cells at each embryonic stage using the methods described in this chapter could represent an interesting alternative.

We believe that the combination of independent approaches using in vitro immortalized epicardial cells, freshly isolated GFP sorted epicardial cells, and *epiWt1KO* cells is required to demonstrate new functions of *Wt1* in the embryonic epicardium (Fig. 3). The present chapter describes diverse strategies for the generation of immortalized epicardial cells from different mice in order to study the role of *Wt1* during epicardium development. It also describes the enzymatic digestion of embryonic GFP hearts from *Wt1GFPKI* mice and control and *epiWt1KO* mice.

1.1 Equipment	1. Dissecting fluorescent stereomicroscope.

1. Dissecting fluorescent stereomicroscope.

2. 33 °C and 37 °C incubators containing 5 % CO_2.

3. Water bath.

4. Microcentrifuge.

5. Thermomixer (Eppendorf).

6. Surgical materials: forceps and needles.

7. Laminar cell culture hood

8. Epifluorescent or confocal microscope for visualizing cells.

9. Plate reader (485 nm excitation and 520 nm filters).

10. FACS machine (FACSAria™).

11. LC480 real time PCR machine (Roche).

2   Materials

2.1 Cell Culture Reagents

1. Gelatin solution: 100 mg of gelatin dissolved in 100 ml of sterile water. Autoclave and store at 4 °C.

2. Trypsin solution: Trypsin diluted 1:10 in Versene (0.48 g/l EDTA in PBS and 6 ml/l of Phenol Red Solution 0.5 % in PBS).

3. Tamoxifen stock solution: dissolve 20 mg tamoxifen in 1 ml of ethanol. Store at –80 °C.

4. Tamoxifen working solution: dilute the tamoxifen stock solution 50 times in DMEM medium without serum. Store at –20 °C.

5. Glutamine solution: l-Glutamine Solution 200 mM (Sigma G7513).

6. Antibiotic solution: Penicillin/Streptomycin.

7. Cell culture condition: Dulbecco's Modified Eagles Medium (DMEM) containing GlutaMAX (Life Technologies), 4.5 g/l d-glucose and pyruvate, and supplemented with 10 % fetal bovine serum, 100 units/ml penicillin, and 100 μg/ml streptomycin. Store at 4 °C.

8. Mouse interferon gamma: Dissolve 1 vial of mouse interferon gamma in DMEM medium without serum at 20 μg/ml. Keep aliquots frozen at –20 °C.

9. PBS (Phosphate Buffered Saline): 138 mM NaCl, 2.7 mM KCl, 8.2 mM $Na_2 HPO_4$, 1.5 mM $KH_2 PO_4$.

2.2 Transfection Reagents

1. Lipofectamine 2000.
2. Optimen medium.
3. CAGGs-CreERT2-IRES-puro R expression construct.

2.3 Immuno-fluorescence Reagents

1. Round glass coverslips coated with 1 % gelatin solution.
2. 2 % Paraformaldehyde solution (PFA): prepare 2 % PFA solution in PBS, pH 7.4. Work in a chemical hood. Keep aliquots frozen at −20 °C.
3. Humidified chamber: prepare a humidified light-protected chamber covered with aluminum foil enough to keep a 24-well plate.
4. Permeabilization solution: 0.1 % Triton X-100 in PBS.
5. Blocking solution: 2 % (w/v) bovine serum albumin (BSA) in PBS.
6. Primary antibody at appropriate dilution in blocking solution.

2.4 Migration Assay

1. Calcein AM: To make 2 mM stock solution, dissolve 1 vial (50 µg) in 30 µl of DMSO.
2. Calcein working solution: Dissolve stock solution to make a 2 µM working solution.
3. 24-well transwell membranes with 8 µm pores.

2.5 FACS Reagents

1. Trypsin solution: Trypsin diluted 1:10 in Versene (0.48 g/l EDTA in PBS and 6 ml/l of Phenol Red Solution 0.5 % in PBS).
2. DMEM culture medium containing GlutaMAX (Life Technologies), 4.5 g/l d-glucose, 1 % pyruvate, and supplemented with 10 % fetal bovine serum, 100 units/ml penicillin, and 100 µg/ml streptomycin. Store at 4 °C.
3. RNAlater buffer solution (Ambion)

2.6 qRT-PCR

1. For Taqman® real time PCR assays use: LC480 2× real time master mix (Roche), RNase/DNase free water, Taqman® probes and endogenous *Gapdh* mouse housekeeping control assay (Roche). Probes and primers are selected according to the universal probe library primer/probe design tool (Roche).
2. For SYBR green real-time assays use: GoTaq 2× real time master mix (Promega), RNase/DNase free water, primers that produce products less than 200 bp (design using Primer3 software), and 18s primers as a housekeeping control (Biomers).

3 Methods

3.1 Mouse Breeding

To generate immortalized epicardial cells *Wt1+/gfp* mice were crossed with the H-2KbtsA58 "immorto" mice carrying a temperature-sensitive simian virus 40 (SV40) large-T antigen 20.

Wt1gfp/+/Immorto⁺/⁻ were mated with *Wt1+/–*, *Wt1loxP/loxP* or CAGG-CreER; *Wt1loxP/loxP* mice in order to generate *Wt1gfp/+* (Control) and *Wt1gfp/–* (*WtlKO*), *Wt1gfp/loxP* (*Wt1loxP* cell lines) or tamoxifen inducible KO (Cre⁺) (*CreER+/Wt1loxP/gfp*) and control cell lines (Cre⁻) (*CreER–/Wt1loxP/gfp*) [3, 7, 8]

3.2 Generation of Mixed Population of Immortalized Epicardial Cells

1. Coat 24-well plates by pipetting 0.5 ml of 1% gelatin solution, allow to stand for at least 30 min and aspirate.

2. Dissect out embryos into sterile PBS and select WT1-GFP positive embryos under a fluorescent stereomicroscope. Fluorescence can be clearly seen in the embryonic kidney as a positive control.

3. Dissect out hearts (also tails for genotyping if needed) and cut out atria with sterile needles.

4. Place GFP+ heart ventricles in a 24-well gelatin dish and incubate. Epicardial cells can be seen migrating out of heart explants onto the surface over the gelatin within 24 h after the procedure.

5. After 48 h, carefully transfer the 24-well plate to the culture hood and remove ventricles with a needle and allow cells to reach confluence and propagate at 33 °C.

6. Cells are propagated at 33 °C in DMEM containing 10% FCS and 20 ng/ml mouse gamma interferon (Peprotech).

3.3 Generation of Cre⁺; Wt1ˡᵒˣᴾ/gfp Stables Clones

1. Day 1: Trypsinize subconfluent *Wt1ˡᵒˣᴾ/gfp* cells and seed at a density of 40,000 cells per cm² in a 24-well plate overnight.

2. Day 2: Transfect each well with 1 μg of CAGGs-CreERT2-IRES-puro R expression construct following lipofectamine 2000 instructions.

3. Day 3: Expand cells by transferring cells onto P100 cell culture dishes.

4. Day 4: Add selection antibiotic (5 μg/ml puromycin).

5. Feed cells with fresh medium containing antibiotics every second day until isolated colonies appear.

6. After 2 weeks, pick healthy colonies with Whatman paper discs and expand them for further analyses.

3.4 Characterization of Immortalized Cells by Immunostaining

1. Trypsinize subconfluent immortalized cells and seed at a density of 40,000 per cm² in a 24-well plate to which sterile coverslips have been coated with gelatine for at least 30 min.

2. Allow cells to grow until desired confluence is reached over the coverslips.

3. Remove medium and fix cells with 2% PFA for 10 min, followed by three washes with PBS.

4. Permeabilize cells for 3 min with PBS containing 0.1 % Triton X-100.

5. Block cells with PBS containing 2 % BSA for at least 1 h at room temperature.

6. Incubate overnight with primary antibody at an optimal dilution.

7. Aspirate primary antibody and wash with PBS three times for 5 min each.

8. Incubate for 1 h with secondary antibody at room temperature in the dark.

9. Wash three times with PBS.

10. Add Vectashield containing DAPI and mount coverslips. Use nail polish to seal the edges of the coverslips.

11. Acquire images using epifluorescence or confocal microscopy.

3.5 Functional Assays

3.5.1 Wound Healing Assay

1. Trypsinize subconfluent immortalized cells and seed at a density of 80,000 cells per cm^2 on a gelatine coated 24-well plate. Leave overnight at 37 °C.

2. Using a P200 pipette tip incise a wound in the central area of the confluent 24-well culture.

3. Gently wash the cells twice with DMEM medium without FCS to remove detached cells.

4. Add fresh warm (37 °C) DMEM medium containing 1 % FCS and the desired additives and conditions.

5. Incubate cells at 37 °C for 24 h and capture images using a live cell imaging system.

3.5.2 Transwell Migration Assay of Immortalized Epicardial Cells

1. Trypsinize subconfluent immortalized cells and seed at a density of 40,000 cells per cm^2 in a T25 flask the day before the experiment. Incubate overnight.

2. Starve cells in culture by adding serum free medium overnight.

3. Coat 24-well transwell membrane inserts with 8 μm pores by adding 200 μl in the apical zone and 900 μl in the basal zone with 1 % gelatin solution. Incubate at 37 °C for 1 h.

4. Wash both sides of the insert with PBS three times.

5. Block membrane by adding 5 % BSA in PBS overnight at 4 °C.

6. Next day wash inserts with sterile water and leave to dry for 3 h inside a hood.

7. Trypsinize starved cells, centrifuge, and resuspend in DMEM medium with 1 % BSA.

8. Seed cells on gelatine coated 24-well transwell membrane inserts at a density of 8×10^5 cells per well. Seeding volume 0.3 ml per insert (upper chamber).

9. Allow cells to migrate towards your "selected conditions" present in the lower chamber (0.9 ml) for 8 h at 37 °C, include a positive control medium containing 10% FCS and negative control with medium without serum.

10. Gently, aspirate medium from both lower and upper chambers and wash twice with PBS.

11. Add Calcein containing solution to each well, 0.1 ml to the upper part and 0.4 ml to the lower part.

12. Incubate cells at 37 °C in a CO_2 incubator for 30 min and wash with PBS.

13. Transfer to a new 24-well plate containing 0.9 ml of DMEM medium with 1% BSA.

14. Read fluorescence in a plate reader (485 nm excitation and 520 nm filters).

3.6 Generation and Analysis of GFP Sorted Epicardial Cells from Wt1GFPKI Mice and Control and epiWt1KO Hearts

1. Dissect out embryos into fresh PBS and select *Wt1GFP* positive embryos using a fluorescent microscope. Fluorescence is clearly seen in the embryonic kidney as a positive control.

2. Dissect hearts (also tails for genotyping if needed) and cut out atria with sterile needles. Take a GFP negative heart as a negative control for fluorescence.

3. Wash dissected ventricles three times with PBS.

4. Warm up trypsin solution: trypsin:versene solution in a 1:10 ratio warmed up to 37 °C.

5. Place GFP heart(s) in a 1.5 ml Eppendorf tube and remove PBS.

6. Add 200 μl of trypsin solution.

7. Place Eppendorfs in a Thermomixer set at 37 °C and mix at 1000 rpm for 10 min.

8. Collect supernatant with dissociated cells into a separate tube containing DMEM medium (with added 10% FCS and 1% Penicillin/Streptomycin) and add fresh trypsin solution. Repeat **steps** 7 and 8 until heart is completely dissociated. Keep supernatant on ice until all dissociated cells are collected.

9. Pass collected cells through a sterile sieving membrane or cell strainer before FACS analysis and sorting.

10. FACS sorting of GFP populations by gating against a littermate GFP negative control.

11. Collect cells directly into RNAlater buffer solution (Ambion) or Trizol, centrifuge gently and store pellet at –80 °C.

3.7 qRT-PCR Quantification

1. Extract RNA from collected cells and measure RNA concentration and quality. We use an RNA extraction kit (Qiagen or Arcturus for very small samples). Store RNA at –80 °C until enough RNA is available to proceed.

2. *Optional. In order to reduce the amount of RNA/samples needed you can amplify the RNA. For RNA quantities of around 5 ng the Arcturus RiboAmp HS-Plus two-round and Turbo labeling kit has been used in our laboratory following the manufacturer's instructions.

3. Convert RNA or amplified RNA into cDNA using Superscript III reverse transcriptase (Invitrogen) following manufacturer's instructions.

4. Sybr Green (Gotaq, Promega) and Taqman (Roche) reaction master mixes for quantification could be used.

5. Select a housekeeping control assay such as 18s or the endogenous mouse *Gapdh* (Roche) for Taqman quantification.

6. Carry out a serial dilution of a control template and dilute samples for quantification.

7. Run qRT-PCR and generate C_t values using an optimized thermal profile.

8. Plot standard curve and read off values from quantified samples.

4   Notes and Useful Tips

1. When making a wound in a wound healing assay use a rapid movement with the tip to ensure a straight wound.

2. When extracting RNA use filter tips over a working surface free of RNase/DNases. RNaseZAP (Sigma) can be used to clean up bench tops.

3. Trypsin solution works well with embryonic mouse hearts up to E16.5; however E13.5 to E16.5 hearts may need gentle pipetting up and down to enable complete dissociation of cells at the final stages of the procedure.

4. When preparing a PCR reaction avoid cross contamination of samples and ensure thorough mixing of reagents to improve quality of results.

References

1. Carmona R, Guadix JA, Cano E et al (2010) The embryonic epicardium: an essential element of cardiac development. J Cell Mol Med 14(8):2066–2072

2. Masters M, Riley PR (2014) The epicardium signals the way towards heart regeneration. Stem Cell Res 13(3 Pt B):683–692

3. Martínez-Estrada OM, Lettice LA, Essafi A et al (2010) Wt1 is required for cardiovascular progenitor cell formation through transcriptional control of Snail and E-cadherin. Nat Genet 42(1):89–93

4. Zhou B, Honor LB, He H et al (2011) Adult mouse epicardium modulates myocardial injury by secreting paracrine factors. J Clin Invest 121(5):1894–1904

5. Van Wijk B, Gunst QD, Moorman AFM et al (2012) Cardiac regeneration from activated epicardium. PLoS One 7(9):e44692

6. Moore AW, McInnes L, Kreidberg J et al (1999) YAC complementation shows a requirement for Wt1 in the development of epicardium, adrenal gland and throughout nephrogenesis. Development 126(9):1845–1857

7. Guadix JA, Ruiz-Villalba A, Lettice L et al (2011) Wt1 controls retinoic acid signalling in embryonic epicardium through transcriptional activation of Raldh2. Development 138(6):1093–1097

8. Velecela V, Lettice LA, Chau Y-Y et al (2013) WT1 regulates the expression of inhibitory chemokines during heart development. Hum Mol Genet 22(25):5083–5095

Chapter 6

Isolation and Colony Formation of Murine Bone and Bone Marrow Cells

Sophie McHaffie and You-Ying Chau

Abstract

Adult homeostasis is dependent on normal *Wt1* expression. Loss of *Wt1* expression in adult mice causes rapid loss of the mesenchymal tissues, fat and bone, amongst other phenotypes. Bone and bone marrow mesenchymal stromal cells can be studied by cell isolation and expansion. The stemness of these cells can then be characterized by carrying out a colony-forming unit-fibroblast assay and observing clonogenic capabilities.

Key words Bone marrow, Bone, Stem cell culture, Mesenchymal, Colony-forming unit fibroblast, Cre

1 Introduction

Wt1 is a major regulator of adult homeostasis. The tamoxifen-inducible ubiquitous knockout of *Wt1* in adult mice results in multiple organ failure within 9 days following tamoxifen-induced deletion [1]. The phenotypes include rapid fat and bone loss; trabecular bone volume is decreased by 30 % and the inner surface of the bone is ragged compared to controls [1]. Adult bone mass is a balance between synthesis from osteoblasts (arising from the mesenchymal stem/progenitors) and turnover by osteoclasts (arising from the hematopoietic progenitors). Increased osteoclast numbers are observed within the mutant bone marrow [1]. In addition, preliminary experiments show that mutant mesenchymal cells are less capable of differentiating into osteoblasts. The size of fat pads and fat vacuoles are also decreased following *Wt1* deletion, as well as adipocyte numbers in bone marrow [1]. Osteoblasts and adipocytes, along with chondrocytes, all differentiate from stromal mesenchymal stem cells (MSCs) found in the bone [2]. Interestingly, around 10 % of Wilms' tumors contain heterologous factors that include fat, bone, and cartilage [3]. A recent study looking at the relationship between MSCs and the mesenchymal properties of Wilms' tumors with *WT1* mutations

Nicholas Hastie (ed.), *The Wilms' Tumor (WT1) Gene: Methods and Protocols*, Methods in Molecular Biology, vol. 1467, DOI 10.1007/978-1-4939-4023-3_6, © Springer Science+Business Media New York 2016

showed that a Wilms' tumor cell line expresses surface proteins specific to human MSCs including CD105, CD90, and CD73 and that are able to differentiate into chondrocytes, osteoblasts, and adipocytes [4]. These findings support the involvement of *Wt1* in MSC biology.

There are compelling parallels between different *Wt1*-expressing mesenchymal cell populations that suggest links with mesenchymal stem/progenitor cells. *Wt1*-expressing mesothelial cells in the developing liver are stellate cell precursors [5–7], while *Wt1* is also expressed in the pancreatic mesothelium and pancreatic stellate cells [1]. The parallels between pancreatic and hepatic stellate cells suggest that pancreatic stellate cells may also be arising from the mesothelium, via epithelial to mesenchymal transition [1, 7, 8]. Stellate cells have spindle-shaped bodies similar in appearance to bone marrow cells cultured under MSC-favoring conditions [9] and are also positive for *nestin* [10], linking them with the *nestin*-expressing MSCs [11]. Stellate cells may originate from both the mesothelium- and bone marrow-derived HSCs and could possibly be another subset of the *Wt1*-expressing cells [6, 12]. Hepatic stellate cells share striking similarities with pericytes [13, 14]. A FACS-sorted pericyte population from the bone marrow was shown to include cells with MSC properties [15]. In the kidney, podocytes, which similarly to pericytes and stellate cells also have a spindle-shaped appearance due to their long processes or "feet", express both *Wt1*, which is a podocyte regulator [16], and *nestin* [17]. In the developing kidney and heart, *nestin* and *Wt1* expressions overlap. *Nestin* is potentially regulated by *Wt1* as its expression is reduced drastically following the loss of *Wt1* in these tissues [18]. *Wt1* is required for mesenchymal to epithelial transition (MET) in the developing kidney as *Wt1* deletion in kidney mesenchyme leads to failure of MET and nephron formation [19]. The opposite is seen in heart development where *Wt1* is required for epithelial to mesenchymal transition (EMT) [20]. Mesenchymal progenitor cells are formed when the epicardial cells undergo EMT. An epicardial-specific *Wt1* knockout resulted in a loss of these mesenchymal progenitor cells [20].

However, the most striking phenotype to support *Wt1*'s involvement with mesenchymal lineages is the effect of *Wt1* deletion [1]. Bone and fat are both mesenchymal derivatives, strongly suggesting that *Wt1* is playing a functional role in the genesis and homeostasis of these mesenchymal tissues, and may even act as a functional marker for a subset of mesenchymal stem or progenitor cells.

There is considerable topical interest in tissue stem and progenitor cells, particularly with regard to potential uses in therapy. Bone marrow is largely split into two halves: the hematopoietic and the non-hematopoietic. The hematopoietic component consists of HSCs, hematopoietic progenitor cells, and their derivatives. The non-hematopoietic component is made up mainly of endothelial and mesenchymal stem cells (MSC) plus their derivatives, including adipocytes, osteoblasts, and chondrocytes [21]. It has been much more difficult to define mesenchymal stem and progenitor cells for different lineages than it has been for the hematopoietic compartment.

The following protocols detail how to isolate bone and marrow cells and how to carry out colony-forming unit-fibroblast assays to characterize the mesenchymal stromal compartment.

2   Protocols

2.1   Isolation of Murine Bone Marrow and Bone Mesenchymal Progenitors

2.1.1   Introduction

Embryonic bone development takes place when a core of prechondrogenic cells is surrounded by stacked osteogenic progenitor cells, all of which are avascular. This central core and surrounding stacked cells differentiate into cartilage to give a cartilage rod or "model". The stacked cells then give rise to osteoblasts [22, 23]. Osteoblasts are located in close proximity to blood vessels with the "back" of the cell toward the capillary and the "front" of the cell secreting osteoid: a collagen type I-rich premineral layer [22, 23]. Vasculature is the dominant factor for the position and survival of the osteoblast cells, unlike chondrogenesis which actively inhibits vascularization [24, 25]. For this reason bone does not replace cartilage, but cartilage is invaded by vascular cells to give the resulting marrow cavity [23], and bone forms independent of the cartilage [24, 25]. In mice, bone development begins with mesenchyme condensing at embryonic day 9.5 (e9.5). By e12 the commitment of mesenchymal cells to the osteogenic lineage occurs, followed by commitment to the chondrogenic lineage on day 13, finishing with vasculature and marrow invasion of the cartilage occurring on days 16–17 of development [25, 26].

Primitive marrow is formed when the chondrocyte core is invaded by vasculature to form the marrow cavity [23]. As previously mentioned, postnatal bone marrow is an organ of two halves: the hematopoietic cells, including the hematopoietic stem cells (HSCs), and the non-hematopoietic cells [27]. The non-hematopoietic cells are also known as the bone marrow stroma, or associated supporting stroma, and this is where the mesenchymal stem cell resides [27]. The bone marrow is the only known organ where two separate stem cells, MSCs and HSCs, with distinct lineage pathways are located and found to interact together to coexist [27].

2.1.2   Materials

1. Culture medium:
   DMEM containing 10% (v/v) fetal calf serum, 1% (v/v) penicillin/streptomycin, 0.5% (v/v) glutamine, and 0.5% (v/v) sodium pyruvate.

2. Sterile dissection kit.

3. 25-gauge needle.

4. 21-gauge needle.

5. 10 mL Syringe.

6. 10 cm Culture dish.

7. Pestle and mortar.

8. Collagenase B (Roche).

9. Rocking chamber heated to 37 °C.

10. 70 micron cell strainer (Falcon).

11. Phosphate-buffered saline (PBS), pH 7.4.

12. Bench centrifuge with swinging bucket rotor.

13. Sterile cell culture plastic pipettes individually wrapped (5, 10, 25 mL).

14. Pipette aid.

15. Sterile conical centrifuge tubes (15 and 50 mL).

16. Cell aspirator.

2.1.3   Methods

2.1.3.1   Isolation of Bone Marrow Cells

1. Euthanize mice by cervical dislocation and dissect out the bilateral femur and tibia.

2. In a sterile culture hood and with a sterile dissection kit remove each end of the long bones and set aside. Carry this out in a 10 cm culture dish. Add a small amount of culture medium to prevent the tissue and bone drying out.

3. Using 8 mL of culture medium flush out the bone marrow from the long bones using the 10 mL syringe and 25-gauge needle.

4. Dissociate the flushed marrow cells using a 21-gauge needle.

2.1.3.2   Isolation of Bone Cells

1. Prepare the collagenase B at a concentration of 3 mg/mL dissolved in culture medium and kept on ice.

2. Crush the pre-flushed long bones and bone ends by pestle and mortar in 10 mL collagenase B until a pulp-like consistency is reached.

3. Transfer the bone pulp and 10 mL collagenase B to a sterile 15 mL tube and incubate at 37 °C for 90 min in a rocking chamber to enable enzymatic digestion.

4. Pass the bone cells through a 70 micron cell strainer into a sterile 50 mL tube.

5. Centrifuge the tube at 300 rcf for 5 min at room temperature in a swinging bucket rotor. Remove the enzyme-containing supernatant by vacuum aspiration and resuspend the cell pellet in pre-warmed culture medium.

2.1.4   Notes

CFU-F assays and MSC isolation are usually carried out using marrow cells flushed from the bone. This protocol uses isolated cells from both marrow and bone which are crushed with a collagenase digest [28]. This extra bone digest step is included as MSCs are located near the endosteum of the bone, in the bone-lining endosteal region, where they interact with bone-lining osteoblasts [29]. Cells in this area are difficult to remove by flushing alone.

3 Colony-Forming Unit-Fibroblast Assay

3.1 Introduction

Colony-forming unit-fibroblast (CFU-F) assays are often used to characterize stromal marrow cells and assess the number of mesenchymal stem and progenitor cells [27, 30, 31]. The bone and fat loss phenotypes seen from the ubiquitous *Wt1* deletion point to the involvement of mesenchymal stromal cells. This makes the CFU-F assay an appropriate tool to investigate its involvement. Adherent stromal cells form colonies which originate from a single cell: the CFU-F [27, 31–34]. There are several methods of obtaining material for CFU-F assays, most commonly the flushing of bone marrow, but also including the crushing of pre-flushed long bones followed by enzymatic digestion [27, 31–34]. The isolation of these cells is covered previously in this chapter.

Proliferation without terminal differentiation, a stem cell characteristic, is demonstrated using CFU-F assays [32], proving that a single cell can result in a colony of cells. Mesenchymal stem cells, or mesenchymal stromal cells (MSCs), are commonly described as spindle-shaped multipotent cells able to self-replicate and generate progenitors that produce a variety of skeletal tissues: bone, cartilage, marrow stroma, fat, ligament, tendon, and connective tissue. MSCs are mainly found in the bone marrow; however they make up a very small proportion of the total number of marrow cells, between 0.01 and 0.001 % [35]. Bone marrow contains MSCs which can undergo chondrogenic, osteogenic, and adipogenic differentiation to form cartilage, bone, and fat, respectively [35, 36]. MSCs are also found in bone fragments which have been crushed and digested with a collagen enzyme. These cells are also able to differentiate into the three main mesenchymal lineages [37].

3.2 Materials

1. Hemocytometer.
2. Sterile 6-well culture plates.
3. MesenCult® media.
4. 0.5 % (w/v) Cresyl violet acetate (Sigma) in methanol: Filter through 25 μm filter paper and store at room temperature.
5. Incubator.

3.3 Methods

1. Count the cells with a hemocytometer.
2. Plate 5×10^5 cells per well of a 6-well culture plate with 2 mL of MesenCult® media per well.
3. Incubate the plates for 48 h to allow adherent cells to attach.
4. Wash with pre-warmed PBS to remove media and nonadherent cells.

5. Add 2 mL pre-warmed MesenCult® to each well and culture.

6. Every 3 days, remove the media and replace with fresh MesenCult® for 10 days. Check that the colonies are not becoming too confluent.

7. Wash plates with PBS.

8. Remove the PBS and stain colonies with 0.5% Cresyl violet acetate solution for 30 min at room temperature.

9. Wash plates with PBS three times, followed by a single wash with distilled H_2O.

10. Remove H_2O and leave to dry.

11. Count colonies with a diameter greater than 1 mm.

3.4   Notes

Higher numbers of colonies form in the bone CFU-F assays compared to the marrow [28, 33, 38]. The trabecular bone is an enriched source of mesenchymal progenitors which corroborates with higher numbers of bone colonies [31, 39].

Due to the bone loss phenotype, the effect of *Wt1* on colony-forming abilities was investigated using mice with a tamoxifen-inducible *Wt1* deletion (CAGG-CreER[T2]; *Wt1loxP/loxP*) [38]. It is difficult to determine whether *Wt1* deletion has any effect on colony formation due to the Cre-only control showing the same trend, potentially masking any gene loss effect [38] (Fig. 1). The results suggest that, at least for colony-forming capabilities, bone and marrow cells are affected by the activated CreER recombinase, rather than *Wt1* deletion. This raises a great concern as to whether activated CreER recombinase is the cause of other phenotypes seen in published studies using this construct and deletion method.

The appropriate Cre-only control should be included if using CFU-F assays in conjunction with the Cre-*loxP* system of gene knockout. It is important to control for not only Cre effects but also gender and tamoxifen [38].

CAGG-CreER[T2] negative;
***Wt1**loxP/loxP*

(i.e. Control)

CAGG-CreER[T2] positive;
***Wt1**loxP/loxP*

(i.e. *Wt1* deletion)

CAGG-CreER[T2] positive

(i.e. Activated CreER recombinase)

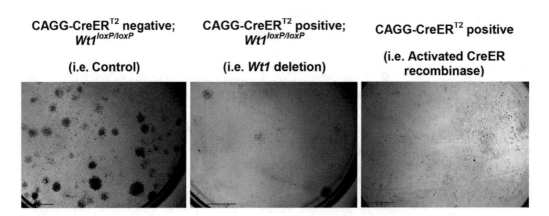

Fig. 1 Activated CreER[T2] recombinase negatively affects colony-forming capabilities

References

1. Chau Y-Y, Brownstein D, Mjoseng H et al (2011) Acute multiple organ failure in adult mice deleted for the developmental regulator, Wt1. PLoS Genet 7(12):e1002404

2. Prockop DJ (1997) Marrow stromal cells as stem cells for nonhematopoietic tissues. Science 276:71–74

3. Royer-Pokora B (2003) Two molecular subgroups of Wilms' tumors with or without *WT1* mutations. Clin Cancer Res 9:2005–2014

4. Royer-Pokora B, Busch M, Beier M et al (2010) Wilms' tumor cells with *WT1* mutations have characteristic features of mesenchymal stem cells and express molecular markers of paraxial mesoderm. Hum Mol Genet 19:1651–1668

5. Ijpenberg A, Pérez-Pomares JM, Guadix JA et al (2007) Wt1 and retinoic acid signalling are essential for stellate cell development and liver morphogenesis. Dev Biol 312:157–170

6. Asahina K, Zhou B, Pu WT et al (2011) Septum transversum-derived mesothelium gives rise to hepatic stellate cells and perivascular mesenchymal cells in developing mouse liver. Hepatology 53(3):983–995, appendix

7. Li Y, Wang J, Asahina K (2013) Mesothelial cells give rise to hepatic stellate cells and myofibroblasts via mesothelial–mesenchymal transition in liver injury. Proc Natl Acad Sci U S A 110(6):2324–2329

8. Masamune A, Shimosegawa T (2009) Signal transduction in pancreatic stellate cells. J Gastroenterol 44(4):249–260

9. Friedman SL (2008) Hepatic stellate cells: protean, multifunctional, and enigmatic cells of the liver. Physiol Rev 88:125–172

10. Lardon J, Rooman I, Bouwens L (2002) Nestin expression in pancreatic stellate cells and angiogenic endothelial cells. Histochem Cell Biol 117(6):535–540

11. Méndez-Ferrer S, Michurina TV, Ferraro F et al (2010) Mesenchymal and haematopoietic stem cells form a unique bone marrow niche. Nature 466:829–834

12. Miyata E, Masuya M, Yoshida S et al (2008) Hematopoietic origin of hepatic stellate cells in the adult liver. Blood 111(4):2427–2435

13. Sato M, Suzuki S, Senoo H (2003) Hepatic stellate cells: unique characteristics in cell biology and phenotype. Cell Struct Funct 28:105–112

14. Bergers G, Song S (2005) The role of pericytes in blood-vessel formation and maintenance. Neuro-Oncology 7(4):452–464

15. Crisan M, Yap S, Casteilla L et al (2008) A perivascular origin for mesenchymal stem cells in multiple human organs. Cell Stem Cell 3(11):301–313

16. Guo J-K, Menke AL, Gubler M-C et al (2002) *WT1* is a key regulator of podocyte function: reduced expression levels cause crescentic glomerulonephritis and mesangial sclerosis. Hum Mol Genet 11(6):651–659

17. Bertelli E, Regoli M, Fonzi L et al (2007) Nestin expression in adult and developing human kidney. J Histochem Cytochem 55:411–421

18. Wagner N, Wagner K-D, Scholz H et al (2006) Intermediate filament protein nestin is expressed in developing kidney and heart and might be regulated by the Wilms' tumor suppressor Wt1. Am J Physiol 291:R779–R787

19. Essafi A, Webb A, Berry RL et al (2011) A Wt1-controlled chromatin switching mechanism underpins tissue-specific *wnt4* activation and repression. Dev Cell 21(3):559–574

20. Martínez-Estrada OM, Lettice LA, Essafi A et al (2010) Wt1 is required for cardiovascular progenitor cell formation through transcriptional control of Snail and E-cadherin. Nat Genet 42:89–93

21. Tocci A, Forte L (2003) Mesenchymal stem cell: use and perspectives. Hematol J 4:92–96

22. Pechak DG, Kujawa MJ, Caplan AI (1986) Morphological and histochemical events during first bone remodeling in embryonic chick limbs. Bone 7:441–458

23. Pechak DG, Kujawa MJ, Caplan AI (1986) Morphology of bone development and bone remodeling in embryonic chick limbs. Bone 7:459–472

24. Caplan AI (1987) Bone development and repair. BioEssays 6(4):171–175

25. Caplan AI (1988) Bone development. In: Wiley J (ed) Cell and molecular biology of vertebrate hard tissues. CIBA Foundation Symposium 136, Chichester, pp 3–21

26. Zelzer E, Olsen BR (2005) Multiple roles of vascular endothelial growth factor (VEGF) in skeletal development, growth, and repair. Curr Top Dev Biol 65:169–187

27. Bianco P, Riminucci M, Gronthos S et al (2001) Bone marrow stromal stem cells: nature, biology, and potential applications. Stem Cells 19:180–192

28. Morikawa S, Mabuchi Y, Kubota Y et al (2009) Prospective identification, isolation, and systemic transplantation of multipotent mesenchymal stem cells in murine bone marrow. J Exp Med 206(11):2483–2496

29. Muguruma Y, Yahata T, Miyatake H et al (2006) Reconstitution of the functional human

hematopoietic microenvironment derived from human mesenchymal stem cells in the murine bone marrow compartment. Blood 107(5):1878–1887

30. Kuznetsov SA, Krebsbach PH, Satomura K et al (1997) Single-colony derived strains of human marrow stromal fibroblasts form bone after transplantation in vivo. J Bone Miner Res 12(9):1335–1347

31. Siclari VA, Zhu J, Akiyama K et al (2013) Mesenchymal progenitors residing close to the bone surface are functionally distinct from those in the central bone marrow. Bone 53(2):575–586

32. Friedenstein AJ, Chailakhjan RK, Lalykina KS (1970) The development of fibroblast colonies in monolayer cultures of guinea-pig bone marrow and spleen cells. Cell Tissue Kinet 3(4):393–403

33. Nakamura Y, Arai F, Iwasaki H et al (2010) Isolation and characterization of endosteal niche cell populations that regulate hematopoietic stem cells. Blood 116:1422–1432

34. Ohishi M, Ono W, Ono N et al (2012) A novel population of cells expressing both hematopoietic and mesenchymal markers is present in the normal adult bone marrow and is augmented in a murine model of marrow fibrosis. Am J Pathol 180:811–818

35. Pittenger MF, Mackay AM, Beck SC et al (1999) Multilineage potential of adult human mesenchymal stem cells. Science 284(5411):143–147

36. Caplan AI (1991) Mesenchymal stem cells. J Orthop Res 9:641–650

37. Guo Z, Li H, Li X et al (2006) In vitro characteristics and in vivo immunosuppressive activity of compact bone-derived murine mesenchymal progenitor cells. Stem Cells 24:992–1000

38. McHaffie SL, Hastie N, Chau Y-Y (2016) Effects of CreER^{T2}, 4-OH tamoxifen, and gender on CFU-F assays. PLoS One 11(2):e0148105

39. Grcevic D, Pejda S, Matthews BG et al (2012) In vivo fate mapping identifies mesenchymal progenitor cells. Stem Cells 30(2):187–196

Chapter 7

Isolation and Fluorescence-Activated Cell Sorting of Murine WT1-Expressing Adipocyte Precursor Cells

Louise Cleal and You-Ying Chau

Abstract

The current global obesity epidemic has triggered increased interest in adipose tissue biology. A major area of attention for many is adipose tissue development. A greater understanding of adipocyte ontogeny could be highly beneficial in answering questions about obesity-associated disease. Recent work has shown that a proportion of mature adipocytes in visceral white adipose tissue are derived from Wt1-expressing adipocyte precursor cells. These adipocyte precursor cells reside within the adipose tissue itself, and are a constituent of the stromal vascular fraction (SVF), along with other, non-adipogenic, cell types. Crucially, heterogeneity exists within the adipocyte precursor population, with only a proportion of cells expressing Wt1. Moreover, it appears that this difference in the precursor cells may influence the mature adipocytes, with Wt1-lineage-positive adipocytes having fewer, larger lipid droplets than the Wt1-lineage negative. Using fluorescence-activated cell sorting, based on specific marker profiles, it is possible to isolate the adipocyte precursor cells from the SVF. Subsequently, this population can be divided into Wt1-expressing and non-expressing fractions, therefore permitting further analysis of the two cell populations, and the mature adipocytes derived from them. In this chapter we outline a method by which adipocyte precursor cells can be isolated, and how, using a specific mouse model, Wt1-expressing and non-expressing cells can be separated.

Key words Adipose tissue, Visceral, Adipocyte precursor, Adipocyte, Stromal vascular fraction, Fluorescence-activated cell sorting, Flow cytometry

1 Introduction

In recent years, interest in adipose tissue biology has substantially increased, driven by the obesity epidemic. Particular focus lies on the developmental origins of adipose tissue and the signaling mechanisms responsible for controlling its development and growth, two areas that remain relatively poorly understood [1].

1.1 Adipose Tissue Overview

In mammals, adipose tissue has traditionally been divided into two types: white adipose tissue (WAT) and brown adipose tissue (BAT). While both are implicated in energy balance, WAT is predominantly involved in the storage and mobilization of triglycerides, while BAT functions to burn fat and increase energy expenditure

Nicholas Hastie (ed.), *The Wilms' Tumor (WT1) Gene: Methods and Protocols*, Methods in Molecular Biology, vol. 1467, DOI 10.1007/978-1-4939-4023-3_7, © Springer Science+Business Media New York 2016

through adaptive thermogenesis [2]. Crucially, WAT has an exceptional capability for expansion, both through increasing adipocyte cell size (hypertrophy) and adipocyte number (hyperplasia), a key factor in the intensifying obesity crisis [3]. A third form of adipose tissue has recently been identified: "beige." "Beige" adipocytes are found within WAT, but display key characteristics of BAT, such as the expression of uncoupling protein-1 (UCP-1): essential for thermogenesis [4].

WAT is further divided into subcutaneous ("good fat") and visceral ("bad fat") depots. Visceral WAT is located within the body cavity, surrounding the major organs, while subcutaneous WAT resides under the skin. Visceral WAT is principally associated with metabolic syndrome and is a large risk factor for the development of cardiovascular disease, diabetes, and certain cancers, while subcutaneous WAT is thought to be protective [1, 5]. In this chapter, the focus is on visceral WAT. The majority of WAT mass can be accounted for by lipid-filled mature adipocytes; however, in terms of cell number, they make up less than half. The remaining cells comprise the stromal vascular fraction (SVF), and include blood, endothelial and mesenchymal cells. Importantly, adipocyte precursor cells reside within this SVF, and it is the presence and differentiation of these cells that determine adipocyte number, both during normal development and in obesity [6].

An important step within the field has been the development of a method by which adipocyte precursor cells can be separated from the non-adipogenic cells that comprise the rest of the SVF. Not only has this meant that it is now possible to isolate the adipocyte precursors, but it has also revealed the identity of the adipogenic SVF cells. Using multicolor flow cytometry, Rodeheffer et al. [7] isolated adipocyte progenitor cells with a specific cell surface marker profile (Lin−CD29+CD34+Sca1+CD24+), going on to show that these cells have the ability to differentiate into functioning WAT in vivo [7]. In addition to this, they went on to identify a pre-adipocyte population, with a slightly different marker profile (Lin−CD29+CD34+Sca1+CD24−) [8]. These cells can form adipocytes, but have a more limited adipogenic potential than the progenitors, and are unable to form fully functioning WAT depots in vivo. Additionally, these pre-adipocyte cells express adipogenic markers, suggesting that they are more committed to the adipocyte lineage than the progenitors [8]. In support of this, they also found that there is an increase in the latter (CD24−) and a decrease in the former (CD24+) populations postnatally, as the cells are further committed to becoming mature adipocytes [8]. Consequently, these cell surface marker profiles are now used to isolate adipocyte precursor cells by fluorescence-activated cell sorting (FACS).

1.2 Wt1 Expression in Adipose Tissue

Wt1 is expressed in the six murine visceral WAT depots: omental, epididymal, mesenteric, pericardial, retroperitoneal, and perirenal, but not in subcutaneous WAT or BAT [9]. Moreover, Wt1 is not expressed in the mature adipocytes, but instead in the adipocyte precursor cells that reside in the SVF of the adult adipose depots [10]. Regarding the marker profiles described above, Chau et al. (2014) showed that 90% of the Wt1-expressing cells in the adult SVF fall into one of these two populations (Lin-CD31-CD29+CD34+), with the large majority (60–90% depending on depot) being in the CD24– pre-adipocyte category [10].

Based on the knowledge that Wt1 is expressed in visceral adipocyte precursor cells, lineage-tracing analysis has been used to investigate whether mature visceral fat arises from Wt1-expressing cells during embryonic and postnatal development [10]. Reporter *mTmG* mice were crossed with knock-in mice expressing tamoxifen-inducible Cre-recombinase at the *Wt1* locus (*Wt1CreERT2*; *mTmG*). With the *mTmG* reporter model, Tomato is ubiquitously expressed prior to Cre-mediated loxP recombination. Recombination leads to the removal of Tomato, causing membranous GFP to be expressed. Crucially, all progeny of the Cre-expressing cells are also labeled [11]. This lineage-tracing revealed that, depending on visceral depot, 28–77% of the mature adipocytes were GFP positive, thus indicating that they were derived from Wt1-expressing precursor cells [10]. In this particular study, tamoxifen was injected into the mother when the embryos were at E14.5, and the adult tissues analyzed at 1.2 years old. Henceforth, with this lineage tracing being reliant on a single dose of tamoxifen, it is likely that these percentages are an underestimate. Further work, involving tamoxifen dosing at 3 weeks old, has also demonstrated that a proportion of mature visceral adipocytes arise from cells expressing Wt1 postnatally [10]. Therefore we know that Wt1-expressing adipocyte precursor cells contribute to mature visceral but not subcutaneous WAT throughout development.

It is well known in the field that molecular differences exist between different WAT depots [2, 12]. In addition to this, with the knowledge that only a proportion of mature visceral adipocytes are derived from Wt1-expressing cells, we now know that within each of the WAT depots, heterogeneous populations of adipocyte precursor cells exist [10]. Moreover, work both in vivo and in an ex vivo culture system indicates that adipocytes derived from Wt1-positive cells have fewer, larger lipid droplets than those in the Wt1-negative lineage, while total lipid content and adipocyte cell size are the same [10], therefore implying that heterogeneity among the adipocyte precursors does influence the mature adipocyte and that Wt1 may have a role in this. In order to further explore the differences between the Wt1-expressing and non-expressing adipocyte precursors, as well as the mature adipocytes derived from these two lineages, it was important to develop a protocol by which these two adipocyte precursor populations could be effectively separated. For this we have utilized the Wt1-green fluorescent protein (GFP) knock-in mouse model, whereby Wt1-expressing cells are labeled with GFP [13].

2   Methods: Fluorescence-Activated Cell Sorting (FACS) Protocol for Isolating Murine Wt1-Expressing Adipocyte Precursor Cells

2.1   Introduction

This protocol was designed to permit the separation of Wt1-expressing (GFP+) and non-expressing (GFP–) adipocyte precursor cells from Wt1-GFP adult mouse visceral WAT depots. Isolated cells can subsequently be used for RNA extraction and gene expression analysis, as well as cell culture and in vitro differentiation. This protocol can either be used to simply separate all Wt1-positive and negative SVF cells, or to firstly isolate specific cells based on the marker profiles outlined by Rodeheffer et al. [7], before going on to separate these based on Wt1 (GFP) expression [7]. Presented here is a description of the tissue isolation, FACS sample preparation, and FACS analysis protocols.

2.2   Materials

1. Sterile dissection kit.
2. Carbon steel surgical blades.
3. 10 cm Culture dish.
4. Collagenase B (Roche).
5. Phosphate-buffered saline (PBS), pH 7.4.
6. Bovine serum albumin (BSA).
7. Penicillin/streptomycin (P/S).
8. 0.22 µM Millex syringe drive filter unit (Millipore).
9. 50 mL Syringe.
10. Rocking chamber heated to 37 °C.
11. 70 µm Nylon cell strainer (Corning).
12. Bench centrifuge with swinging bucket rotor.
13. Sterile cell culture plastic pipettes individually wrapped (5, 10, 25 mL).
14. Pipette aid.
15. Sterile conical centrifuge tubes (15 and 50 mL).
16. Cell aspirator.
17. Fetal calf serum (FCS).
18. FACS buffer: PBS, 5 % (v/v) FCS, 1 % (v/v) P/S.
19. 5 mL Polystyrene round-bottom tube with cell strainer cap (35 µm) (Corning).
20. Biotin mouse lineage panel (containing lineage markers: CD3e, CD11b, CD45R (B220), Gr-1, Ly-76) (BD Biosciences).
21. Antibodies (*see* Table 1).
22. OneComp eBeads (eBioscience).
23. Culture medium: Dulbecco's modified Eagle medium 1× (DMEM), 10 % (v/v) fetal calf serum, 1 % (v/v) penicillin/streptomycin, 0.5 % (v/v) sodium pyruvate (if culturing sorted cells).

Table 1
Markers and fluorochromes used in the flow cytometry panel for the isolation of adipocyte precursors, including dilutions and excitation/emission wavelengths [6]

Antibody	Gene name	Supplier	Fluorochrome	Excitation laser (nm)	Emission (nm)	Dilution[a]
CD31	Platelet/endothelial cell adhesion molecule 1	eBioscience	PerCP-eF710	488 (Blue)	710	1:100
CD29	Integrin β1	eBioscience	APC	637–647 (Red)	660	1:100
CD24	Heat-stable antigen	eBioscience	eF780	633–647 (Red)	780	1:200
CD34	Cluster differentiation hematopoietic progenitor cell antigen	Biolegend	PE-Cy5	488 (Blue)	670	1:50
Sca-1	Stem cell antigen-1	Biolegend	Pacific Blue	405 (Violet)	455	1:160
Streptavidin[b]		eBioscience	PerCP-Cy5.5	488 (Blue)	690	1:340

[a]Dilutions are a recommendation based on our work. The user should determine the optimal dilution for different antibodies, fluorochromes, and FACS machines

[b]Secondary antibody to detect the biotinylated primary antibodies of the mouse lineage panel

24. TRIzol® Reagent (Invitrogen) (if extracting RNA from sorted cells).

2.3   Methods

2.3.1   Isolation of Stromal Vascular Fraction Cells

1. Euthanize mice by cervical dislocation and dissect out required adipose depots.

2. Dissolve collagenase B at a concentration of 1 mg/mL in sterile PBS containing 4 mg/mL bovine serum albumin and 1% (v/v) penicillin/streptomycin (*see* **Note 1**).

3. In a 10 cm culture dish, using carbon steel surgical blades, chop the fat pads into 1–2 mm pieces (*see* **Note 2**).

4. Transfer the chopped fat tissue and 5–10 mL collagenase B solution into a 15 mL tube and incubate at 37 °C for 1 h in a rocking chamber.

5. Shake the samples vigorously by hand to obtain a single-cell suspension.

6. Filter the suspension through a 70 μm nylon cell strainer into a 50 mL Falcon tube.

7. Centrifuge the tube at $300 \times g$ for 5 min at 4 °C in a swinging bucket rotor.

8. Using vacuum aspiration, remove the supernatant containing the enzyme and mature adipocytes (*see* **Note 3**).

9. Resuspend the stromal vascular fraction (SVF) cell pellet in 1 mL FACS buffer.

2.3.2 FACS Sample Preparation/Antibody Staining

1. If sorting based on cell surface marker profiles, dilute required antibodies to appropriate concentrations in FACS buffer (Table 1; suggested antibody concentrations). Follow the manufacturer's instructions for diluting antibodies from the biotin mouse lineage panel (*see* **Note 4**).

2. Filter the SVF suspension (from Subheading 2.1.9) into a 5 mL polystyrene round-bottom tube with cell strainer cap (35 μm) (*see* **Note 5**).

3. Centrifuge the tube at $300 \times g$ for 5 min at 4 °C in a swinging bucket rotor (*see* **Note 6**).

4. Tip off the supernatant and resuspend the pellet in the appropriate antibody staining solution (~100 μL). Incubate the suspension in the dark at room temperature for 15 min (*see* **Note 7**). If simply sorting all Wt1-positive and Wt1-negative cells, so NOT antibody staining, pellet can be resuspended in ~150 μL FACS buffer, and go directly to **step 7**.

5. To wash, add 3 mL FACS buffer to each sample and centrifuge at $300 \times g$ for 5 min at 4 °C. Tip off the supernatant and repeat the staining procedure for secondary/additional antibodies if required.

6. Once staining is complete, resuspend the final pellet in ~150 μL FACS buffer. The cells are now ready for FACS.

7. FACS-separated cells will be collected into either 1.5 mL Eppendorf tubes or 15 mL Falcon tubes. If sorted cells are to be cultured in vitro, these tubes should be filled with culture media prior to sorting. Alternatively, if RNA is to be extracted from the sorted cells, they can be sorted directly into 500 μL TRIzol® Reagent.

2.3.3 FACS/Flow Cytometry

1. We use a BD FACSAria II laser sorter/analyzer to sort and analyze our SVF samples along with BD FACSDiva and FlowJo software.

2. Compensation: When performing multicolor flow cytometric analysis (as described here), it is important that any potential overlap between the emission spectra of two or more fluorochromes is eliminated. This overlap can occur when more than one detector is capable of measuring a particular fluorescent dye. If this step is not carried out correctly it may be the case that a population of cells negative for an antigen of interest will appear positive, due to spillover of the fluorescent signal from another fluorescent antibody with a similar emission spectra. This compensation can be carried out using the single-color compensation controls (antibody-capture beads and SVF cells) outlined in Table 2. Each bead/cell sample is stained with just

Table 2 Proposed sample setup for the isolation of adipocyte precursors [14]

Single-color compensation controls (capture beads/cells)	Lin (biotin mouse lineage panel)	Streptavidin PerCP-Cy5.5	CD31 PerCP-eF710	CD29 APC	CD24 eF780	CD34 PE-Cy5	Sca-1 Pacific Blue
Beads—unstained	-	-	-	-	-	-	-
Beads—Lin-SA.PerCP-Cy5.5	+	+	-	-	-	-	-
Beads—CD31-PerCPeF710	-	-	+	-	-	-	-
Beads—CD29-APC	-	-	-	+	-	-	-
Beads—CD24-eF780	-	-	-	-	+	-	-
Beads—CD34-PECy5	-	-	-	-	-	+	-
Beads—Sca1-PB	-	-	-	-	-	-	+
SVF cells—unstained	-	-	-	-	-	-	-
SVF cells—Lin-SA.PerCP-Cy5.5	+	+	-	-	-	-	-
SVF cells—SA.PerCP-Cy5.5	-	+	-	-	-	-	-
SVF cells—CD31-PerCPeF710	-	-	+	-	-	-	-
SVF cells—CD29-APC	-	-	-	+	-	-	-
SVF cells—CD24-eF780	-	-	-	-	+	-	-
SVF cells—CD34-PECy5	-	-	-	-	-	+	-
SVF cells—Sca1-PB	-	-	-	-	-	-	+
Fluorescence-minus-one controls							
SVF cells—Lin-SA.PerCP-Cy5.5	-	-	+	+	+	+	+
SVF cells—CD31-PerCPeF710	+	+	-	+	+	+	+
SVF cells—CD29-APC	+	+	+	-	+	+	+
SVF cells—CD24-eF780	+	+	+	+	-	+	+
SVF cells—CD34-PECy5	+	+	+	+	+	-	+
SVF cells—Sca1-PB	+	+	+	+	+	+	-
Test samples: SVF cells (all markers)	+	+	+	+	+	+	+

one of the fluorescent antibodies from the multicolor panel. The beads/cells are then gated on to gain the single-color controls for each dye [6, 14].

3. Fluorescence-minus-one (FMO) controls: To support the compensation controls, and ensure that any observed fluorescent signal has arisen from the antibody of interest only, FMO controls should be carried out. For each fluorescent antibody used, a sample of SVF cells should be stained with all other antibodies in the panel, excluding the one that has been compensated for. This FMO control and the experimental sample (stained with the entire panel of antibodies) should now be analyzed using the same compensation settings (those set up for the antibody being verified). If the compensation settings are correct, a signal should be observed for the antigen of interest in the experimental sample only, and not in the FMO control. If a fluorescent signal is observed in the FMO control, this is the result of a signal from another antibody spilling over, and the compensation settings should be adjusted in order to eliminate this [6]. *See* Table 2 for the suggested FMO control setup.

4. Regarding data acquisition, typically we begin by generating a forward scatter height (FSC-H) vs. forward scatter area (FSC-A) plot to select for singlets and remove doublets. Subsequently, this population of cells is gated on side scatter area (SSC-A) vs. FSC-A to remove debris. This main population of cells is then gated further, including all the fluorescent parameters, in order to obtain the required cell populations (Fig. 1a). When sorting into Wt1+ (GFP+) and Wt1- (GFP-) fractions, it is important that the GFP gate is established on a sample of SVF cells negative for GFP (Fig. 1b).

3 Notes

1. Allow for 5–10 mL of collagenase solution for digestion of one adipose depot. If sorted cells are to be cultured, collagenase solution should be sterilized before use, by filtration through a syringe-driven filter unit (0.22 μM).

2. If sorted cells are to be cultured, all procedures from and including **step 3** must be carried out in a sterile culture hood (where possible), using sterile conditions.

3. The cells of the SVF will pellet at the bottom of the Falcon tube, while the mature adipocytes will float to the top of the supernatant.

4. For all antibodies listed in Table 1, approximately 100 μL of staining solution is sufficient to stain the SVF from one adipose depot, although exact volumes should be determined by the individual user.

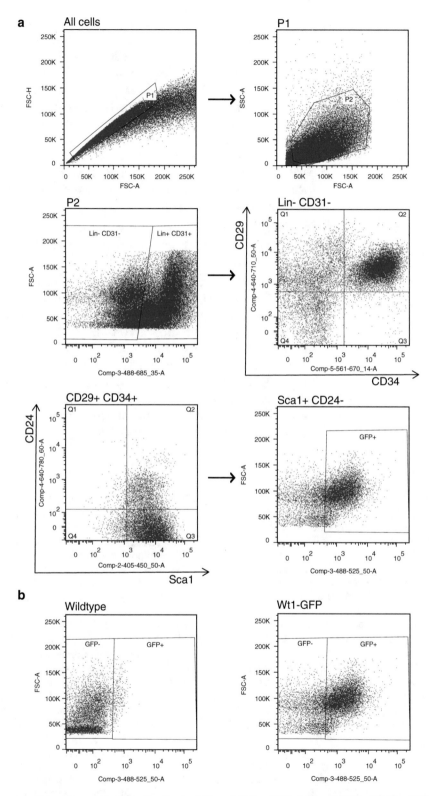

Fig. 1 Example flow cytometry gating for the isolation of Wt1+ (GFP+) Lin− CD31− CD29+ CD34+ Sca1+ CD24− pre-adipocytes from the stromal vascular fraction (**a**). A non-GFP-expressing cell sample should be used to establish the GFP+ gate (**b**)

5. If sorting cells based on a specific marker profile, compensation and fluorescence-minus-one controls must also be included. For each marker used, filter 2× 100 μL of the cell suspension into two separate 5 mL polystyrene round-bottom tubes with cell strainer caps (35 μm). One of these samples should be incubated with one antibody only (single-color compensation sample), and the other should be incubated with all antibodies being used, except the one being compensated for (fluorescence-minus-one sample), as outlined in Table 2. Additionally, for each marker used, 7 μL of OneComp eBeads should be incubated with an individual antibody, and treated as one of the compensation samples.

6. If cells are to be used for culture and must remain in sterile conditions, the FACS tube cell strainer cap should be replaced with a snap cap prior to centrifugation.

7. If sorting cells based on a specific marker profile (i.e.: Lin-CD29+CD34+Sca1+CD24−), primary antibodies from the biotin mouse lineage panel should be added to the cells first (made up into one solution according to the manufacturer's protocol). Unlike the other antibodies (Table 1), those in the lineage panel are not conjugated to a fluorophore, but are biotinylated, so a secondary streptavidin fluorochrome conjugate must be added in a second incubation (streptavidin PerCP-Cy5.5). Following this, all other required antibodies (Table 1) can be added in a single step.

References

1. Sanchez-Gurmaches J, Guertin DA (2013) Adipocyte lineages: tracing back the origins of fat. Biochim Biophys Acta 1842:340–351

2. Billon N, Dani C (2012) Developmental origins of the adipocyte lineage: new insights from genetics and genomics studies. Stem Cell Rev Rep 8:55–66

3. Tang QQ, Lane MD (2012) Adipogenesis: from stem cell to adipocyte. Annu Rev Biochem 81:715–736

4. Rosen ED, Spiegelman BM (2014) What we talk about when we talk about fat. Cell 156:20–44

5. Bergman RN, Kim AP, Catalano KJ et al (2006) Why visceral fat is bad: mechanisms of the metabolic syndrome. Obesity 14:16S–19S

6. Church CD, Berry R, Rodeheffer MS (2014) Isolation and study of adipocyte precursors. Methods Enzymol 537:31–46

7. Rodeheffer MS, Birsoy K, Friedman JM (2008) Identification of white adipocyte progenitor cells in vivo. Cell 135:240–249

8. Berry R, Rodeheffer MS (2013) Characterization of the adipocyte cellular lineage in vivo. Nat Cell Biol 15:302–309

9. Chau Y-Y, Brownstein D, Mjoseng H et al (2011) Acute multiple organ failure in adult mice deleted for the developmental regulator Wt1. PLoS Genet 7:e1002404

10. Chau Y-Y, Bandiera R, Serrels A et al (2014) Visceral and subcutaneous fat have different origins and evidence supports a mesothelial source. Nat Cell Biol 16:367–375

11. Muzumdar MD, Tasic B, Miyamichi K et al (2007) A global double fluorescent Cre reporter mouse. Genesis 45:593–605

12. Tchkonia T, Lenburg M, Thomou T et al (2007) Identification of depot-specific human fat cell progenitors through distinct expression profiles and developmental gene patterns. Am

J Physiol Endocrinol Metab 292:E298–E307

13. Hosen N, Shirakata T, Nishida S et al (2007) The Wilm's tumor gene WT1-GFP knock-in mouse reveals the dynamic regulation of WT1 expression in normal and leukemic hematopoiesis. Leukemia 21:1783–1791

14. Bradford JA, Clarke ST (2011) Panel development for multicolour flow-cytometry testing of proliferation and immunophenotype in hMSCs. Meth Mol Biol 698:367–385

Chapter 8

In Vivo Assays for Assessing the Role of the Wilms' Tumor Suppressor 1 (Wt1) in Angiogenesis

Richard J. McGregor, R. Ogley, PWF Hadoke, and Nicholas Hastie

Abstract

The Wilms' tumor suppressor gene (*WT1*) is widely expressed during neovascularization, but it is almost entirely absent in quiescent adult vasculature. However, in vessels undergoing angiogenesis, *WT1* is dramatically upregulated. Studies have shown *Wt1* has a role in both tumor and ischemic angiogenesis, but the mechanism of *Wt1* action in angiogenic tissue remains to be elucidated. Here, we describe two methods for induction of in vivo angiogenesis (subcutaneous sponge implantation, femoral artery ligation) that can be used to assess the influence of *Wt1* on new blood vessel formation. Subcutaneously implanted sponges stimulate an inflammatory and fibrotic response including cell infiltration and angiogenesis. Femoral artery ligation creates ischemia in the distal hindlimb and produces an angiogenic response to reperfuse the limb which can be quantified in vivo by laser Doppler flowmetry. In both of these models, the role of *Wt1* in the angiogenic process can be assessed using histological/immunohistochemical staining, molecular analysis (qPCR) and flow cytometry. Furthermore, combined with suitable genetic modifications, these models can be used to explore the causal relationship between *Wt1* expression and angiogenesis and to trace the lineage of cells expressing *Wt1*. This approach will help to clarify the importance of *Wt1* in regulating neovascularization in the adult, and its potential as a therapeutic target.

Key words Angiogenesis, Ischemia, Cardiovascular disease, Wilms' tumor, *Wt1*

1 Introduction

The Wilms' tumor suppressor gene (*Wt1*) is a transcription factor which has recently been implicated in angiogenesis; neovascularization from pre-existing blood vessels. The angiogenic response, whilst essential to tumor growth in cancer, is also triggered by arterial occlusion and hypoxia, and hence, can contribute to reperfusion of ischemic tissues in cardiovascular disease, reducing ischemic injury [1, 2]. Therefore, increasing the speed or magnitude of the angiogenic response is of considerable therapeutic interest to improving outcomes in a number of cardiovascular conditions including, myocardial infarction, stroke and peripheral limb ischemia.

Nicholas Hastie (ed.), *The Wilms' Tumor (WT1) Gene: Methods and Protocols*, Methods in Molecular Biology, vol. 1467,
DOI 10.1007/978-1-4939-4023-3_8, © Springer Science+Business Media New York 2016

Despite being integral to embryogenesis, *Wt1* expression is notably sparse in the healthy adult organism, with expression only in a few cell types. *Wt1* is largely absent from non-regenerating adult vasculature (except for reports of low expression in a few smaller arteries [3]) but is up-regulated in endothelial cells, fibroblasts and pericytes in vasculature undergoing angiogenesis [4–6]. Furthermore, following induction of myocardial infarction (MI) in rats, *Wt1* is expressed in the coronary vasculature of the ischemic tissue, yet not in the adjacent healthy tissue [6]. In order to assess the role of *Wt1* in new vessel formation, angiogenesis can be induced in a number of in vivo models.

A simple, reproducible method of inducing angiogenesis is the well-described model of subcutaneous sponge implantation [7, 8]. In brief, polyurethane sponges are implanted subcutaneously in vivo and become infiltrated by a number of cell types (including fibroblasts, immune cells and endothelial cells), with angiogenesis occurring to provide a blood supply. Sponges are routinely harvested 20 days after implantation (when considerable angiogenesis has occurred) but can be retrieved at any time deemed suitable. Angiogenesis in these sponges can be measured in vivo (e.g. Using Fluorescence Molecular Tomography) and ex vivo (e.g. by measuring hemoglobin or by histological analysis). Mechanisms underlying angiogenesis can be assessed using immunohistochemistry, quantitative PCR and FACs to isolate cell populations. Angiogenesis in this model can be manipulated by pharmacological treatment (systemic or directly administration into the sponge [7]) or by impregnation of the sponge with an appropriate cell population in Matrigel prior to implantation [9].

Ischemic angiogenesis can be assessed using a model of femoral artery ligation [10]. Reperfusion in this model comprises a combination of proximal collateral formation (arteriogenesis) and distal angiogenesis [11]. Experiments are routinely maintained for between 4 and 28 days following induction of ischemia and laser Doppler analysis during the experiment allows a quantitative measure of the time-dependent restoration of blood flow. Tissues can be harvested at appropriate time-points for analysis of vascular density (using histology/immunohistochemistry), cell populations (FACS) and measurement of transcript expression (real time PCR). As with the sponge implantation model, the angiogenic response to hindlimb ischemia can be modulated by pharmacological manipulation [12] or cell administration [13].

Both these in vivo models of angiogenesis (sponge implantation, hindlimb ischemia) can be applied to rodent models of disease [14, 15] and to genetically modified animals [7]. When carried out using mice with tissue-specific *Wt1* KO, data from these models provides information on the functional effect of *Wt1* on angiogenesis and reperfusion whilst subsequent analyses (qPCR, histology, cell sorting) of sponge and muscle tissue allows insights into the mechanisms underlying the influence of *Wt1* on angiogenesis.

All methods described herein can be applied to genetically modified mice, to provide further insight into the actions of *Wt1* in vivo. $Wt1^+$ cells can be traced using *Wt1* reporter mice (such as the *Wt1*-GFP or *Wt1*. Cre-ERT2; mTmG mouse lines) [16, 17] revealing the translocation of these cells and the site of *Wt1* influence. Insight into the effect of *Wt1* on recovery from ischemia can be deduced using mice with inducible knockout of *Wt1* from specific cells (e.g. the vascular endothelium) [18] and quantification of the angiogenic response as outlined above.

2 Materials

Prepare and store all reagents at room temperature (RT) using dH_2O for preparation if necessary, unless otherwise stated.

2.1 Subcutaneous Sponge Implantation

A comprehensive list of all equipment required to undertake the procedure is outlined below. All surgical tools should be autoclaved prior to use.

1. Blunt tip serrated forceps (0.8×0.7 mm).
2. Hemostats (12.5 cm).
3. Surgical scissors (22 mm straight tip).
4. Wound closure clips (1.75×7.5 mm).
5. Electric shaving clippers.
6. Polyurethane sponge ($0.5 \times 0.5 \times 1$ cm).
7. Sterile surgical drapes.
8. Heated mat.
9. Autoclave tape.
10. Anesthetic rig with medical-grade O_2 supply.
11. CO_2 chamber with CO_2 supply.

2.2 Femoral Artery Ligation

A comprehensive list of all equipment required to undertake the procedure is outlined below. All surgical tools should be autoclaved prior to use.

1. Standard tip fine forceps (0.1×0.06 mm).
2. 2× Angled tip fine forceps (0.1×0.06 mm).
3. Blunt tip serrated forceps (0.8×0.7 mm).
4. Haemostats (12.5 cm).
5. Surgical scissors (22 mm straight tip).
6. Fine surgical scissors (3 mm straight tip).
7. Scalpel.
8. Straight bulldog clips (28 mm).

9. Wire wound retractor.

10. 5-0 silk suture thread.

11. 5-0 nonabsorbable monofilament sutures, 19 mm 3/8 circle reverse cutting needle.

12. Electric shaving clippers.

13. Sterile surgical drapes.

14. Sterile H_2O for injections.

15. Heated mat.

16. Autoclave tape.

17. Surgical microscope.

18. Anesthetic rig with medical-grade O_2 supply.

19. CO_2 chamber with CO_2 supply.

20. MoorLDI2-HIR laser Doppler.

21. MoorLDI V6 software.

2.3 Solutions and Reagents for Surgical Procedures

1. Sterile H_2O for injections.

2. PBS solution.

3. Isoflurane.

4. Vetergesic (buprenorphine).

5. Povidone Iodine solution.

6. EMLA cream.

7. 1% lidocaine solution.

8. Paraformaldehyde (4% in PBS).

9. Ethanol (70% in dH_2O).

2.4 Materials for Isolating GFP+ Cells from Sponges Using FACS

1. Leibovitz's L-15 Medium (Invitrogen, UK).

2. Primary tissue culture hood (Ultimat Biological Safety Cabinet, Medical Air Technology Ltd., UK).

3. 60-mm Petri dish.

4. Scalpel blades.

5. PBS.

6. BSA (4 mg/mL, Sigma-Aldrich, UK).

7. Collagenase B (Roche, UK).

8. Stuart SI_3OH hybridization Oven (Bibby Scientific Ltd., UK).

9. 10% Fetal calf serum.

10. 100, 70 and 40 μm sterile cell strainers (Scientific Laboratory Supplies Limited, England).

11. Red Blood Cell lysis buffer (Biolegend, UK).

12. 50 mL centrifuge tubes.

2.5 Components for RNA Extraction and cDNA Synthesis

1. Ultra Turrax homogenizer (Fisher Scientific, UK).
2. Centrifuge.
3. Techne™ TC-512 thermal cycler (Fisher Scientific, UK).
4. Nanodrop spectrophotometer.
5. 2 mL Eppendorf tubes.
6. RNase-free water.
7. Chloroform.
8. GelRed™ (Biotium, USA).
9. 1× TAE buffer.
10. Agarose.
11. QIAzol® Lysis Reagent (Qiagen, UK).
12. RNeasy® Mini Kit (Qiagen, UK).
13. Quantitect® Reverse Transcription Kit (Qiagen, UK).

3 Methods

3.1 Subcutaneous Sponge Implantation

1. Anesthetize mice with inhaled isoflurane (5 %) in O_2 and maintain anesthesia thereafter at 2–3 % isoflurane in O_2.
2. Remove a roughly 3 cm^2 area of fur from the dorsal neck region using clippers, with the midpoint centered between the scapulae.
3. Sterilize exposed skin using Povidone Iodine solution.
4. Inject (subcutaneous) the analgesic Vetergesic (buprenorphine) diluted 1:10 in sterile H_2O at a dose of 0.05 mg/kg body weight.
5. Cover the animal with sterile drapes and make a 1.5 cm horizontal incision between the scapulae using a scalpel.
6. Using blunt dissection with hemostat forceps, subcutaneously extend the incision with the point of the blunt forceps facing away from the body cavity by inserting and opening the forceps to create two tunnels extending caudally over the left and right hindquarters.
7. Insert one 0.5×0.5×1 cm sterile polyurethane sponge into each subcutaneous pocket, with the longest axis of the sponge lying parallel to the body.
8. Close the wound using wound clips and apply EMLA cream topically.
9. Allow mice to recover from anesthetic on a heated mat and monitor over the course of the experiment.
10. Cull mice by CO_2 asphyxiation at desired time points.
11. Expose sponges by cutting from the site of incision in an anterior–posterior direction and then across as necessary (Fig. 1).

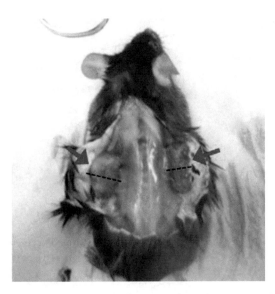

Fig. 1 Exposed subcutaneous sponges in situ 21 days after implantation. Sponges are indicated by *red arrows* and the *dotted line* represents the axis along which sponges were cut for processing

12. Excise sponges by cutting through the membrane between the sponge and the muscle or skin, keeping the points of the scissors facing away from the sponge to avoid damage while peeling away the skin.

13. Sponges can then be cut in half across the shortest axis.

14. Sponges can then be; preserved in 4 % paraformaldehyde in PBS at 4 °C overnight, then placed in 70 % ethanol; or snap frozen on dry ice and stored at −80 °C prior to further analysis.

3.2 Extraction of RNA from Subcutaneous Sponge and cDNA Synthesis

1. Remove sponge samples from −80 °C and homogenize in 700 μL QIAzol® Lysis Reagent in a suitable Eppendorf tube for 2 min or until of a uniform consistency.

2. Divide the sample equally between two further Eppendorf tubes and add a further 350 μL of QIAzol® Lysis Reagent to each.

3. Using an Ultra Turrax homogenizer (Fisher Scientific) homogenize each sample for 1 min and leave for 5 min.

4. Add 200 μL of chloroform to each sample and leave to stand for 2 min at RT.

5. Centrifuge samples at $12,000 \times g$ and 4 °C for 15 min.

6. Combine aqueous fractions from the same sample and carry out RNA extraction using an RNeasy Mini Kit as per manufacturer's instructions. Store RNA at −80 °C.

7. Determine RNA concentration and integrity using a Nanodrop spectrophotometer and GelRed™ agarose gel electrophoresis.

8. Using the quantities determined by the Nanodrop spectropho-tometer, dilute each sample to a final concentration of 0.5 ng/μL in 12 μL using RNase-free water.

9. Synthesize cDNA from RNA using a Quantitect® Reverse Transcription Kit as per manufacturer's instructions, a Techne TC-512 thermal cycler and a reaction mix of 20 μL.

10. Store cDNA at −20 °C prior to qPCR analysis.

3.3 Isolating GFP+ Cells from Subcutaneous Sponges Using FACS

1. Cull mice by asphyxiation in CO_2, and remove the sponges and kidneys immediately, placing them in separate falcon tubes con-taining Leibovitz's L-15 Medium. The kidneys of the experi-mental mice in these experiments act as positive tissue controls as the glomeruli are known to express *Wt1* in the GFP+ mice.

2. Under a primary tissue culture hood transfer the sponges into a 60-mm Petri dish, and disrupt as finely as possible using for-ceps and scalpel blades.

3. Resuspend tissue homogenate in 10 mL prewarmed PBS plus BSA (4 mg/mL) with 1 mg/mL Collagenase B per sample.

4. Next, incubate the samples for 45 min at 37 °C in a hybridiza-tion oven.

5. Stop the digestion process by adding 15 mL Leibovitz's L-15 Medium containing 10% FCS.

6. Pass the digested sponge through a 100 μm sterile cell strainer into a 50 mL centrifuge tube; permitting the removal of any undigested fibrous tissue. Pass the resulting suspension through a 70 μm sterile cell strainer to remove contaminating tubular fragments.

7. Wash the sieved cells by centrifugation ($10,000 \times g$, 5 min).

8. Discard the supernatant and re-suspended the pellet in 1 mL Red Blood Cell lysis buffer and leave for 3 min at room temperature.

9. Wash the pellet by adding 15 mL PBS and centrifuging for a further 5 min at $10,000 \times g$.

10. Discard the supernatant and re-suspend the pellet in 1 mL PBS containing 2% FCS.

11. Finally, filter the sample through a 40 μm sterile cell strainer prior to FACS.

12. In our lab FACS was performed using the BD FACSAri™ II System (BD Biosciences, UK) equipped with five lasers and fluorescent detectors. Once **steps 1–11** have been performed to isolate the cells from GFP+ and GFP- mice sponge and kid-ney, prepare them as single cell suspensions in PBS/5% FCS. Incubate the cells in the dark at 4 °C for 15 min with the appropriate antibody combinations, with 5 min PBS/5% FCS

washes between stainings. Create sorting gates using sponge and kidney cells from GFP⁻ mice. Isotype control antibodies and OneComp eBeads (Catalogue ♯01-1111, eBioscience, UK) act as negative controls. Perform analysis using FlowJo Software Version 7.6.5 (TreeStar Inc., USA).

3.4 Induction of Hindlimb Ischemia

1. Anesthetize mice with inhaled isoflurane (5 %) in O_2 and maintain anesthesia thereafter at 2–3 % isoflurane in O_2.

2. Remove fur from the ventral surfaces of both hindlimbs extending up to the lower abdomen.

3. Immobilize mice (supine) on a non-reflective surface and secure hindlimbs parallel to the tail.

4. Using a laser Doppler scanner and Moor LDI software (5.3) carry out a preoperative laser Doppler scan, with the scan region comprising the whole of both hindlimbs and the corresponding length of tail.

5. Following completion of the laser Doppler scan, sterilize exposed skin of the left hindlimb by rubbing with Povidone Iodine solution.

6. Inject (subcutaneously) the analgesic Vetergesic (buprenorphine) diluted 1:10 in sterile H_2O at a dose of 0.05 mg/kg body weight.

7. In the supine position, on a heated mat, cover the animal with sterile drapes and secure the limbs extended with tape. Perform the rest of the surgical procedure using a surgical microscope at appropriate magnification.

8. Using fine forceps and surgical scissors make a 1 cm incision down the medial thigh, starting at the mid-point of the inguinal ligament.

9. Using blunt dissection with fine forceps, separate the subcutaneous fat to reveal the femoral vessels.

10. Secure the surgical field with a small retractor and topically apply 1 % lidocaine liquid to lubricate the field and cause arterial dilatation.

11. Displace the femoral nerve inferiorly to ensure it is not damaged.

12. Superior to the popliteal artery apply a temporary ligation with 5-0 suture silk to the femoral artery and vein, controlling tension by securing with a bulldog clip.

13. Isolate the femoral artery from the vein distal to this ligation using blunt dissection to reveal a section of femoral artery ~20 mm in length.

14. Apply two permanent double-knotted permanent ligatures to the femoral artery using 5-0 suture silk, first proximally, then distally.

15. Remove the temporary ligation and transect the femoral artery between the knots, 5 mm inferior to the proximal and superior

to the distal knots, respectively, using fine surgical scissors. Remove the ~10 mm length of femoral artery.

16. Close the skin using 5/0 nonabsorbable monofilament sutures and apply EMLA cream topically.

17. Allow mice to recover from anesthetic on a heated mat and monitor over the course of the experiment.

18. Perform a postoperative laser Doppler scan to confirm ablation of blood flow in the left hindlimb (Fig. 2) and then further laser Doppler scans to monitor hindlimb reperfusion at appropriate intervals (usually, 3, 7, 14, 21, 28 days) until termination of the experiment.

19. Carry out postexperimental color quantification of laser Doppler images using MoorLDI software (5.3).

3.5 Tissue Extraction Post-Hindlimb Ischemia

1. After 28 days and completion of all laser Doppler scans, cull mice by asphyxiation in CO_2.

2. Using forceps and surgical scissors, remove the skin from the left and right hindlimbs. All following stages are carried out on both the left and right hindlimbs.

3. Using blunt dissection on the medial thigh expose the adductor muscle. Isolate from other muscles and transect as distally and proximally as possible using fine scissors.

4. Isolate the gastrocnemius muscle from the lower limb and transect as proximally and distally as possible using fine scissors.

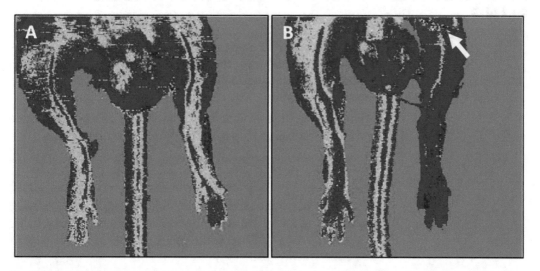

Fig. 2 Representative laser Doppler scans of mouse hindlimbs. Laser Doppler imaging (**a**) preoperatively and (**b**) postoperatively reveal abolition of blood flow in the left hindlimb following femoral artery ligation and reactive hyperemia in the right hindlimb and tail. Color from *red* to *dark blue* represents speed of blood flow and *arrow* indicates distal site of femoral artery ligation

5. Remove, using blunt dissection, the small section of dark brown muscle clearly visible on the inner gastrocnemius.

6. Cut both muscles in half across the shortest axis. Fix half of each muscle in 4 % paraformaldehyde in PBS at 4 °C overnight, then place in 70 % ethanol. Freeze the other half at –80°c prior to further analysis.

3.6 RNA Extraction from Muscle Tissue and cDNA Synthesis

1. Remove muscle samples from –80 °C and homogenize in 800 µL QIAzol® Lysis Reagent in a suitable Eppendorf tube for 2 min or until of uniform consistency.

2. Add 200 µL of chloroform to each sample and leave to stand for 2 min at R.T.

3. Centrifuge samples at $12,000 \times g$ and 4 °C for 15 min.

4. Carry out RNA extraction using an RNeasy Mini Kit as per manufacturer's instructions. Store RNA at –80 °C.

5. Determine RNA concentration and integrity using a Nanodrop spectrophotometer and GelRed™ agarose gel electrophoresis.

6. Using the quantities determined by the Nanodrop spectrophotometer dilute each sample to a final concentration of 0.5 ng/µL in 12 µL using RNase-free water.

7. Synthesize cDNA from RNA using the Quantitect® Reverse Transcription Kit as per manufacturer's instructions, a Techne TC-512 thermal cycler and a reaction mix of 20 µL.

8. Store cDNA at –20 °C prior to qPCR analysis.

4   Notes

1. It is possible to investigate the effect of different drugs or factors on angiogenesis in the subcutaneous sponge implantation model, by impregnating sponges with these factors prior to insertion [7, 9].

2. Sponges can be compacted with the hemostat forceps for ease of implantation, as they will expand once securely in situ.

3. On removal of sponges, differential impregnation of sponges by blood vessels, at different time points, or due to different treatments/genotypes is often evident by visual inspection. Furthermore, when fixing sponges in 4 % paraformaldehyde, sponges pre-implantation or those with relatively little organic tissue will float, while sponges with a high density of organic tissue sink.

4. Due to its thin wall, the femoral vein is relatively fragile and easily punctured, especially when attempting to separate it from the femoral artery. The risk of rupturing the vein can be reduced by keeping the point of the forceps pointing away

from the vein and towards the artery, which is, by comparison, less prone to rupture.

5. In the event of rupture of the femoral artery or vein, hemostasis can usually be achieved by application of gentle pressure to the site of bleeding with a sterile cotton bud.

6. In the event of persistent or recurrent bleeding from the femoral vein, it may be necessary to ligate the femoral artery without complete separation of the artery from the vein. In this instance, cut each end of the artery proximal and distal to the ligations and remove as much of the artery as possible. Transect remaining section of artery along its length with fine scissors to prevent any recovery of blood flow.

7. The femoral artery branches at a number of points close to the site of ligation. Variation in the local anatomy between mice can influence the possible placement of the distal ligature.

8. The extent of hindlimb perfusion, at baseline and during experiments, inevitably varies between mice, especially due to size and weight of the mouse. To eliminate this variation and obtain a clearer representation of the relative change in blood flow, it is advisable to express hindlimb perfusion as a ratio relative to the tail perfusion [19]. It is also possible to use the right hindlimb to normalize values, but reactive postoperative hyperemia may act as a confounding factor.

9. When extracting RNA from tissues and following initial centrifugation to separate solutions, if only a small amount of aqueous phase is present, with a large amount of white, colloidal phase, add another 200 µL of Qiazol reagent and repeat centrifugation.

10. Suggested histochemical and immunohistochemical stains for assessment of sponges and hindlimb muscle tissue include; Hematoxylin and Eosin (H&E) staining for general tissue morphology; triple immunostaining for CD31 (endothelial cells), α-smooth muscle actin (αSMA) (smooth muscle cells, fibroblasts, pericytes and myofibroblast) and the nuclear stain DAPI; CD31 immunoperoxidase (DAB) staining for visualization and quantification of vessels; picrosirius red collagen staining; F4.80 DAB staining for macrophages; *Wt1*/CD31/αSMA/DAPI staining; *Wt1* DAB staining.

Acknowledgment

R.O. is funded by a British Heart Foundation studentship and RMcG by a Wellcome-Trust-funded ECAT research fellowship. The authors are grateful for support from the Edinburgh British Heart Foundation Centre for Research Excellence (CoRE).

References

1. Carmeliet P, Jain RK (2011) Molecular mechanisms and clinical applications of angiogenesis. Nature 473(7347):298–307. doi:10.1038/nature10144

2. Khurana R, Simons M, Martin JF, Zachary IC (2005) Role of angiogenesis in cardiovascular disease: a critical appraisal. Circulation 112(12):1813–1824. doi:10.1161/CIRCULATIONAHA.105.535294

3. Vasuri F, Fittipaldi S, Buzzi M et al (2012) Nestin and WT1 expression in small-sized vasa vasorum from human normal arteries. Histol Histopathol 27(9):1195–1202

4. Katuri V, Gerber S, Qiu X et al (2014) WT1 regulates angiogenesis in Ewing Sarcoma Oncotarget 15:5(9) 2436–49

5. Dohi S, Ohno S, Ohno Y et al (2010) WT1 expression correlates with angiogenesis in endometrial cancer tissue. Anticancer Res 3192:3187–3192

6. Wagner K, Wagner N, Bondke A, Nafz B (2002) The Wilms' tumor suppressor Wt1 is expressed in the coronary vasculature after myocardial infarction 1. FASEB J:1117–1119. doi:10.1096/fj.01

7. Small GR, Hadoke PWF, Sharif I et al (2005) Preventing local regeneration of glucocorticoids by 11beta-hydroxysteroid dehydrogenase type 1 enhances angiogenesis. Proc Natl Acad Sci U S A 102(34):12165–12170. doi:10.1073/pnas.0500641102

8. Andrade SP, Fan TP, Lewis GP (1987) Quantitative in-vivo studies on angiogenesis in a rat sponge model. Br J Exp Pathol 68(6):755–766

9. Barclay GR, Tura O, Samuel K et al (2012) Systematic assessment in an animal model of the angiogenic potential of different human cell sources for therapeutic revascularization. Stem Cell Res Ther 3(4):23. doi:10.1186/scrt114

10. Niiyama H, Huang NF, Rollins MD, Cooke JP (2009) Murine model of hindlimb ischemia. J Vis Exp 23:2–4. doi:10.3791/1035

11. Limbourg A, Korff T, Napp LC, Schaper W, Drexler H, Limbourg FP (2009) Evaluation of postnatal arteriogenesis and angiogenesis in a mouse model of hind-limb ischemia. Nat Protoc 4(12):1737–1748, Available at: http://dx.doi.org/10.1038/nprot.2009.185

12. Emanueli C, Minasi A, Zacheo A et al (2001) Local delivery of human tissue kallikrein gene accelerates spontaneous angiogenesis in mouse model of hindlimb ischemia. Circulation 103(1):125–132. doi:10.1161/01.CIR.103.1.125

13. Dar A, Domev H, Ben-Yosef O et al (2012) Multipotent vasculogenic pericytes from human pluripotent stem cells promote recovery of murine ischemic limb. Circulation 125(1):87–99. doi:10.1161/CIRCULATIONAHA.111.048264

14. Biscetti F, Pitocco D, Straface G et al (2011) Glycaemic variability affects ischaemia-induced angiogenesis in diabetic mice. Clin Sci (Lond) 121(12):555–564. doi:10.1042/CS20110043

15. Chau Y-Y, Bandiera R, Serrels A et al (2014) Visceral and subcutaneous fat have different origins and evidence supports a mesothelial source. Nat Cell Biol 16(4):367–375. doi:10.1038/ncb2922

16. You D, Cochain C, Loinard C et al (2008) Hypertension impairs postnatal vasculogenesis role of antihypertensive agents. Hypertension 51(6):1537–1544. doi:10.1161/HYPERTENSIONAHA.107.109066

17. Hosen N, Shirakata T, Nishida S et al (2007) The Wilms' tumor gene WT1-GFP knock-in mouse reveals the dynamic regulation of WT1 expression in normal and leukemic hematopoiesis. Leukemia 21(8):1783–1791. doi:10.1038/sj.leu.2404752

18. Wagner K-D, Cherfils-Vicini J, Hosen N et al (2014) The Wilms' tumour suppressor Wt1 is a major regulator of tumour angiogenesis and progression. Nat Commun 5:5852. doi:10.1038/ncomms6852

19. Kirkby NS, Duthie KM, Miller E et al (2012) Non-endothelial cell endothelin-B receptors limit neointima formation following vascular injury. Cardiovasc Res 95(1):19–28. doi:10.1093/cvr/cvs137

Chapter 9

Multiphoton Microscopy for Visualizing Lipids in Tissue

Martin Lee and Alan Serrels

Abstract

Visualizing the appearance of fat droplets and adipocytes in tissue can be realized using a label-free imaging method known as coherent anti-Stokes Raman spectroscopy (CARS). CARS is a nonlinear optical technique that allows label-free imaging of a material with contrast based on the same vibrational signatures of molecules found in Raman spectroscopy. CARS can be combined with other single and multiphoton imaging modes such as second harmonic generation and two-photon fluorescence to image a broad variety of biological structures.

Here we describe the construction of a multiphoton microscope that will enable the study of both fluorescently labeled and unlabeled tissue. This has been used to monitor the contribution of Wt1 expressing cells towards the visceral fat depots during gestation.

Key words Multiphoton, CARS, SHG, Lipids, Raman, Microscopy

1 Introduction

The need to understand complex biological processes in cells and tissue has seen advanced fluorescent microscopy become a central component of the research strategy in many laboratories. Throughout this chapter we will focus on one aspect of this, namely multiphoton microscopy, and describe in detail how to setup and use an imaging system for two-photon fluorescence, second harmonic generation, and coherent anti-Stokes Raman spectroscopy. Further, we will provide insights into the benefits of this approach for imaging tissue, with particular focus on the function of WT1 in adipocytes.

With advances in laser technology and commercialization of user-friendly imaging systems, multiphoton microscopy has rapidly become more accessible to researchers in biomedicine. As a highly customizable and versatile imaging tool, it can be setup to offer both label-dependent (i.e., fluorescence) and label-free imaging of samples depending upon the specific requirements of the user. The most common form of multiphoton microscopy used is two-photon excitation fluorescence (TPEF), which, instead of using a single

Nicholas Hastie (ed.), *The Wilms' Tumor (WT1) Gene: Methods and Protocols*, Methods in Molecular Biology, vol. 1467,
DOI 10.1007/978-1-4939-4023-3_9, © Springer Science+Business Media New York 2016

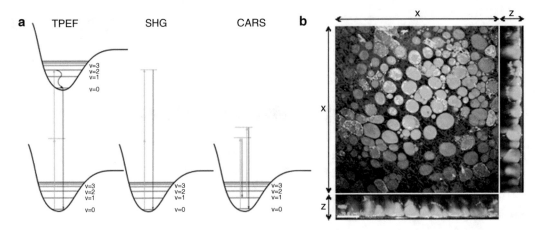

Fig. 1 Multiphoton energy diagrams and imaging. (**a**) Energy diagrams for two-photon fluorescence, second harmonic generation, and coherent anti-Stokes Raman scattering. In TPEF the energy from the two absorbed photons (*green*) raises an electron to an excited state; relaxation to the ground state emits a fluorescent photon (*blue*). In SHG there is no excited state, with the transition occurring via a virtual energy level. In the CARS process, the initial pump (*green*) and probe (*red*) photons stimulate a vibration from which the probe photon (typically degenerate with the pump photon) inelastically scatters. (**b**) Adipose tissue imaged by all three methods simultaneously. TPEF (*green*) shows the fluorescently labeled cells; CARS (*cyan*) tuned to image the CH2 stretch that occurs in lipids. SHG (*red*) shows the capsular collagen mesh that covers the tissue

photon to excite a fluorophore, relies on the near simultaneous absorption of two photons each containing half the required energy [1] (Fig. 1a). Given that the probability of simultaneous absorption of two photons is relatively small, a very high photon flux is required. Spatially, this is achieved through the use of a high numerical aperture lens, which results in a smaller focal spot with increased photon density. Further, temporal modulation of the laser beam through the use of pulsed laser sources results in delivery of a laser pulse with a high peak power. This increases the photon density and therefore the chances of simultaneous absorption of two photons [2] while maintaining a low average power required to preserve sample viability. This inherent dependence on two photons means that the intensity of the fluorescence emission scales quadratically with the excitation power, rather than linearly as is the case with one-photon fluorescence. For this reason, multiphoton techniques are often referred to as nonlinear optical microscopy.

The use of two or more higher wavelength, lower energy photons, confers several benefits over conventional one-photon microscopy. Firstly, as the intensity of the beam decreases away from the focal point, the probability of a two-photon absorption drops rapidly. This results in inherent optical sectioning as little fluorescence is generated outside of the focal point. Thus two-photon microscopy does not require a confocal pinhole, making it possible to reduce the distance of the light path between the back aperture of the objective lens and the detector, therefore minimizing signal loss [3]. The benefits of this restricted excitation further extend to reduced photobleaching and phototoxicity, preserving fluorophores outwith the focal spot and increasing sample viability. Secondly, the longer wavelength used for two-photon excitation is far away from the emission wavelength, enabling easier separation of the emission signal with filters. Lastly, when compared to single-photon excitation, two-photon excitation exhibits superior deep tissue imaging on many samples for several reasons. The lack of a confocal pin hole allows scattered emission fluorescence to be collected whereas in standard confocal these photons would be rejected by the pin hole; photons are also less likely to be absorbed by fluorophores outside of the focal spot so photons are able to penetrate deeper; and the use of longer wavelength photons also allow for better depth penetration than standard fluorescence as the degree of light scattering is inversely proportional to the fourth power of the light wavelength [4].

For the reasons listed above, TPEF has become the technique of choice for high-resolution deep tissue imaging, and its use for intra-vital microscopy has helped make important contributions to our understanding of complex biological processes in vivo. The major drawback of this approach is that it requires the use of a fluorophore to label a protein or structure of interest. While application of exogenous fluorescent dyes represents a relatively easy method for labeling structures of interest, e.g., blood vessels, in general fluorescent probes must be expressed either through the use of vector-based expression systems or through transgenic modification of the host-organisms genome. These latter approaches are in general both time-consuming and expensive, and result in labeling only discrete structures or cell populations that represent a small fraction of the complex environment found in tissue. Furthermore, fluorescent dyes may exhibit limited tissue penetration, and fluorophores in general are subject to photobleaching. This said, TPEF represents a powerful technique for interrogating complex biology. However, there is a need to complement it with other multiphoton techniques that can illuminate additional features and provide greater context within the image. Such complementary techniques include Second Harmonic Generation (SHG), Third Harmonic Generation (THG), and Coherent anti-Stokes Raman Scattering (CARS), which unlike TPEF generate image contrast based on structural or chemical properties intrinsic to the sample (Fig. 1b).

Second Harmonic Generation (SHG) shares many of the same features as TPEF microscopy and can be realized using the same imaging setup. For this reason it is routinely used alongside TPEF. However, the way in which the emission signal is generated is mechanistically different than in TPEF. Rather than simultaneous absorption of two-photons as in TPEF, SHG uses two-photons to induce a polarization in the material, resulting in their conversion to a single photon with exactly half the wavelength and double the energy (Fig. 1a). The lack of absorption helps reduce phototoxicity and bleaching of signal [5]. As a second order nonlinear polarization, this process can only occur in a medium lacking a center of symmetry, and in biological imaging this can be observed in structural protein arrays such as collagen, myosin, and tubulin [6]. Thus, SHG represents a label-free imaging modality for visualizing the abundance and structural composition of the extracellular matrix found in many tissues types and disease states.

Another set of techniques that are complementary to both TPEF and SHG are those based on vibrational microscopy, such as Raman spectroscopy. These techniques allow for chemically selective imaging and commercial Raman microscopes have been adapted for confocal imaging to allow depth profiling [7]. Raman scattering relies on the inelastic scattering of a photon where the energy lost is used to excite the molecule to a higher vibrational energy. As different molecules have unique Raman vibrations, they can be imaged across a cell or tissue of interest and a chemical map generated [8]. However, acquisition of Raman spectra is slow, often requiring milliseconds per pixel. Coherent anti-Stokes Raman scattering is a nonlinear technique that uses two synchronized laser beams, termed the pump and Stokes beams, that interact via a four wave mixing process to produce an anti-Stokes photon (Fig. 1a). When the frequency difference between the pump and Stokes beams is tuned to match a Raman resonance, the CARS signal is significantly enhanced allowing video rate imaging [9]. CARS has shown promise in imaging a variety of lipid and protein rich structures including adipocytes, blood, nerve fibers, lipid droplets, and cells [10]. In general, microscopes designed for CARS imaging are inherently capable of TPEF and SHG. Therefore these technologies can be integrated onto a single imaging system, and when acquired simultaneously can provide a more complete image of the tissue environment. The design and construction of such an imaging system is described in detail below.

CARS imaging has many potential applications in biomedical research, and as a label-free imaging modality it is clinically translatable using an endoscopy-based approach. In preclinical research it is routinely used to study aspects of lipid biology, and when combined with TPEF and SHG it represents a powerful tool for basic and translational research focussed on fat. As an example of this, we will focus on its application in understanding the role of Wt1 in visceral fat formation. Cells expressing Wt1, a zinc-finger transcription factor, have been shown to contribute significantly towards the visceral fat depots during gestation and a subset of visceral white adipose tissue continue to arise from Wt1-expressing cells. Multiphoton microscopy provides an excellent tool to examine this as the formation of lipid droplets can be monitored using CARS. Lipid droplets generate strong CARS signals when probed at the CH_2 stretch 2845 cm^{-1} and CARS microscopy has helped to shed new light on lipid research [11]. Wt1 expression can be monitored using a knock-in mouse expressing tamoxifen-inducible Cre recombinase at the Wt1 promoter locus crossed with a reporter mTmG. After Cre-mediated loxP recombination, a membranous GFP is expressed allowing genetic marking of CreER-expressing cells, driven by Wt1 promoter activity, and allows subsequent tracing of these cells and their progeny [12].

2 Materials

2.1 Microscope

1. Olympus FV1000-MPE with mini scanhead.
2. Olympus XLPlan N 25× 1.05NA objective lens.
3. Olympus 690 Turret Dichroic in U-MF2 cube unit.
4. Emission filters (32 mm diameter): Semrock: FF01-440/40, FF03-525/50; Chroma: ET605/75 m, ET687/95 m. Emission Dichroic Mirrors (44 mm × 32 mm × 1.5 mm with corners cut) Chroma: LM01-466, t640lpxr.in FV10-MROPT filter cube and Semrock FF552-Di02 in FV10MP-SDMOPT slide in dichroic holder.
5. Stage: Prior Scientific: H117 Proscan flat top motorized scanning stage.

2.2 Laser

1. APE picoEMERALD CARS laser source with AOM.

2.3 Optical Table and Components

1. Mechanical Shutter: Uniblitz: VS14 Optical shutter; Thorlabs: TR75/M universal post, UPH50/M universal post holder.
2. Optical Table: Thorlabs: PTP603—Set of four standard duty passive legs; PTM51504—Standard optical table.
3. Beam Expander: Thorlabs: AC254-200-B, AC127-050-B lenses; TR75/M×2 universal post, UPH50/M×2 universal post holder, CP11/M SM05 cage plate, CP90F removable cage plate, CP02/M SM01 cage plate, ER12×4 cage rods.
4. Optical Path: Thorlabs: BB1-E03×6 dielectric mirrors, AHWP05M-980×2 Achromatic half-wave plates, POLARIS-K1-H×7 mirror mounts, RSP1/M×2 Rotation mounts, TR75/M×10 universal post, UPH50/M×9 universal post holder, LB1 beam block, RA90 right angle clamp; Edmund Optics: #49–872 Polarizing beam splitter; Newport: UPA-CH1 Cube holder.

2.4 Tools

1. Beam viewing and profiling: Thorlabs: BP209-VIS/M beam profiler, VRC5 IR detector card, PM100D energy meter, S121C photodiode power sensor; FJW: Find-R-Scope Infrared viewer.

3   Methods

3.1   Microscope Construction

A multiphoton microscope is mainly comprised of a laser scanning confocal microscope adapted for the near IR, coupled with a pulsed laser source. A number of additional elements can be added to improve the flexibility of the system.

1. **Laser**

   For the setup described here, an APE picoEMERALD laser system was used to provide two spatially and temporally aligned laser beams. A tunable beam between 720 and 980 nm with 5–6 ps pulse width and 80 MHz repetition rate was used as the pump beam in the CARS process whilst a fixed 1064 nm, 7 ps, 80 MHz repetition rate laser was used as a Stokes beam. The APE picoEMERALD is software controlled from a remote panel PC allowing easy tuning and temporal alignment (*see* **Note 1**).

2. **Microscope**

   An Olympus FV1000 scan unit on an IX81 frame with Prior Scientific H117 stage was used in the build. The microscope included four non descanned PMTs to allow acquisition of multiple imaging modalities and fluorescence channels with high efficiency. At least one PMT should have good red sensitivity as the CARS process generally produces photons around the 660 nm wavelength. Silver or gold coated mirrors ensure high IR reflectivity on mirror components throughout the system.

3. **Optomechanics**

   Before placing any components on an optical table, careful planning should be taken in the design of the optical path. Modeling the table and components in a CAD program such as AutoCAD or Solidworks can help identify space and access issues on the table (Fig. 2a).

   Optical components are very sensitive to dirt and oils that reside on hands and should always be handled with appropriate latex or nitrile gloves, and held using the edges, or with tweezers or forceps.

   Mirrors should be placed first on the table and aligned using a sighting laser that uses a visible beam with a low power output. Mirror angles should be kept 45° to avoid generating elliptical beam shapes, and the beam focused on the center of the mirror. After the mirrors are placed and aligned, additional optical components can be added and aligned so as not to disturb the beam path. This should be started at the furthest point from the laser source. After all of the optical components are in place and aligned with the sighting laser, the IR laser beam should be manually checked one optical component at a time, starting with the mirror nearest the laser source and working towards the microscope body. Appropriate beam

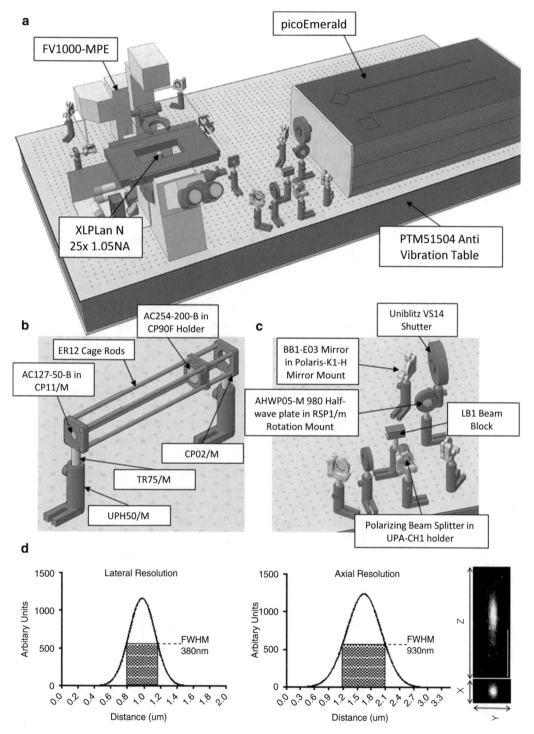

Fig. 2 Microscope design. (**a**) Layout of a multiphoton microscope on a 2 m × 1 m optical table modeled using AutoCAD. (**b**) Diagram of a 4× beam expander used to expand the laser beam to overfill the objective back aperture. (**c**) Diagram of the manual power control, consisting of a half-wave plate and polarizing beam splitter. (**d**) Microscope resolution is calculated using the FWHM of sub-diffraction-sized fluorescent beads

blocks should be used to minimize unwanted laser scattering that may occur from unaligned beams. The beam can be followed around the table using a laser viewing card (Thorlabs VRC5) or an IR viewer (FJW Find-R-Scope). Finally the beam alignment through the microscope can be optimized by using a photodiode sensor placed over a slide to measure the light emitted by the objective (Thorlabs S121C).

Caution: Proper protective eye wear must be worn when aligning lasers and laboratory controls including interlocks should be used to ensure the safety of the workers and visiting personnel (*see* **Note 2**).

4. **Beam Telescope**

The back aperture of the microscope objective should be slightly overfilled to maintain diffraction-limited optical performance; this may not match up with the beam size of the laser so optics are used to expand or contract the beam size before insertion into the microscope. The microscope frame often has a beam expander after the scanning mirror, so any magnifications should be calculated with this kept in mind. The laser beam will diverge as it exits the laser so the actual beam size entering the telescope should be used, rather than the manufacturer's specifications. This can be measured by a beam profiler along the laser path (Thorlabs BP209-VIS/M) and the optimal spot for a beam expander can be located. In our setup the laser beam is measured as having a 1.1 mm diameter after 1 m from the laser aperture. The objective has a 15.2 mm back aperture whilst the microscope has a 3.6× beam expander after the scanning mirrors. A 4× beam expander is built using lenses with focal lengths of 50 mm and 200 mm, respectively. The magnification of a Keplerian telescope can be calculated as the ratio of the focal lengths of the two lenses used. The lenses are separated by the sum of their focal lengths, but due to the divergence of the laser beam small adjustments might need to be made to ensure the output beam is perfectly collimated and this can be made using the beam profiler to measure the divergence of the beam at several points after the beam expander. The final beam size of 15.84 mm slightly overfills the objective lens (*see* **Note 3**).

5. **Beam Intensity Control**

The setup described here utilizes a half-wave plate on a rotation mount, which when rotated alters the polarization of the light prior to passing through a polarizing beam splitter. By changing this polarization it is possible to ascertain fine control over laser power, as light of a given polarization will be redirected from the light path onto a beam dump. Such an approach provides an important means of manually controlling laser power, and can be used as an alternative, or a safety backup, to laser power control provided in the APE picoEMERALD software (*see* **Note 4**).

6. Objective Lens

When performing combined CARS/TPEF imaging, it is important that the objective lens has a high numerical aperture, low chromatic aberration, and good transmission of light in the near IR. For physiological imaging, a water immersion lens will minimize spherical aberration when samples are immersed in an aqueous medium and may not be directly in contact with the cover glass. If the objective lens, such as that described here, has a corrective collar, then this must be adjusted to match the thickness of the cover glass used. This will ensure optimal performance in terms of image brightness and resolution (*see* **Note 5**).

7. Filter Cube

Design of the filter setup within the filter cubes requires careful consideration of which fluorophores will be used, and what excitation and emission characteristics they have. The filters selected must offer sufficient blocking of the excitation light, high transmission of the emission light, and have a bandwidth that minimizes spectral bleed through when used in conjunction with other fluorophores. An example of a setup used for four channel simultaneous detection of GFP, tdTomato, CARS (CH_2 stretch), and SHG from tissue removed from an mTmG mouse is shown in Fig. 3.

3.2 Optimizing CARS Imaging

Aligning, optimizing, and validating the CARS imaging is an essential step in the microscope build. Both the pump and Stokes beams in the CARS process need to be aligned individually, and then synchronized temporally to generate an optimal CARS image.

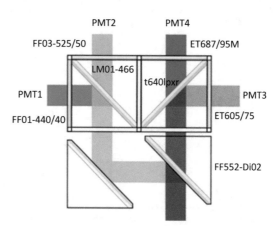

Fig. 3 Filter block layout. Four non-descanned photomultiplier tubes are used which allows SHG, CARS, and two fluorescent channels to be imaged at once. In this setup broad emission filters are used for flexible choices on fluorophores used; however these filters can be replaced with tighter emissions if bleed through is a concern

1. Laser adjustment can be made using a power meter set at the tip of the objective lens. Set the scanning field to the highest zoom possible and start scanning with the pump beam. Adjust the final two mirrors to achieve maximum laser power on the detector. Repeat using the Stokes beam and the alignment mirrors in the laser.

2. Place a strong CARS emitting sample (solid paraffin) on to a No. 1.5 coverslip and mount on the microscope. Tune the pump laser to 816.8 nm. Adjust the delay between the two lasers until the maximum signal is obtained (*see* Fig. 4a).

3. Record the signal and power relationship between the pump and Stokes beams (Fig. 4b, c). A CARS signal should be found to be linearly proportional to the Stokes beam, and quadratically proportional to the pump beam. No signal should be detectable when either laser power is at 0 mW (*see* **Note 6**).

4. Verify the wavelength dependence of the signal by collecting a spectral sweep. This is done by tuning the pump laser in short steps across a known vibrational resonance. With paraffin the

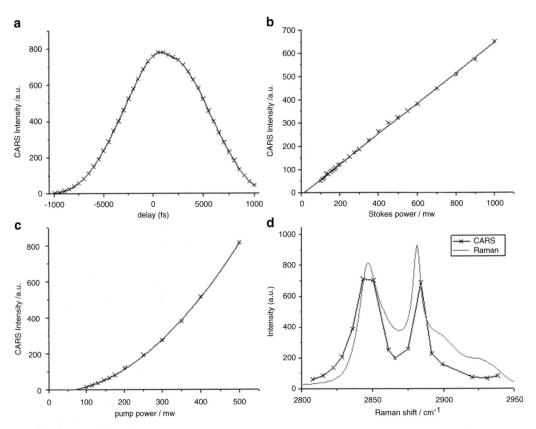

Fig. 4 CARS optimization and validation. (**a**) Temporal overlap is maximized using a strong CARS emitting object. (**b** and **c**) The dependence of the CARS signal on the pump and Stokes wavelengths is calculated, ensuring a linear trend with the Stokes laser, and quadratic trend with the pump laser. (**d**) CARS spectra overlaid on a Raman spectra of paraffin, ensuring vibrational resonance dependence of the signal

2800–3000 cm^{-1} region can be scanned by tuning from 805 to 820 nm. The CARS spectrum should follow a similar pattern to the Raman spectrum (Fig. 4d).

3.3 Imaging a Sample

1. Harvest tissue of interest from mouse, keeping at 4 °C in PBS.
2. Place tissue on glass bottomed dish and keep hydrated with PBS.
3. Mount sample on microscope using appropriate immersion media on the objective lens. Check that any correction collars are aligned to match the thickness of the glass.
4. Tune pump laser to 816.8 nm to monitor the CH$_2$ stretch (Raman wavelength 2845 cm^{-1}) to allow detection of lipid droplets in the CARS channel. Anti-Stokes photons are generated at ≈663 nm, SHG at ≈408 nm (*see* **Note 7**).
5. Adjust imaging parameters for best effects. Low image intensity should be adjusted firstly by raising PMT voltages, then increasing pixel dwell times, and finally by adjusting the laser power. Low laser powers help minimize sample damage and photobleaching.
6. Check for unwanted fluorescence bleed through or other effects in the PMT channels by both temporally desynchronizing pump and Stokes beams, illuminating with beams independently and tuning away from the Raman resonance to an off-resonance image at 830 nm.
7. Capture Image (Fig. 5).

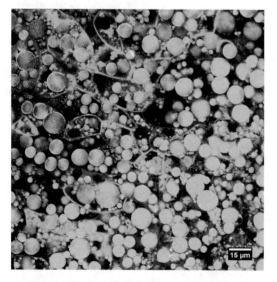

Fig. 5 Image of Wt1 labeled explants. Image of lipid droplets in epididymal appendage explants (Wt1^{CreERT2}; mTmG/+) cultured in adipogenesis differentiation medium. Wt1-derived adipocytes (GFP—*green*), neighboring adipocytes (tdTomato—*red*), and lipid droplets (CARS—*cyan*)

4 Notes

1. The most important component of a multiphoton system is the laser source. Pulsed laser sources provide high peak powers required to generate nonlinear effects, whilst retaining a low overall average power to prevent thermal damage. Pulsed laser sources are available from a range of laser manufacturers to suit a variety of budgets and applications. Typically the most important feature to look at is the output wavelength as this limits the selection of fluorophores that can be used in the system. A laser that is tunable from 700 to 1000 nm will cover blue, green, and yellow fluorophores, whilst red and far red fluorophores require excitation in the far infrared (>1100 nm). Pulse duration is another factor to consider with shorter pulses providing increased excitation efficiency, which makes them favorable for TPEF, SHG, and THG applications. In the case of CARS microscopy however, the pulse duration directly affects the spectral resolution of the vibrational imaging as well as the nonresonant background [13]. Picosecond pulses are preferred here as they offer higher spectral sensitivity and lower background levels.

2. Special care must be taken when working with Class IV lasers, and reference to local laser safety policies should always be considered. Coherent laser light, both direct from the laser source, and specular scattering can be of sufficient intensity to cause eye damage. Further, these laser beams are of sufficient power to burn skin and clothing, as well as ignite volatile substances. Laser paths should be kept at low heights and contained within a controlled room with restricted access. When possible the light path should be enclosed to minimize risk.

3. Using a lens-based system allows the telescope objective lens to be swapped out for different beam magnifications to match a range of microscope objective lenses. Lenses, however, are not free from chromatic aberration, so the best possible performance would be obtained using a reflective beam expander which exhibits virtually no chromatic aberration.

4. Although manual beam control is not necessary and can be removed from the build, it does allow for another beam path to be created. This can be used to add a new path for a small objective lens, or the addition of an adaptive optics element whilst still offering a clean path for comparison.

5. In order to ensure diffraction limited images, optical components such as mirrors and lenses must be clean, and interfering optical elements such as differential interference contrast prisms should be removed from the light path. The resolution of the constructed system should be regularly checked to ensure optimal alignment and maximum image quality is maintained. This can be done by measuring the point spread

functions of subresolution beads (Fig. 2d) [14]. The theoretical resolution for a multiphoton image can be calculated using the following formulas [15]:

$$FWHM(xy) = 2\sqrt{\ln(2)}\frac{0.325\lambda}{\sqrt{2}\ NA^{0.91}}$$

$$FWHM(z) = 2\sqrt{\ln(2)}\frac{0.532\lambda}{\sqrt{2}\left(n-\sqrt{n^2-NA^2}\right)}$$

6. Sources of unwanted signal can include the pump and Stokes beams themselves if the filters used do not sufficiently block the IR region. Extra shortpass filters can be added to filter sets to offset this. Another source of unwanted signal in the CARS channel can be due to fluorescent bleed through, particularly when red and far red fluorophores are used. This often presents itself as a signal that remains when one of the beams are turned off, but may be due to fluorescence arising from the interaction of both beams. It is possible to separate out CARS photons from fluorescent photons by using lifetime imaging if contaminating fluorescences are unavoidable [16].

7. To convert from the pump wavelength to the wavenumber probed by the CARS system, the difference in the pump and Stokes photons, in wavenumbers, needs to be calculated.

$$\text{Wavenumber probed} = \frac{10^7}{\text{Pump wavelength (nm)}} - \frac{10^7}{\text{Stokes wavelength (nm)}}$$

To calculate the wavelength of the emitted CARS photon, the difference between two pump photons and one Stokes photons is calculated in wavenumbers and then converted back to wavelength

$$\text{CARS wavelength (nm)} = \frac{10^7}{\frac{2\times10^7}{\text{Pump wavelength}} - \frac{10^7}{\text{Stokes wavelength (nm)}}}$$

Acknowledgements

For support in building the microscope we would like to thank: Cancer Research UK (grant C157/A12753), The College of Medicine and Veterinary Medicine at the University of Edinburgh, The Medical Research Council Human Genetics Unit, the Caledonia Events Committee (CRUK grant C157/A16508), and the Clerk Maxwell Cancer Fund. This work was supported by

Cancer Research UK (program grant C157/A15703) and the European Research Council Advanced Investigator Grant (grant number 294440 Cancer Innovation to M.C.F.).

References

1. Wollman AJM, Nudd R, Hedlund EG et al (2015) From Animaculum to single molecules: 300 years of the light microscope. Open Biol 5(4):150019. doi:10.1098/Rsob.150019

2. Denk W, Strickler J, Webb W (1990) Two-photon laser scanning fluorescence microscopy. Science 248(4951):73–76. doi:10.1126/science.2321027

3. Oheim M, Michael DJ, Geisbauer M et al (2006) Principles of two-photon excitation fluorescence microscopy and other nonlinear imaging approaches. Adv Drug Deliv Rev 58(7):788–808. doi:10.1016/j.addr.2006.07.005

4. Benninger RKP, Piston DW (2013) Two-photon excitation microscopy for the study of living cells and tissues. Curr Protoc Cell Biol. doi:10.1002/0471143030.cb0411s59

5. Campagnola PJ, Dong CY (2011) Second harmonic generation microscopy: principles and applications to disease diagnosis. Laser Photon Rev 5(1):13–26. doi:10.1002/lpor.200910024

6. Mohler W, Millard AC, Campagnola PJ (2003) Second harmonic generation imaging of endogenous structural proteins. Methods 29(1):97–109. doi:10.1016/s1046-2023(02)00292-x

7. Tague T (2007) Infrared and Raman microscopy: complimentary or redundant techniques? Microsc Microanal 13(S02):1696–1697. doi:10.1017/s1431927607074855

8. Stewart S, Priore RJ, Nelson MP et al (2012) Raman imaging. Annu Rev Anal Chem 5(1):337–360. doi:10.1146/annurev-anchem-062011-143152

9. Evans CL, Potma EO, Puoris'haag M et al (2005) Chemical imaging of tissue in vivo with video-rate coherent anti-Stokes Raman scattering microscopy. Proc Natl Acad Sci 102(46):16807–16812. doi:10.1073/pnas.0508282102

10. Lee M, Downes A, Chau Y-Y et al (2015) In vivo imaging of the tumor and its associated microenvironment using combined CARS/2-photon microscopy. IntraVital 4(1):e1055430. doi:10.1080/21659087.2015.1055430

11. Le TT, Yue S, Cheng JX (2010) Shedding new light on lipid biology with coherent anti-Stokes Raman scattering microscopy. J Lipid Res 51(11):3091–3102. doi:10.1194/jlr.R008730

12. Chau Y-Y, Bandiera R, Serrels A et al (2014) Visceral and subcutaneous fat have different origins and evidence supports a mesothelial source. Nat Cell Biol 16(4):367–375. doi:10.1038/ncb2922

13. Cheng J-x, Volkmer A, Book LD et al (2001) An epi-detected coherent anti-Stokes Raman scattering (E-CARS) microscope with high spectral resolution and high sensitivity. J Phys Chem B 105(7):1277–1280. doi:10.1021/jp003774a

14. Cole RW, Jinadasa T, Brown CM (2011) Measuring and interpreting point spread functions to determine confocal microscope resolution and ensure quality control. Nat Protoc 6(12):1929–1941. doi:10.1038/nprot.2011.407

15. Zipfel WR, Williams RM, Webb WW (2003) Nonlinear magic: multiphoton microscopy in the biosciences. Nat Biotechnol 21(11):1369–1377. doi:10.1038/nbt899

16. Slepkov AD, Ridsdale A, Wan H-N et al (2011) Forward-collected simultaneous fluorescence lifetime imaging and coherent anti-Stokes Raman scattering microscopy. J Biomed Opt 16(2):021103. doi:10.1117/1.3490641

Chapter 10

Function and Regulation of the *Wilms' Tumor Suppressor 1 (WT1)* Gene in Fish

Birgit Perner, Thomas J.D. Bates, Uta Naumann, and Christoph Englert

Abstract

The *Wilms' tumor suppressor gene Wt1* is highly conserved among vertebrates. In contrast to mammals, most fish species possess two *wt1* paralogs that have been named *wt1a* and *wt1b*. Concerning *wt1* in fish, most work so far has been done using zebrafish, focusing on the embryonic kidney, the pronephros. In this chapter we will describe the structure and development of the pronephros as well as the role that the *wt1* genes play in the embryonic zebrafish kidney. We also discuss Wt1 target genes and describe the potential function of the Wt1 proteins in the adult kidney. Finally we will summarize data on the role of Wt1 outside of the kidney.

Key words Pronephros, Mesonephros, Zebrafish, Glomerulus, Podocyte, Regeneration, Kidney

1 Introduction

Wt1 genes are highly conserved among vertebrates. Mammalian *Wt1* encompasses ten exons [1] one of which, namely exon 5, is alternatively spliced. An additional alternative splicing event occurs at the end of exon 9, leading to the insertion of the tripeptide KTS. While the latter is conserved (albeit it is KPS in fugu) in all species where *Wt1* has been found to date, exon 5 is missing in fish [2,3]. Moreover, and in contrast to mammals, reptiles, and amphibians fish possess two *wt1* paralogs that have been named *wt1a* and *wt1b* [4,5], whilst in the rainbow trout three *wt1* genes have been reported [6]. A fish-specific splicing event is alternative splicing of exon 4, which we have recently shown [7].

While *wt1* genes have been described in a number of different fish species, most attention has been given to zebrafish, which serves as an eminent model in developmental biology and, increasingly, also in biomedical research [8]. The majority of Wt1-related studies in zebrafish have focused on the pronephros, which serves as the embryonic kidney in fish. Later in development, the mesonephric kidney forms and in teleost fish the mesonephros represents the final stage of kidney development, persisting throughout life

Nicholas Hastie (ed.), *The Wilms' Tumor (WT1) Gene: Methods and Protocols*, Methods in Molecular Biology, vol. 1467, DOI 10.1007/978-1-4939-4023-3_10, © Springer Science+Business Media New York 2016

[9]. In this chapter, we summarize the regulation and function of the wt1 genes in fish with an emphasis on the zebrafish pronephros. However, we will also touch on the possible role of Wt1 in other fish organs as well as in regeneration.

2   The Zebrafish Pronephros

2.1   Composition

The zebrafish pronephros is an anatomically simple organ consisting of a single pair of excretory units called nephrons. Each nephron shares a common glomerulus, where the blood is filtered [10]. A key component of the blood filter is the slit diaphragm, formed between interdigitating projections (foot processes) of specialized epithelial cells termed podocytes [10]. Further, the zebrafish pronephric nephron is made up of the following elements: a short neck region, a segmented tubule for selective reabsorption and secretion, and a duct that terminates in the cloaca [11]. Despite this simple composition, differentiation and organization of the pronephric nephron are similar to that of the kidney in higher vertebrates [12, 13].

2.2   Morphogenesis

Pronephros development can be divided into four stages, specification (12 h post-fertilization, hpf), epithelialization (16–24 hpf), segment maturation (24–40 hpf), and angiogenesis (40–48 hpf) [14]. Pronephric progenitors arise from the intermediate mesoderm at early stages of somitogenesis, whereby axial position within the pronephric field predicts cell fate. Areas destined to develop into glomerular, neck, and tubular cells are arranged in an anterior to posterior fashion and correspond roughly with overlapping but discrete expression domains of the transcription factor-encoding genes *wt1a*, *pax2a*, and *sim1a* [15]. After the intermediate mesoderm has adopted a nephric fate, epithelialization of the pronephros commences. The stage of nephron segment maturation gives rise to the pronephric glomerulus and tubule. The angiogenesis stage is characterized by invasion of angiogenic sprouts from the dorsal aorta into the glomerulus, resulting in the formation of capillary loops. Remarkably, the central glomerulus functions as a blood filter already at around 48 hpf [10, 16].

3   *Wt1a* and *Wt1b* Expression During Pronephros Development

In situ hybridization analysis showed that *wt1a* and *wt1b* are expressed in overlapping, but not identical patterns [4]. *Wt1a* is first detectable at 10–11 hpf as two stripes in the intermediate mesoderm and remains in a stripe-like manner until 14 hpf. After becoming more diffuse, the stripes condense at around 24 hpf. Thereafter, *wt1a* expression appears as two dots, which later (36–50 hpf) merge [4, 17]. Expression of *wt1b* initiates 3 h after the first appearance of *wt1a* and is restricted to a caudal subdomain of the *wt1a* expressing field in the intermediate mesoderm. Although the two dot-like domains of *wt1b* expression migrate towards the midline between 24 and 35 hpf, they never merge completely and a central gap remains [4, 18].

Both *wt1a* and *wt1b* are markers of podocyte progenitors within the intermediate mesoderm. However, the broad domain of *wt1a* expression does not only mark renal precursors. Only cells next to the third somite were found to become podocyte precursors [4, 11, 18], while another fraction of *wt1a* expressing cells marks the primordium of the interrenal organ. The latter is the teleost homologue of the mammalian adrenal gland and is located close to the pronephric primordium at 24 hpf. It has been shown that *nr5a1a* expressing interrenal precursor cells arise from the *wt1a* expression domain but do not co-express *wt1b* or *pax2a* [18, 19]. In contrast, the restricted expression of *wt1b* specifically defines the location of podocyte progenitors [4, 11]. Expression of both *wt1* paralogs persists during formation and differentiation of the glomerulus and in mature podocytes [4, 15, 18].

4   Function of Wt1a and Wt1b

Morpholino knockdown studies have shown that Wt1a plays a very early and fundamental role in pronephros formation. *Wt1a* morphant embryos do not express mature podocyte markers (*nephrin*, *podocin*, *podocalyxin*), indicating that depletion of Wt1a disrupts glomerular morphogenesis and differentiation [18–21]. A combinatorial knockdown approach, together with biochemical assays, revealed that Wt1a cooperates with FoxC1/2 transcription factors and the Notch mediator Rbpj to regulate podocyte fate. Embryos injected with morpholinos against *wt1a*, *foxc1a*, or *rbpj* develop fewer podocytes but a simultaneous knockdown of any two of these genes induced a complete lack of glomerulogenesis [18].

Concerning the role of Wt1b inconsistent results have been reported. In one case, *wt1b* morphants were described to possess normal podocytes and simultaneous depletion of *wt1a* and *wt1b* did not induce additional effects on podocyte number and differentiation in comparison to the single *wt1a* knockdown [18]. In another study, however, it was demonstrated that while knockdown of *wt1b* is compatible with initial formation of glomerular structures, at 48 hpf *wt1b* morphant embryos develop pronephric cysts and subsequent pericardial edema [21]. Transcript levels of podocyte markers *nephrin* and *podocin* were detectable but in a reduced manner, suggesting that podocyte differentiation had occurred and the filtration unit is at least in part present in *wt1b* morphants. Together with the finding that knockdown of both *wt1* genes caused defects that were stronger than in either case alone, it has been concluded that Wt1a and Wt1b fulfill different functions in the development of the zebrafish pronephros. One possible explanation for the discrepancy could be the application of different morpholinos and/or the use of different amounts.

As mentioned above, the *wt1a* expression profile suggests a role in interrenal development. Contradictory findings have been reported regarding the effect of *wt1a* knockdown on *nr5a1a* expressing interrenal progenitors. Initial studies had shown a reduced size of interrenal primordia in *wt1a* morphants [19], while a later report showed an increased number of *nr5a1a* expressing cells following *wt1a* knockdown [18]. However, *nr5a1a* positive cells were completely absent in *wt1a/fox1a* double morphant embryos, suggesting that Wt1a and Fox1a work together in the specification of the interrenal gland [18].

5   Regulation of *Wt1a/b* Expression

In zebrafish, the occurrence of podocyte progenitor cells that express *wt1a* and *wt1b* is dependent on balanced retinoic acid (RA) signaling [11, 22, 23]. RA is an important morphogen, playing a role in the development and patterning of many tissues. Both synthesizing and degrading enzymes control its local concentration [24, 25]. RA signaling is activated when RA binds to heterodimers of the RA receptor (RAR) with the partner protein retinoic X receptor (RXR). A combination of deletion analysis and stable as well as transient transgenesis revealed the presence of an enhancer element approximately 4 kb upstream of the *wt1a* gene, which is necessary for its proper expression in the intermediate mesoderm. This element is highly conserved between fish and mammals, is bound by RAR/RXR complexes, and mediates responsiveness to RA in vivo and in cell culture [26]. Moreover, both knockdown and mutation of *aldh1a2*, encoding an RA synthesizing enzyme, lead to reduced expression of *wt1a* and *wt1b*, while expression of both paralogs was completely absent following suppression of RA signaling by application of DEAB, an inhibitor of RA synthesis [11, 23]. RA is also involved in pronephric segmentation. Inhibition of RA signaling causes a loss of proximal segments and expansion of distal ones [11, 23]. Thus, an RA deficiency, either genetically or chemically induced, blocks the formation of podocytes, suggesting a fundamental role of RA in nephrogenesis by facilitating podocyte and proximal tubule specification and suppression of distal tubular fates [11, 23].

The homeobox transcription factors Cdx1a and Cdx4 were also found to be important regulators of zebrafish pronephros segmentation [11]. Cdx-deficient embryos exhibit a posterior expansion of *wt1a* expression [11, 27] indicative of a pronephric positioning defect. Cdx transcription factors act via regulating RA activity along the embryonic axes [11].

Other factors acting downstream of retinoic acid signaling but upstream or in parallel to Wt1a and the Notch pathway during podocyte formation are the HNF1β paralogs Hnf1ba and Hnf1bb [28]. In *hnf1ba/b* deficient embryos, the expression domain of *wt1a* and *wt1b* was found to be expanded to regions corresponding to the future neck and proximal tubule [28, 29]. Deficiencies in *hnf1ba/b* also caused ectopic expression of *nephrin* and *podocin*, suggesting that Hnf1b transcription factors are important in restricting a podocyte fate. Furthermore, it was found that knock-down of *wt1a* and *rbpj* in *hnf1ba/b* deficient embryos resulted in complete absence of *wt1b* expression, demonstrating that Wt1a and Notch signaling are required for ectopic podocyte formation in *hnf1ba/b* deficient embryos [28].

To restrict the domain of *wt1a* expression, and thus podocyte development appropriate expression of the transcription factor gene *pax2a* is essential [30]. During pronephric development, *wt1a* and *pax2a* are initially co-expressed in neck cells, which arise adjacent to podocytes [18]. Later, only *wt1a* expression persists in the glomerulus, while *pax2a* can be detected in the neck region, the tubule, and the forming cloaca [10, 30]. Zebrafish embryos harboring mutations in *pax2a* display caudally expanded *wt1a* expression and failed tubulogenesis [30], while *wt1a* deficiency causes decreased level of *pax2a* expression [18]. Taken together, these date suggest a *pax2a/wt1a* regulatory interplay, which is important for the demarcation of glomerular and tubular progenitors during nephron patterning.

6   Wt1 Target Genes

A recent report suggests a regulatory network in which *wt1a* expression is induced by RA, followed by a Wt1a-dependent induction of *odd-skipped related 1* (*osr1*) in podocyte progenitors [22]. *Osr1* encodes a zinc finger transcription factor, which is required for podocyte and proximal tubule formation in zebrafish. Embryos deficient of *osr1* were found to express *wt1a* but in a scattered pattern. The Wt1a-positive cells do not fuse at the midline and fail to express the podocyte marker *nephrin* indicating that the podocyte progenitors are arrested in an immature state [31]. These data show that the expression of *wt1a* is not dependent on Osr1. On the other hand, it has been reported that *osr1* expression was absent in embryos deficient in RA signaling as well as in *wt1a* morphants, indicating that Osr1 acts downstream of *wt1a* as an effector of podocyte differentiation [22].

A genome-wide expression profiling analysis using a human cell line with inducible *Wt1* has led to the discovery of a number of WT1-induced genes, among them *CXXC5* [32, 33]. *CXXC5* encodes a negative regulator of the WNT/β-Catenin signaling pathway in vitro as well as in zebrafish and was renamed *WID*

(Wt1-induced inhibitor of Dishevelled [33]). Depletion of Wid in zebrafish gave rise to malformed embryonic kidneys with large cysts in the glomerular-tubular region, implicating a role for Wid in pronephrogenesis [33].

By a ChIP-Seq approach using mouse glomeruli as starting material, we have recently identified novel Wt1 target genes that mediate its function in podocyte differentiation and maintenance, among them Nphs2 (encoding podocin), Mafb, and Magi2. The zebrafish genome harbors single *nphs2* and *magi2* genes and two *mafb* orthologues [34]. *Nph2*, *magi2*, and *mafba* but not *mafbb* are expressed in the glomerular region of the pronephros [12, 18, 21, 34], and are significantly decreased in *wt1a* and *wt1b* deficient embryos. Furthermore, inactivation of *nph2*, *magi2*, and *mafba* disrupts normal pronephros development, suggesting that like Podocin, Mafba, and Magi2 regulate zebrafish pronephros development.

7   Wt1 Function in the Adult Kidney

Whilst both Wt1a and Wt1b play a vital role during pronephric development [21], these factors seem also involved in mesonephric neonephrogenesis and regeneration [35, 36]. While the mammalian kidney can respond to damage with dedifferentiation and repopulation of damage tissue [37], the zebrafish has an extraordinary ability to perform neonephrogenesis, or to form new tubules. This process can be followed and visualized by the help of respective transgenic lines, e.g., *wt1a:EGFP* or *wt1b:EGFP* transgenic zebrafish [26]. The *wt1b:EGFP* fish line shows new GFP-positive populations at 12 days post-fertilization (dpf), involved in the formation of the new nephrons of the mesonephros [36]. The *wt1b*-positive populations described are initially organized in clusters, which undergo a mesenchymal-epithelial transition (MET), form a luminal structure, with nephrons that have GFP-positive glomeruli, which subsequently express the podocyte differentiation marker *podocin*. To study regeneration of the fish kidney one often uses the nephrotoxic antibiotic Gentamicin [35, 38]. Five days post-injury (5 dpi) there is an increase in proliferative (PCNA-positive) Wt1b-positive tubules, evidence that regenerative mesonephric neonephrogenesis appears to recapitulate normal stages of nephron development [36].

With the discovery of adult neonephrogenesis, next came the concept of adult progenitors, cells that give the kidney the ability to regenerate [35]. When investigating the processes of new nephron formation in more detail, the authors describe the role of Wt1b-positive and Lhx1a-positive populations, the fish orthologues of the mammalian kidney-related transcription factors [39, 40]. Single Lhx1a-positive cells were discovered, as well as renal vesicles that were Wt1b-/Lhx1a-positive. Gentamicin-induced kidney damage increased the numbers of Wt1b-/Lhx1a-positive cells, but it was noted that *wt1b* expression was only activated following cellular aggregation, whilst *lhx1a* was expressed in single cells before this. When transplanted, the single Lhx1a-positive cells were able to form new nephrons, whilst there was no engraftment when transplanting the Wt1b-/Lhx1a-positive renal vesicles. These results suggest that Lhx1a-positive cells are nephron progenitors in the zebrafish kidney, whilst *wt1b's* later expression in renal vesicles indicates a different role during formation, but not initiation of new tubules.

In addition to playing a role in tubular regeneration, it is also suggested that Wt1b plays a role in glomerular repair in the adult zebrafish [41]. Utilizing podocyte-specific (*pod:NTRmCherry*) expression of a bacterial nitroreductase enzyme (NTR), which has the ability to cause the prodrug metronidazole (Mtz) to become toxic, cell ablation was performed. Following Mtz treatment, transgenic fish have defective glomerular filtration. After damage, cells are able to repair and retain their function, and interestingly Wt1b-positive cells are found in the glomeruli of fully differentiated nephrons, suggesting a restarted developmental cycle in the glomeruli [41].

Studies in the zebrafish pronephros and the adult mammalian kidney suggest an evolutionarily conserved role for *Wt1* genes [21, 34, 42]. This hypothesis is also supported by the expression of *wt1* in renal vesicles 14 days after kidney damage in medaka [43]. This response highlights a functional conservation across fish species, something that has also been shown in relation to splice isoforms [7].

8   Wt1 in Other Organs

As well as playing important roles in the kidney, *Wt1* genes are also linked to cardiac development. During formation of the heart, the endocardium (mesothelial lining of heart), myocardium (cardiac muscle), and pericardium (heart sac) are organized. The pericardium arises from the dorsally located proepicardium organ (PEO) and migrates over the surface of the heart. The use of *wt1* transgenic reporter lines highlighted Wt1a as a more complete marker of the epicardial cells during embryogenesis [44, 45] . In previous experiments, before the distinction between *wt1a* and *wt1b*, *wt1* expression was found surrounding the heart at 4 dpf [46]. This resembles presumably Wt1a activity, due to lack of Wt1b signal, a result that has been subsequently confirmed. At 3 dpf, during the development of the heart, *wt1b* is expressed in the myocard covering epicardial cells, with additional colocalization with *cmlc2* in deeper cardiac muscle cells [47].

While cardiac injury in mammals leads to scarring, zebrafish can also regenerate significant portions of the heart after cardiac injury [48]. In the adult zebrafish heart, Wt1b persists in a subset of epicardial cells, plus in sparsely found intramyocardial cells, which are likely to be hematopoietic [47]. Following both mild (scratching) and severe (puncture/resection/cryoinjury) cardiac injury, *wt1b* expression is found in and around the injury site, with some Wt1b-positive cells being proliferative [47, 49, 45] showing a role for Wt1b during heart regeneration.

9   Outlook

Much of what we have learned about the function of Wt1 in fish is based on expression studies, transgenic lines, and morpholino-mediated knockdown experiments. From those studies a conserved role for Wt1 primarily in development of the kidney has emerged. However, fish offer the opportunity to study the function of Wt1's role beyond development, namely in regeneration. With the development of inducible and tissue-specific knockouts in zebrafish [50] and the advent of sophisticated genome editing tools like CRISPR/ Cas, we will undoubtedly learn about novel functional aspects of this fascinating transcription factor in and outside of the kidney.

References

1. Haber DA, Sohn RL, Buckler AJ et al (1991) Alternative splicing and genomic structure of the Wilms' tumor gene WT1. Proc Natl Acad Sci U S A 88:9618–9622

2. Kent J, Coriat AM, Sharpe PT et al (1995) The evolution of WT1 sequence and expression pattern in the vertebrates. Oncogene 11:1781–1792

3. Miles C, Elgar G, Coles E et al (1998) Complete sequencing of the Fugu WAGR region from WT1 to PAX6: dramatic compaction and conservation of synteny with human chromosome 11p13. Proc Natl Acad Sci U S A 95:13068–13072

4. Bollig F, Mehringer R, Perner B et al (2006) Identification and comparative expression analysis of a second wt1 gene in zebrafish. Dev Dyn 235:554–561

5. Kluver N, Herpin A, Braasch I et al (2009) Regulatory back-up circuit of medaka Wt1 co-orthologs ensures PGC maintenance. Dev Biol 325:179–188

6. Brunelli JP, Robison BD, Thorgaard GH (2001) Ancient and recent duplications of the rainbow trout Wilms' tumor gene. Genome 44:455–462

7. Schnerwitzki D, Perner B, Hoppe B et al (2014) Alternative splicing of Wilms' tumor suppressor 1 (Wt1) exon 4 results in protein isoforms with different functions. Dev Biol 393:24–32

8. Goessling W, North TE (2014) Repairing quite swimmingly: advances in regenerative medicine using zebrafish. Dis Model Mech 7:769–776

9. Gilbert SF (2003) Developmental biology. Sinauer Associates, Sunderland, MA, p xvii, 838 pp

10. Drummond IA, Majumdar A, Hentschel H et al (1998) Early development of the zebrafish pronephros and analysis of mutations affecting pronephric function. Development 125:4655–4667

11. Wingert RA, Selleck R, Yu J et al (2007) The cdx genes and retinoic acid control the positioning and segmentation of the zebrafish pronephros. PLoS Genet 3:e189

12. Kramer-Zucker AG, Wiessner S, Jensen AM et al (2005) Organization of the pronephric filtration apparatus in zebrafish requires Nephrin, Podocin and the FERM domain protein Mosaic eyes. Dev Biol 285:316–329

13. Wingert RA, Davidson AJ (2008) The zebrafish pronephros: A model to study nephron segmentation. Kidney Int. 73:1120–1127

14. Drummond IA, Davidson AJ (2010) Chapter 9—zebrafish kidney development. In: William H, Detrich MW, Leonard IZ (eds) Methods in cell biology. Academic Press, New York, pp 233–260

15. Serluca FC, Fishman MC (2001) Pre-pattern in the pronephric kidney field of zebrafish. Development 128:2233–2241

16. Drummond I (2003) Making a zebrafish kidney: a tale of two tubes. Trends Cell Biol 13:357–365

17. Huang C-J, Wilson V, Pennings S et al (2013) Sequential effects of spadetail, one-eyed pinhead and no tail on midline convergence of nephric primordia during zebrafish embryogenesis. Dev Biol 384:290–300

18. O'Brien LL, Grimaldi M, Kostun Z et al (2011) Wt1a, Foxc1a, and the Notch mediator Rbpj physically interact and regulate the formation of podocytes in zebrafish. Dev Biol 358:318–330

19. Hsu HJ, Lin G, Chung BC (2003) Parallel early development of zebrafish interrenal glands and pronephros: differential control by wt1 and ff1b. Development 130:2107–2116

20. Kroeger PT, Wingert RA (2014) Using zebrafish to study podocyte genesis during kidney development and regeneration. Genesis 52:771–792

21. Perner B, Englert C, Bollig F (2007) The Wilms' tumor genes wt1a and wt1b control different steps during formation of the zebrafish pronephros. Dev Biol 309:87–96

22. Tomar R, Mudumana SP, Pathak N et al (2014) osr1 is required for podocyte development downstream of wt1a. J Am Soc Nephrol 25:2539–2545

23. Wingert RA, Davidson AJ (2011) Zebrafish nephrogenesis involves dynamic spatiotemporal expression changes in renal progenitors and essential signals from retinoic acid and irx3b. Dev Dyn 240:2011–2027

24. Duester G (2008) Retinoic acid synthesis and signaling during early organogenesis. Cell 134:921–931

25. Ross SA, McCaffery PJ, Drager UC et al (2000) Retinoids in embryonal development. Physiol Rev 80(3):1021–1054

26. Bollig F, Perner B, Besenbeck B et al (2009) A highly conserved retinoic acid responsive element controls wt1a expression in the zebrafish pronephros. Development 136:2883–2892

27. Davidson AJ, Ernst P, Wang Y et al (2003) cdx4 mutants fail to specify blood progenitors and can be rescued by multiple hox genes. Nature 425:300–306

28. Naylor RW, Przepiorski A, Ren Q et al (2013) HNF1β is essential for nephron segmentation during nephrogenesis. J Am Soc Nephrol 24:77–87

29. Sun Z, Hopkins N (2001) vhnf1, the MODY5 and familial GCKD-associated gene, regulates regional specification of the zebrafish gut, pronephros, and hindbrain. Genes Dev 15:3217–3229

30. Majumdar A, Lun K, Brand M et al (2000) Zebrafish no isthmus reveals a role for pax2.1 in tubule differentiation and patterning events in the pronephric primordia. Development 127:2089–2098

31. Mudumana SP, Hentschel D, Liu Y et al (2008) Odd skipped related1 reveals a novel role for endoderm in regulating kidney versus vascular cell fate. Development 135:3355–3367

32. Kim H-S, Kim MS, Hancock AL et al (2007) Identification of novel Wilms' tumor suppressor gene target genes implicated in kidney development. J Biol Chem 282:16278–16287

33. Kim MS, Yoon SK, Bollig F et al (2010) A novel Wilms' tumor 1 (WT1) target gene negatively regulates the WNT signaling pathway. J Biol Chem 285:14585–14593

34. Dong L, Pietsch S, Tan Z et al (2015) Integration of cistromic and transcriptomic analyses identifies Nphs2, Mafb, and Magi2 as Wilms' tumor 1 target genes in podocyte differentiation and maintenance. J Am Soc Nephrol 26(9):2118–2128

35. Diep CQ, Ma D, Deo RC et al (2011) Identification of adult nephron progenitors capable of kidney regeneration in zebrafish. Nature 470:95–100

36. Zhou W, Boucher RC, Bollig F et al (2010) Characterization of mesonephric development and regeneration using transgenic zebrafish. Am J Physiol Renal Physiol 299:F1040–1047

37. Kusaba T, Lalli M, Kramann R et al (2014) Differentiated kidney epithelial cells repair injured proximal tubule. Proc Natl Acad Sci U S A 111:1527–1532

38. Salice CJ, Rokous JS, Kane AS, Reimschuessel R (2001) New nephron development in goldfish (Carassius auratus) kidneys following repeated gentamicin-induced nephrotoxicosis. Comp Med 51(1):56–59

39. Haber DA, Buckler AJ, Glaser T et al (1990) An internal deletion within an 11p13 zinc finger gene contributes to the development of Wilms' tumor. Cell 61:1257–1269

40. Kobayashi A, Kwan KM, Carroll TJ et al (2005) Distinct and sequential tissue-specific activities of the LIM-class homeobox gene Lim1 for tubular morphogenesis during kidney development. Development 132:2809–2823

41. Zhou W, Hildebrandt F (2012) Inducible podocyte injury and proteinuria in transgenic zebrafish. J Am Soc Nephrol 23:1039–1047

42. Gebeshuber CA, Kornauth C, Dong L et al (2013) Focal segmental glomerulosclerosis is induced by microRNA-193a and its downregulation of WT1. Nat Med 19:481–487

43. Watanabe N, Kato M, Suzuki N et al (2009) Kidney regeneration through nephron neogenesis in medaka. Dev Growth Differ 51:135–143

44. Peralta M, Steed E, Harlepp S et al (2013) Heartbeat-driven pericardiac fluid forces contribute to epicardium morphogenesis. Curr Biol 23:1726–1735

45. Peralta M, González-Rosa JM, Marques IJ, Mercader N (2014) The epicardium in the embryonic and adult zebrafish. J Dev Biol 2: 101–116

46. Serluca FC (2008) Development of the proepicardial organ in the zebrafish. Dev Biol 315:18–27

47. Kikuchi K, Gupta V, Wang J et al (2011) tcf21+ epicardial cells adopt non-myocardial fates during zebrafish heart development and regeneration. Development 138:2895–2902

48. Poss KD, Wilson LG, Keating MT (2002) Heart regeneration in zebrafish. Science 298:2188–2190

49. Itou J, Akiyama R, Pehoski S et al (2014) Regenerative responses after mild heart injuries for cardiomyocyte proliferation in zebrafish. Dev Dyn 243:1477–1486

50. Hans S, Kaslin J, Freudenreich D et al (2009) Temporally-controlled site-specific recombination in zebrafish. PLoS One 4:e4640

Chapter 11

Immunofluorescence Staining of Wt1 on Sections of Zebrafish Embryos and Larvae

Birgit Perner and Christoph Englert

Abstract

Immunohistochemistry is one of the most powerful tools for direct visualization of distribution and localization of gene products. The presented protocol provides an opportunity to determine the localization patterns of Wt1 in zebrafish via antibody staining.

Key words Wt1, Kidney, Cryosectioning, Immunohistochemistry, Pronephros

1 Introduction

This protocol has been optimized to enable immunolabeling of Wt1-positive cells on sections of zebrafish embryos or larvae (Fig. 1). It is important to note that the Wt1 antibody is only appropriate for unfixed frozen and shortly postfixed samples. The protocol includes instructions for cryostat embedding and sectioning. To suppress pigmentation, embryos should be raised in embryo water with PTU.

2 Materials

1. Embryo water: *0.3× Danieau's* medium (30 % of 1× Danieau's medium; 1× Danieau's medium: 58 mM NaCl, 0.7 mM KCl, 0.4 mM $MgSO_4$, 0.6 mM $Ca(NO_3)_2$, 2.5 mM HEPES, do not add methylene blue.

2. Embryo water with PTU: 0.003 % 1-Phenyl-2-thiourea (PTU) in embryo water (1:100 dilution of a 0.3 % stock stored at 4 °C, which needs to be warmed to 65 °C for a while because PTU recrystallizes).

3. Tricaine solution: 0.02 % Tricaine (Ethyl 3-aminobenzoate methanesulfonate salt) in embryo water.

Nicholas Hastie (ed.), *The Wilms' Tumor (WT1) Gene: Methods and Protocols*, Methods in Molecular Biology, vol. 1467, DOI 10.1007/978-1-4939-4023-3_11, © Springer Science+Business Media New York 2016

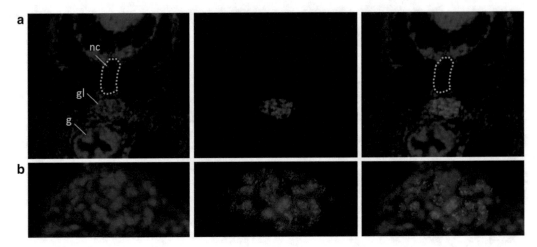

Fig. 1 Cross section of a 4-day-old zebrafish larvae labeled with a Wt1 antibody (*red*) and counterstained with Hoechst (*blue*). (**a**) Overview images (20× objective). Wt1-positive cells are detectable in the glomerular region. (**b**) Higher magnification images (40× objective) of the glomerulus. *nc* notochord, *gl* glomerulus, *g* gut

4. Infiltration mixture: 50 % Frozen section medium and 20 % sucrose in PBS.

5. Frozen section medium: Richard-Allan Scientific™ NEG 50™ (Thermo Scientific).

6. PBT: 1× PBS, 0.2 % Tween 20, pH: 7.5.

7. Blocking buffer: 2 % BSA, 10 % normal goat serum in PBT.

8. Wt1 antibody solution: Rabbit polyclonal IgG (C-19, Santa Cruz Biotech), 1:500 in blocking buffer.

9. Secondary antibody/Hoechst solution: Alexa-488 or Alexa-564 F(ab)2 fragment of goat anti-rabbit IgG (Life Technologies), 1:1000 and Hoechst stock solution, 1:1000 in blocking buffer.

10. Hoechst stock solution: 5 mg Bis-Benzimide H33258 (Sigma) in 1 ml H_2O.

11. Mounting medium: Prolong Gold Antifade Reagent (Life Technologies).

3 Methods

3.1 Processing Embryos for Cryosectioning

1. Collect embryos or larvae of desired age and anesthetize them by replacing the embryo water with tricaine solution.

2. Transfer them with a Pasteur pipette into a small dish with infiltration mixture (*see* **Note 1**).

3. Remove the remaining embryo water and infiltrate the fish for 15–30 min (*see* **Note 2**).

4. Transfer 1–5 embryos or larvae to handmade aluminum foil mold filled with frozen section medium and arrange them with a small pipette tip between top and bottom of the mold (*see* **Note 3**).

5. Freeze the mold on dry ice (*see* **Note 4**).

6. Wrap it in cling foil and transfer it to –80 °C, where it can be stored (*see* **Note 5**).

3.2 Sectioning

1. Cut 10–20 μm sections at a cryostat at –20 °C, transfer them to slides (Superfrost Plus, Thermo Scientific), and allow them to dry at RT (*see* **Note 6**).

2. Store the slides in a slide box at –80 °C until needed.

3.3 Immuno-histochemistry

1. Put the slide box on dry ice, take out only the slides you want to use, and let them dry at RT for 30 min (*see* **Note 7**).

2. Fix the sections with freshly made 4 % paraformaldehyde (PFA) in 1× PBS for 10 min at RT (*see* **Note 8**).

3. Wash five times for 5 min in PBT.

4. Incubate with blocking buffer at RT for 1 h (*see* **Note 9**).

5. Exchange to the Wt1 antibody solution.

6. Incubate the slices inside a humidified box at 4 °C overnight.

7. Wash slices five times for 5 min in PBT.

8. Apply the secondary antibody/Hoechst solution (*see* **Note 10**).

9. Incubate inside a humidified box at RT for 1 h.

10. Wash five times for 5 min in PBT.

11. Coverslip slides with 50 μl mounting medium.

12. To allow the mounting medium to cure, keep slides horizontally at 4 °C for at least 24 h.

13. Slides can be stored in a slide box at –20 ° C (*see* **Note 11**).

4 Notes

1. Try to take up the embryos or larvae with as little tricaine solution as possible.

2. Dip the fish with a small pipette tip into the infiltration mixture and remove the drop of tricaine solution from the surface of the medium with a pipette.

3. Mark one side of the mold (side lengths approximately 15×15×15 mm). Align the embryos or larvae next to each other, so that their heads are located close to the marked mold wall. To prevent that the animals are located at the edge of a section (which may cause tissue disruption) arrange the animals approximately in the middle between top and bottom of the mold. Remove air bubbles with a pipette.

4. Prepare a flat surface of dry ice. Avoid slow freezing, which would favor formation of ice crystals that harm tissue integrity.

5. Several molds can be stored together in a sealable plastic bag.

6. Stick the opposite side of the marked mold wall with frozen section medium to the sample holder that means sectioning will be performed from head to tail. Check the quality of the sections under a preparation microscope. Mark those sections you want to use for immunohistochemistry (e.g. optimal sections of the kidney region).

7. Do not freeze thawed slides again.

8. Dissolve PFA powder (Sigma) in 1× PBS, stir on a hot plate heating up for 5 min to 65–68 °C (no hotter), add 2 N NaOH until PFA solution becomes clear, and adjust to pH 7 with 2 N HCl.

9. Always use freshly prepared blocking buffer.

10. Prepare fresh blocking buffer.

11. For long-term storage seal slides with nail polish.

Chapter 12

Fluorescence-Activated Cell Sorting (FACS) Protocol for Podocyte Isolation in Adult Zebrafish

Thomas J.D. Bates, Uta Naumann, and Christoph Englert

Abstract

Zebrafish is becoming a very important model for studying human diseases. The conserved structure of the nephrons in the kidney allows the user to answer questions relating to study human kidney disorders. *Wt1a*-expressing podocytes are the most important cells within the glomeruli of adult zebrafish. In order to understand the molecular characteristics of these cells, within damage models, we have established a method for isolating them.

Key words Podocytes, Wt1a, FACS, RNA isolation, qPCR

1 Introduction

When analyzing kidney function in adult zebrafish, it is sometimes necessary to perform tissue-specific gene expression analysis. This protocol was developed to allow the isolation of GFP-positive cells from the adult zebrafish kidney (*wt1a:EGFP*) and thus gives the user the ability to obtain podocytes for RNA isolation and qPCR. Here you will find a detailed explanation of the tissue isolation, FACS sample preparation, and subsequent analysis.

2 Materials

1. Fish water: 25 l ddH$_2$O, 2.5 g sea salt, 4.95 g CaSO$_4$, 1 mg NaHCO$_3$.

2. Tricaine stock: 2.5 g Tricaine, 50 ml dH$_2$O.

3. Tricaine solution: 2 ml Tricaine stock, 250 ml fish water.

4. HBSS.

5. Sterile cell culture PBS.

6. Collagenase II (20 mg/ml).

Nicholas Hastie (ed.), *The Wilms' Tumor (WT1) Gene: Methods and Protocols*, Methods in Molecular Biology, vol. 1467, DOI 10.1007/978-1-4939-4023-3_12, © Springer Science+Business Media New York 2016

7. Dispase 4 %.

8. FACS buffer: Sterile PBS, 2 % FCS, 2 mM EDTA.

9. Fetal calf serum (FCS).

3 Methods

3.1 Kidney Isolation

1. Fish are euthanized in tricaine solution for 5 min, until the heart stops beating.

2. Firstly, remove the head, with a cut just behind the eyes (*see* **Note 1**).

3. Lay fish ventral side up, and make a cut from the cloaca towards the left gill, along the body wall. Repeat for the right side of the body.

4. Next fold ventral back towards head, taking attached organs. Remove remaining organs with fine forceps (*see* **Note 2**).

5. The zebrafish kidney adheres to the dorsal wall of the zebrafish body cavity. It is distinguishable from muscle, by its distinctive grey color. Podocytes can be visualized on a simple fluorescent microscope (Fig. 1a).

6. Kidney tissue is removed using two pairs of fine forceps (*see* **Note 3**). Starting at the most posterior region, start to remove the kidney tissue.

7. When you have isolated the whole kidney, place onto a glass petri dish (*see* **Note 4**). Using a sterile scalpel blade, macerate the kidney tissue lightly, and carefully transfer to a sterile 5 ml Eppendorf tube.

3.2 FACS Sample Preparation

1. Add 1 ml HBSS (+100 μl Collagenase) and incubate tubes for 1 h at 37 °C.

2. Place a 100 μl cell strainer on top of a sterile 50 ml Falcon tube.

3. Using a 1 ml pipette, add the whole sample (plus any remaining tissue) onto the cell strainer. Using a plunger from a 2 ml syringe, gently push any remaining tissue through the cell strainer.

4. Add 1 ml of sterile PBS to the filter, to wash the filter (*see* **Note 5**).

5. Centrifuge samples at $300 \times g$ for 5 min at 4 °C.

6. Remove supernatant, and resuspend pellet in 1 ml sterile PBS (+25 μl Collagenase II and 3 μl Dispase) and incubate tubes for 1 h at 37 °C.

7. Add 100 μl FCS to samples, to stop digestion.

8. Again, centrifuge samples at $300 \times g$ for 5 min at 4 °C.

9. Resuspend pellet in 500 μl of FACS buffer. 10 μl of cell suspension is put onto a cytometer to check the quality of population (Fig. 1b).

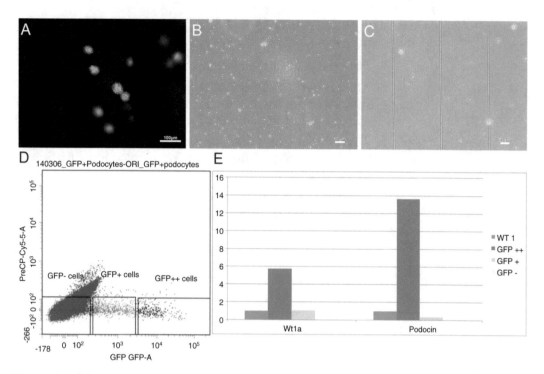

Fig. 1 FACS of Wt1a podocytes. (**a**) *wt1aE:GFP* fish exhibit a positive signal in the glomeruli of adult zebrafish. (**b**) Very few GFP+ve cells are seen when analyzing unsorted whole-kidney mass. (**c**) Following stringent FACS, a higher proportion of GFP+ve cells is achieved. (**d**) Sorting gates are shown that can distinguish cells into three groups, based upon GFP intensity. (**e**) qPCR data suggests that GFP++ are podocytes, as they express high levels of *wt1a* and *podocin*

3.3 FACS Analysis

1. Samples were sorted based on GFP fluorescence (*see* **Note 6**) using a 100 μl nozzle at 20 psi.

2. Isolated cells were checked under a normal fluorescent microscope (Fig. 1c, d), and then centrifuged at $300 \times g$ for 5 min at 4 °C.

3. Total RNA was isolated from the cells with a MagMax Total RNA Isolation kit (*see* **Note 7**), and standard qPCR (Fig. 1e) was possible after this.

4   Notes

1. After decapitation, it is best to blot any blood away. This often hinders dissection of kidney tissue.

2. This should be done delicately; if possible, one should not rip/tear organs.

3. This takes some practice, and is often initially learned using fixed tissue.

4. Place the petri dish on ice, to keep samples cool at all times.

5. There is normally an accumulation of sample on the underside that does not drip into the Falcon tube. This can be retrieved with a 1 ml pipette after the 1 ml of PBS has been added.

6. To set up the FACS machine for detecting, a GFP–ve kidney is initially analyzed. This allows for correct identification of GFP+ve cells.

7. This kit is from Ambion, but any kit that allows RNA isolation from low cell numbers should suffice.

Chapter 13

In Vitro Transcription to Study WT1 Function

Stefan G.E. Roberts

Abstract

In vitro transcription methods using mammalian nuclear extracts have been available for over 30 years and have allowed sophisticated biochemical analyses of the transcription process. This method has been extensively used to study the basic mechanisms of transcription, allowing the identification of the general transcription factors and elucidation of their mechanisms of action. Gene-specific transcriptional regulators have also been studied using in vitro transcription. This has facilitated the identification of their cofactors and provided information on their function that is invaluable to facilitate their study in a more physiological setting. Here we describe the application of in vitro transcription methods to study the mechanism of action of WT1. Coupling transcription assays with methods to purify transcription complexes, and protein affinity chromatography, has provided insights into how WT1 can both positively and negatively regulate transcription.

Key words WT1, BASP1, Transcription, Nuclear, Promoter, Histone, Affinity chromatography

1 Introduction

WT1 is a zinc-finger protein that plays a central role in development and tumorigenesis (reviewed in ref. 1). The four zinc fingers of WT1 can interact with DNA sequence elements with a consensus 5′-GCGGGGGCG-3′ and thus a major function of WT1 is to act as a transcription factor [2]. Alternative splicing of WT1 generates several isoforms and one of the alternative forms contains an additional three amino acids (KTS) between the third and fourth zinc fingers. This +KTS form of WT1 can also bind to RNA and in addition form complexes with several splicing factors (reviewed in ref. 3). Thus, WT1 likely has roles at multiple events in the gene expression process. Although there is still substantial evidence for a role for the +KTS form of WT1 in transcription, experimental analysis of transcription has traditionally focused on the −KTS WT1 isoforms.

WT1 has been shown to regulate the expression of several genes involved in cell growth, apoptosis, and differentiation (reviewed in ref. 1). WT1 can activate or repress the transcription rate of several genes and the actual outcome is dependent on both

Nicholas Hastie (ed.), *The Wilms' Tumor (WT1) Gene: Methods and Protocols*, Methods in Molecular Biology, vol. 1467,
DOI 10.1007/978-1-4939-4023-3_13, © Springer Science+Business Media New York 2016

cell type and cell context. Early studies showed that WT1 contains both transcriptional repression (R, residues 71–180) and activation (A, residues 180–245) domains [4–6], and that within the repression domain a specific region, the suppression domain (SD; residues 71–101), acts to silence the transcriptional activation domain ([7]; Fig. 1a). WT1 also contains a second transcriptional activation domain that is specific to the splice isoforms containing the 17 amino acids encoded by exon 5 ([8]; Fig. 1a).

WT1 exhibits complex transcriptional regulatory functions. Indeed, in addition to acting through its own DNA-binding

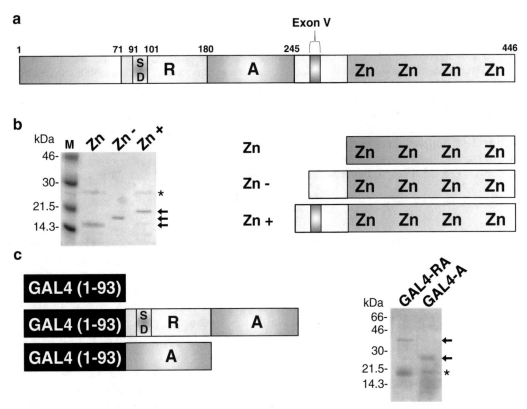

Fig. 1 Preparation of 6XHIS-tagged WT1 proteins. (**a**) Schematic of WT1. Specifically, the isoforms that lack the KTS insertion are shown for simplification. R is the transcriptional repression domain, A is the transcriptional activation domain, SD is the suppression domain. The zinc fingers are indicated (Zn). The 17-amino-acid region encoded by exon V and alternatively spliced is indicated. Amino acid numbering denotes the WT1 form that contains exon V but lacks the KTS insertion. (**b**) At right a schematic of WT1 derivatives containing the zinc finger region alone, and the zinc finger region in addition to N-terminal sequences that either lacks or contains the 17AA insertion. At left a Coomassie-stained gel is shown that contains these purified fusion proteins. *Arrows* denote the specific WT1 derivatives and contaminants are indicated by an *asterisk*. Molecular weight markers (kDa) are shown at left. These data are from Richard et al. [8]. (**c**) At left a schematic of GAL4 (residues 1–93)-WT1 fusion proteins is shown that contain the transcriptional repression (R) and transcriptional activation (A) regions. At right a Coomassie-stained gel is shown of purified GAL4-RA and GAL4-A fusion proteins. *Arrows* denote the specific WT1 derivatives and contaminants are indicated by an *asterisk*. Molecular weight markers (kDa) are shown at left. These data are from McKay et al. [7]

domain, WT1 can also be recruited to the promoter of a gene by interacting with other DNA-binding proteins, for example steroidogenic factor 1 [9] and the tumor suppressor p53 [10]. The intricate transcriptional regulatory activities, acting as either a transcriptional activator or repressor, suggest that WT1 likely also interacts with different cofactors to elicit distinct outcomes. Indeed, WT1 can interact with several other proteins to direct the final transcriptional outcome. WT1 binds to the histone acetyl transferase CBP [11] to effect acetylation of histone tails at the promoter. In contrast, when WT1 associates with the transcriptional corepressor BASP1 it can recruit histone deacetylases [12], and/or recruit the CTCF protein to modulate chromatin architecture [13]. Moreover, WT1 can act with menin and recruit the DNA methyltransferase DNMT1, which leads to modification of both histone tails and DNA through methylation [14]. Thus, the disparate transcriptional regulatory activities of WT1 can lead to multiple effects on the local environment surrounding gene promoters and ultimately in the regulation of transcriptional activity. These functions are further complicated by the multiple forms of WT1 that arise from alternative splicing which alters the WT1 interactome and results in distinct transcriptional outcomes (reviewed in ref. 1).

While the analysis of the function of transcription factors in cell culture systems yielded much information, the use of in vitro transcription methods has the potential to allow a more mechanistic analysis of function and the identification of cofactors functionally rather than through interaction alone. RNA interference and chromatin immunoprecipitation (ChIP) have greatly facilitated the analysis of transcription factors in living cells, but there are still aspects of in vitro transcription analysis that can be exploited to dissect the mechanism of action of WT1. In this chapter I will provide methods for in vitro transcription analysis and demonstrate how it can be exploited to shed light on WT1 function.

2 Materials

2.1 Nuclear Extract Preparation

1. 10× Phosphate-buffered saline (PBS): 1.37 M NaCl, 27 mM KCl, 100 mM Na_2HPO_4, 18 mM KH_2PO_4.

2. Hypotonic buffer: 10 mM N-[2-hydroxyethyl] piperazine-N'-[2-ethanesulfonic acid] (HEPES) pH 7.6, 1.5 mM $MgCl_2$, 10 mM KCl, 1 mM dithiothreitol (DTT), and 1 mM phenylmethanesulfonyl fluoride (PMSF).

3. Dounce Homogenizer (ThermoFisher Scientific, Waltham, MA).

4. Nuclear lysis buffer: 20 mM HEPES pH 7.6, 25% (v/v) glycerol, 0.42 M NaCl, 5 mM $MgCl_2$, 0.2 mM ethylenediaminetetraacetic acid (EDTA), 1 mM DTT, and 1 mM PMSF.

5. Buffer D: 20 mM HEPES pH 8, 100 mM KCl, 0.2 mM EDTA, 20% (v/v) glycerol, 0.5 mM DTT, 0.2 mM PMSF.

2.2 Preparation of His-Tagged Proteins

1. H-buffer: 20 mM Tris(hydroxymethyl)aminomethane (TRIS)–HCl pH 8.0, 1 M NaCl, 10 mM β-mercaptoethanol, 20 mM Imidazole, 10% (v/v) glycerol, 0.1% (v/v) Nonidet-P40 (NP40).

2. Misonix S-4000 Sonicator with the ¼ inch horn (Misonix, Farmingdale, NY).

3. Ni-NTA agarose (Qiagen, Valencia, CA).

4. H-buffer with imidazole: 20 mM Tris(hydroxymethyl)aminomethane (TRIS)–HCl pH 8.0, 1 M NaCl, 10 mM β-mercaptoethanol, 20 mM imidazole, 10% (v/v) glycerol, 0.1% (v/v) Nonidet-P40 (NP40), 0.3 M imidazole.

5. Buffer D: 20 mM HEPES pH 8, 100 mM KCl, 0.2 mM EDTA, 20% (v/v) glycerol, 0.5 mM DTT, 0.2 mM PMSF.

2.3 In Vitro Transcription

1. 100 mM $MgCl_2$.

2. 10 mM rNTP mix (containing 10 mM each of ATP, CTP, GTP, and UTP). Store in aliquots at –20 °C for several months.

3. Stop solution: 125 mM Tris–HCl pH 7.5, 12.5 mM EDTA, 150 mM NaCl, 1% (w/v) SDS.

4. Proteinase K (2 mg/ml in H_2O): Can be stored in aliquots for >1 year at –20 °C.

5. Phenol/chloroform (2:1 v:v).

6. 3 M Sodium acetate pH 5.2: Dissolve sodium acetate in H_2O and adjust the pH with glacial acetic acid.

7. Propan-2-ol.

8. 80% Ethanol (v/v in H_2O).

9. 5× Hybridization buffer: 0.2 M Piperazine-N,N'-bis[2-ethanesulfonic acid] (PIPES) pH 6.4, 5 mM EDTA, 2 M NaCl.

10. γ32P-ATP (3000 Ci/mmol; Perkin Elmer, Waltham, MA).

11. 0.5 M Ammonium acetate in H_2O.

12. 5× RT buffer: 250 mM Tris–HCl pH 8.3, 370 mM KCl, 20 mM $MgCl_2$.

13. 10 mM dNTP mix (10 mM each of dATP, dTTP, dCTP, and dGTP): Store in aliquots at –20 °C for several months.

14. 0.1 M DTT (in H_2O): Store in aliquots at –20 °C for several weeks.

15. AMV reverse transcriptase.

16. Loading dye: 95% (v/v) Formamide, 0.09% (w/v) bromophenol blue, and 0.09% (w/v) xylene cyanol.

17. 10% Denaturing polyacrylamide gel (20 cm×20 cm, 0.4 mm thick, gel).

2.4 Immobilized DNA Template

1. Immobilization buffer: 1 M NaCl, 10 mM Tris–HCl pH 8.0, 0.005 % (v/v) Tween.

2. Streptavidin magnetic beads (Life Technologies, Grand Island, NY).

3. Transcription buffer: 12 mM HEPES pH 8.0, 12 % (v/v) glycerol, 60 mM KCl, 0.12 mM EDTA pH 8.0, 7.5 mM $MgCl_2$, and 0.5 mM DTT.

4. Magnetic separation rack (Life Technologies, Grand Island, NY).

5. Standard SDS-PAGE protein mini-gel system.

2.5 Functional Identification of WT1 Cofactors

1. Buffer D: 20 mM HEPES pH 8, 100 mM KCl, 0.2 mM EDTA, 20 % (v/v) glycerol, 0.5 mM DTT, 0.2 mM PMSF.

2. 2 ml Disposable plastic columns (ThermoFisher Scientific, Waltham, MA).

3. Protein precipitation solution: 100 % (w/v) Trichloroacetic acid/0.4 % (w/v) sodium deoxycholate.

4. Acetone.

5. 4× SDS-PAGE loading buffer: 200 mM Tris–HCl (pH 6.8), 400 mM DTT, 8 % (w/v) SDS, 40 % (v/v) glycerol, 0.4 % (w/v) bromophenol blue.

3 Methods

3.1 Preparation of Nuclear Extracts That Are Competent for In Vitro Transcription

The standard method for the preparation of transcription-competent nuclear extracts was developed by Dignam et al. [15]. A non-adherent HeLa cell line is used to grow cells in bulk, typically yielding greater than 1 g of cells. All steps are performed with chilled buffers on ice.

1. The cells are harvested by mild centrifugation at $2300 \times g$ for 2 min. Remove the media and estimate the packed cell volume (PCV).

2. The cells are washed two consecutive times in 1× PBS to remove the remains of the growth medium. To do this, resuspend the cells in 20× PCV of 1× PBS, fully (but gently) dispersing the cells, then centrifuge at $2300 \times g$ for 20 min, and discard the supernatant. Repeat.

3. The cells are resuspended in 5× packed cell volumes (PCV) of hypotonic buffer. The cells are left to swell on ice for 20 min and then harvested at $2000 \times g$ for 10 min.

4. The swollen cells are resuspended in 2× PCV of hypotonic buffer and transferred to a Dounce homogenizer. After five strokes in the Dounce homogenizer using the tight pestle the disrupted cells are immediately centrifuged at $2300 \times g$ for 10 min (see **Note 1**).

5. The upper cytoplasmic layer is discarded (but can also be used for other purposes). The nuclear pellet is resuspended in 1.5 volumes of nuclear lysis buffer. Use a pipette tip with the end clipped to widen the bore and take care not to cause frothing (*see* **Note 2**). The tube is placed on a rocker at 4 °C for 30 min.

6. Remove the nuclear debris by centrifugation at $16,000 \times g$, 4 °C, for 30 min. The supernatant is then dialyzed against two changes of Buffer D over 3 h.

7. The nuclear extract is then centrifuged at $16,000 \times g$, 4 °C, for 30 min to remove any precipitate that has formed during dialysis. Aliquot and store at –80 °C. Nuclear extracts can be stored at –80 °C for several months without losing significant activity. After removing from the –80 °C freezer, the nuclear extract should be centrifuged at $16,000 \times g$ for 20 min before use (*see* **Note 3**).

The above protocol is useful for large-scale preparation of nuclear extracts, but frequently it is either necessary or convenient to prepare nuclear extracts from cells grown on a smaller scale. For preparation of nuclear extracts from smaller volumes of non-adherent cells, or adherent cells grown on tissue culture plates, a modified method can be employed [16].

1. After harvesting the cells and washing them in PBS twice to remove the culture medium the cells are resuspended in 1× PCV of hypotonic buffer, transferred to a microtube, and placed on ice for 15 min.

2. Pre-wash a 1 ml syringe with hypotonic buffer and then draw the suspended cells into the syringe. Place a 23 Gauge needle onto the syringe and force the cells through the needle into a microtube. Draw the cells back into the syringe and repeat a further four times. Then, immediately microfuge the cells at $15,000 \times g$ for 20 s (*see* **Note 1**).

3. Discard the supernatant and resuspend the nuclear pellet in 2/3 PCV of nuclear lysis buffer. The method then follows the remainder of the method for large-scale preparations.

For transcriptional competence it is important to obtain nuclear extracts with a high protein concentration. Routinely we aim for 10 mg/ml, but we have been able to obtain transcription signals with extracts as low as 1 mg/ml protein concentration.

3.2 Preparation of Recombinant WT1 Proteins

Full-length WT1 proteins have proved difficult to produce. One way around this problem has been to produce sections of WT1 either alone or as fusion proteins. We took an approach to prepare histidine-tagged WT1 derivatives that lack regions at the N-terminus of WT1 [7]. Several vectors are available commercially to produce histidine-tagged proteins that can be rapidly purified using nickel-agarose beads. The N-terminal region of WT1 is largely responsible for difficulties in purifying the intact protein or fragments. However, the C-terminal region does not pose significant problems and purification of WT1 derivatives composed of C-terminal regions is straightforward. For example, we have previously purified WT1 sections encompassing the C-terminal region that either lack or contain the 17 additional amino acids encoded by exon 5 that are present only in specific isoforms of WT1 ([8]; Fig. 1b). These derivatives contain the zinc finger region of WT1 (and thus possess intrinsic DNA-binding activity) in addition to more central regions of the protein which harbor transcriptional regulatory function.

The N-terminal region of WT1 is more problematic in purification from *E. coli*, but the solubility can be enhanced by generating fusion proteins. For example, we have purified 6XHIS-tagged GAL4 (1-93)-fusion proteins that contain the repression (R) and activation (A) regions of WT1 (Fig. 1c). The study of GAL4-fusion proteins that contain the transcriptional regulatory regions of WT1 can facilitate mechanistic studies of the function of specific motifs. Although such studies are highly derivatized, subsequent experiments using full-length WT1 in cells can then be used to validate the results. The 6XHIS-tagged WT1 proteins (both native and GAL4-fusion) were purified by Nickel-NTA affinity chromatography using a method based on Reece et al. [17]. The protocol uses a 1 l culture of bacteria in which expression of the His-tagged protein has been induced. Intact WT1 and GAL4 are zinc-finger proteins and thus it is important to induce protein synthesis after the addition of $ZnCl_2$ to the growth media to a final concentration of 100 μM. Solubility of the proteins is also aided by limiting the production using short induction times (typically 2 h) at 30 °C.

1. Resuspend the *E. coli* pellet in 10 ml of H-buffer. Ensure that the bacteria are fully resuspended with no clumps and then sonicate the suspended bacteria to rupture the cells (*see* **Note 4**). We use a Misonix S-4000 with the ¼ in. horn with a medium setting, using 6×30 s sonication procedure (*see* **Note 5**). The cell debris are then pelleted at $16,000 \times g$ for 20 min.

2. The supernatant which contains the soluble proteins from the *E. coli* is transferred to a fresh tube. Add 0.5 ml Ni-NTA-agarose (preequilibrated in H-buffer). Place the sample on a rocking table at 4 °C for 30 min to allow the His-tagged protein to bind to the Ni-NTA agarose.

3. Collect the Ni-NTA agarose by centrifugation at $1000 \times g$ for 1 min. Wash briefly with 12 ml of H-buffer and collect the beads as above. Wash for 10 min in H-buffer at 4 °C. Repeat.

4. Load the Ni-NTA agarose into a small disposable column (*see* **Note 6**). Wash the column with 10 ml H-buffer.

5. Elute the His-tagged protein in 2 ml of H-buffer containing 0.3 M imidazole (*see* **Note 7**).

6. The eluted protein is dialyzed into 1 l of buffer D to remove the imidazole. The purified protein is aliquoted and can be stored at −80 °C for over 1 year.

3.3 *In Vitro Transcription Method Using Primer Extension*

In vitro transcription methods involve incubating nuclear extract with a DNA template containing a promoter sequence and ribonucleotides, followed by analysis of the transcripts that are produced. Detection of transcripts can be achieved either by using radioactive UTP in the transcription reaction or by using a ^{32}P-labeled primer and primer extension to detect the transcripts. We have employed the latter technique because the reaction conditions are less complex and it also provides the additional benefit of transcription start site mapping [18, 19].

1. A typical in vitro transcription reaction contains

   25 μl nuclear extract (optimally at a concentration of 10 mg/ml)

   3 μl 100 mM $MgCl_2$

   1 μl DNA template (200 ng)

   3 μl rNTP mix (containing 10 mM each of ATP, CTP, GTP, and UTP)

   8 μl H_2O

   Further proteins can be added to the reaction (for example, activators or repressors), reducing the water accordingly (*see* **Note 8**).

2. The transcription reaction is incubated at 30 °C for 1 h. 160 μl of stop solution is then added and then 5 μl of 2 mg/ml Proteinase K. Place the reaction at 55 °C for 15 min.

3. Add 60 μl of phenol/chloroform (2:1), briefly vortex, and microfuge at 15,000g for 5 min. Keep the supernatant (*see* **Note 9**).

4. Add 60 μl of chloroform, briefly vortex, and then microfuge at 15,000g for 3 min.

5. The final supernatant is added to 10 μl of 3 M sodium acetate pH 5.2 and then 200 μl of propan-2-ol. Vortex briefly, then incubate on dry ice or in the −80 °C freezer for 10 min, and collect the nucleic acid pellet in a microfuge at 15,000g for 10 min.

6. Wash the pellet with 100 μl of 80 % ethanol. Allow the pellet to air-dry for 2 min.

7. The nucleic acid pellet is resuspended in 20 μl of 1× hybridization buffer. 2 ng of ^{32}P-labeled primer is added. Annealing of the primer to the RNA is performed at 37 °C overnight (*see* **Note 10**).

8. 160 μl of 0.5 M ammonium acetate is added and then 200 μl of propan-2-ol. Vortex briefly and then incubate on dry ice (or at –80 °C) for 10 min to precipitate the nucleic acid. Collect the precipitate in the microfuge at 15,000g for 10 min.

9. Wash the pellet in 80% ethanol and then air-dry. The pellet is resuspended in 6 μl of nuclease-free H_2O, 2 μl of 5xRT buffer, 1 μl of dNTPs (containing 10 mM each of dATP, dCTP, dTTP, dGTP), 1 μl of 0.1 M DTT, and 1 μl (1 unit) of AMV reverse transcriptase. Place the reaction at 42 °C for 1 h to allow primer extension to take place.

10. Add 10 μl of loading dye. Heat the samples at 95 °C for 2 min and resolve on a 10% denaturing polyacrylamide gel (we typically use a 20 cm×20 cm, 0.4 mm thick, gel). Run the bromophenol blue 2/3 of the way along the gel and this will retain the unincorporated oligonucleotide on the gel, sufficiently spaced from the reverse-transcribed products. After drying the gel, the ^{32}P-labeled products are visualized by autoradiography or phosphorimaging.

3.4   Transcriptional Regulation by WT1 In Vitro

The DNA template used in the in vitro transcription assays needs to contain a promoter region that encompasses a transcriptional start site that is recognized by RNA polymerase II and the general transcription factors. Frequently, viral promoters are used because of the robust signals that are generated in transcription assays, but we have found that cellular promoters can also be effectively used in such assays [19, 20]. The adenovirus E4 (AdE4) promoter contains a functional TATA motif and initiator sequence and functions robustly in in vitro transcription, producing two distinct clusters of transcripts generated from tandem initiation sites [19]. Figure 2a shows a schematic of the AdE4 core promoter linked to a group of five GAL4 DNA recognition sites (G5E4T). Multiple GAL4 sites will facilitate the binding of several transcriptional activator proteins to produce the synergy required for robust transcriptional activation [21]. The transcript from this DNA template will ultimately be analyzed using a specific primer that will anneal to the RNA and correspond to approximately 40 bases downstream of the transcription initiator.

Incubation of the G5E4T template with HeLa cell nuclear extract as outlined above produces a low level of transcription (Fig. 2b). When GAL4 protein is included in the reaction, transcription initiated from the AdE4 promoter is unchanged. GAL4 (residues 1–93) is able to dimerize and bind to a consensus GAL4 DNA-binding sequence, but it lacks any domains that can regulate transcription. A GAL4 fusion protein that contains both the repression and activation domains of WT1 (GAL4-RA) was also unable to elicit a transcriptional response at the G5E4T DNA template [7]. In contrast, a GAL4-fusion protein containing the WT1 activation domain alone

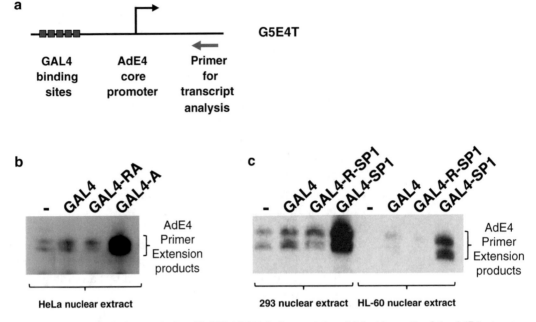

Fig. 2 In vitro transcription analysis with GAL4-WT1 fusion proteins. (**a**) A schematic of the AdE4 core promoter linked to five GAL4 DNA-binding sites (G5E4T). The *red arrow* indicates the site containing the sequence recognized by the primer used to perform primer extension analysis. (**b**) Section of a gel to analyze E4 transcripts. In vitro transcription assays were performed with the G5E4T DNA template, HeLa nuclear extract, and the GAL4 derivatives indicated (and shown in Fig. 1c). E4 transcripts form a doublet. These data are from McKay et al. [7]. (**c**) Section of a gel to analyze E4 transcripts. In vitro transcription assays were performed with the G5E4T DNA template. Nuclear extract prepared from either HEK293 or HL-60 cells was used in in vitro transcription with a GAL4, a GAL4-fusion protein containing GAL4 (1-93) linked to the WT1 repression domain linked to the SP1 transcriptional activation domain, or a GAL4-fusion protein linked to the SP1 transcriptional activation domain

(GAL4-A) was able to stimulate transcription of the G5E4T template. Thus, even though GAL4-RA contains a transcriptional activation domain, it is unable to elicit transcriptional activation. This is due to an inhibitory effect of the repression (R) domain. Indeed, the WT1 repression domain has the capacity to inhibit a heterologous transcriptional activation domain [7, 22]. In Fig. 2c we show transcription assays performed with the G5E4T DNA template in nuclear extracts prepared from two different cell types (human embryonic kidney 293 cells and leukemic HL-60 cells). These nuclear extracts were prepared using the small-scale method as described above. While a GAL4-fusion protein containing the SP1 transcriptional activation domain (GAL4-SP1) is able to stimulate transcription, when the WT1 repression domain (R) is fused to the SP1 activation domain (GAL4-R-SP1), the activity of the SP1 activation domain is repressed. These data, in combination with others, led to the proposal that the WT1 repression domain acts to suppress transcriptional activation by recruiting a transcriptional corepressor [6, 7, 22].

The above analysis of WT1 transcription function employed a GAL4-fusion approach to overcome solubility problems with the WT1 N-terminal regions when proteins are prepared from *E. coli*. We have also studied WT1 derivatives that contain the WT1 DNA-binding region and also segments of the transcriptional regulatory domains of WT1 ([8]; Fig. 1b). For these experiments, the GAL4 DNA-binding sites in the G5E4T DNA template were replaced with five consensus WT1 recognition elements (5′-GCGGGGGCG-3′) to produce W5E4T. While mammalian extracts do not contain any DNA-binding proteins that recognize the GAL4 DNA-binding site, there are several mammalian factors that recognize a DNA-binding site similar to that bound by WT1. Thus, transcription assays comparing the baseline activity of G5E4T and W5E4T DNA templates in a HeLa cell nuclear extract show that W5E4T has a high transcriptional activity (Fig. 3a). HeLa cells do not contain detectable WT1 and so the high activity of W5E4T in HeLa nuclear extract is likely due to other transcriptional activators that can bind to the WT1 recognition motif. This high activity will interfere with analysis and we therefore took the approach to remove these factors from the HeLa nuclear extract by fractionation over a column containing immobilized DNA motifs of the WT1 site. These extracts were devoid of high baseline activity. Using the fractionated HeLa nuclear extract it is now possible to analyze the transcriptional activity of WT1 derivatives that contain the natural WT1 DNA-binding region. Such studies allowed the identification of a second transcriptional activation domain that requires the 17AA encoded by exon V of the WT1 gene (compare WT1 Zn+ and WT1 Zn– that contain and lack the 17AA, respectively; [8]; Fig. 3b).

3.5 Purification of Transcription Complexes

In vitro transcription measures RNA production from a promoter construct. This functional measure is useful to assess the effect of proteins on transcription rate. It is also possible to explore some of the underlying mechanisms that are involved in the transcription changes. This is achieved by purifying the transcription complexes and requires the immobilization of the promoter DNA template [23–25]. The promoter region and regulatory sites of G5E4T or W5E4T (or other promoters) are amplified by PCR in which one of the primers is biotinylated at the 5′ end. Such primers are commercially available from several sources. The biotinylated DNA fragment can then be attached via the biotin moiety to streptavidin-coated beads as follows:

1. Incubate the biotinylated DNA with magnetic beads in 1 ml of immobilization buffer for 2 h at room temperature. Use 0.08 pmol of promoter DNA per 2 μl of magnetic streptavidin beads (*see* **Note 11**).

2. Wash the beads three times in immobilization buffer by placing the tube in a magnetic rack, allowing the beads to collect

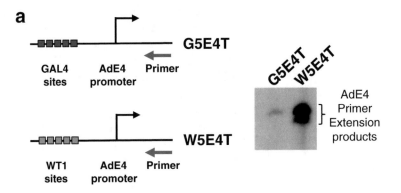

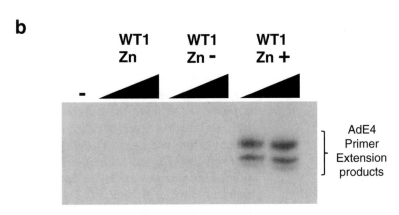

Fig. 3 Analysis of transcriptional regulation by WT1 derivatives. (**a**) At left, a schematic of the G5E4T DNA template (as shown in Fig. 2a), and the same DNA template in which the five GAL4 DNA-binding sites have been replaced with five WT1 DNA-binding sites (W5E4T). At right, an in vitro transcription reaction was performed with G5E4T and W5E4T DNA templates and HeLa cell nuclear extracts. These data are from Richard et al. [8]. (**b**) An in vitro transcription reaction using HeLa cell nuclear extract that had first been depleted of factors that interact with the WT1 DNA-recognition site. The assays contained 6XHIS-tagged WT1 proteins as indicated and also shown schematically in Fig. 1b. AdE4 extension products are indicated. These data are from Richard et al. [8]

and aspirating the supernatant (*see* **Note 11**). Resuspend the beads in fresh immobilization buffer by gentle pipetting.

3. After the final wash, resuspend the beads in 1× PBS such that 2 μl of the solution contains approximately 0.08 pmol of DNA fragment (*see* **Note 12**).

4. To form transcription complexes assemble the following components:

25 μl Nuclear extract (optimally at a concentration of 10 mg/ml)

3 μl 100 mM $MgCl_2$

2 μl Magnetic bead/DNA template

10 μl H_2O

5. Incubate at 30 °C for 1 h, keeping the beads in suspension by gentle pipetting every 10 min.

6. Add 1 ml of transcription buffer containing 0.0003 % NP40 (*see* **Note 13**). The beads are then harvested using a magnetic rack.

7. Wash the beads three times in 1 ml of transcription buffer containing 0.0003 % NP40.

8. Resuspend the beads containing purified complexes in 40 μl of transcription buffer.

Such purified transcription complexes are functional, and will undergo transcription when rNTPs are added. Alternatively, the purified complexes can be resolved by SDS-PAGE and immunoblotted to detect the level of specific factors and therefore monitor their recruitment to the promoter.

Figure 4 shows an immunoblot of purified transcriptional complexes formed on an immobilized promoter DNA template in the absence or presence of a transcriptional activator protein. The purified complexes were immunoblotted with antibodies against the TBP subunit of TFIID, TFIIB, or RNA polymerase II. The data show that the activator protein stimulates the recruitment of TFIIB and RNA polymerase II, but has only a modest effect on TFIID recruitment. Analysis of complexes in this way can yield valuable information on the effects of transcriptional regulators on the recruitment of other factors to the promoter and therefore on their mechanism of action. Indeed, the transcriptional activation function of WT1 has been associated with both TFIID [8] and TFIIB [7], suggesting a role in their recruitment to the promoter during the stimulation of transcription.

3.6 Functional Identification of WT1 Cofactors

In vitro transcription assays coupled with analysis in cells allows the identification of the domains within a transcription factor that play a role in regulating the transcription machinery. Using these methods, we identified a discrete region of WT1 (residues 71–101) that is responsible for inhibiting the transcriptional activation domain [7]. We termed this region of WT1 the suppression domain (SD), because it specifically suppressed transcriptional activation domains rather than directly repressing the RNA polymerase II complex. Site-directed mutagenesis of the WT1 suppression domain coupled with in vitro transcription assays identified key phenylalanine residues (F92 and F100) that are critical to mediate inhibition of a transcriptional activation domain [22]. Due to the mechanism of action it was most likely that the suppression domain functioned by interacting with a nuclear protein to mediate its effects.

Protein affinity chromatography coupled with SDS-PAGE and protein stains can be used to identify interaction partners for a protein of interest. The availability of mutant-derivative proteins can provide a correlation between the ability of a protein to bind and a functional effect that is affected by the mutation. In addition, protein affinity

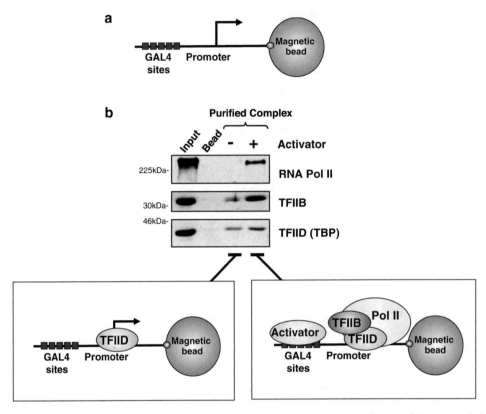

Fig. 4 Experiments with immobilized DNA templates can be used to analyze recruitment of the transcriptional machinery. (**a**) A promoter DNA template is immobilized onto streptavidin-coated magnetic beads via a biotin moiety. The beads can then be incubated with nuclear extract, and then washed to remove unbound factors. (**b**) The content of the complexes is analyzed here by immunoblotting against candidate factors. Magnetic beads containing nonspecific DNA is used as a control (bead). Example immunoblots are shown exploring the effect of an activator protein (GAL4) in the recruitment of RNA polymerase II (pol II), TFIIB, and TFIID (through the TBP subunit) to the promoter. Below the autoradiograms the content of the complexes is shown diagrammatically

chromatography can be used to specifically deplete factors from a nuclear extract that can then be tested in transcription analysis to determine if depletion of such factors has an effect on transcription.

We used protein affinity chromatography to analyze the WT1 suppression domain [22]. Large-scale preparation of GST or GST linked to the WT1 suppression domain (residues 71–101) allowed the assembly of affinity columns containing 2 mg of purified protein linked to 1 ml of glutathione agarose (Fig. 5). In addition we produced a GST fusion protein containing a WT1 suppression domain in which the phenylalanine residues at positions 92 and 100 were substituted with alanine (F92A/F100A). Immobilized GST-fusion proteins were prepared as described [18]. In vitro transcription assays had demonstrated that F92A/F100A mutations rendered the suppression domain as nonfunctional [22]. Nuclear proteins that interact with the WT1 suppression domain were identified as follows;

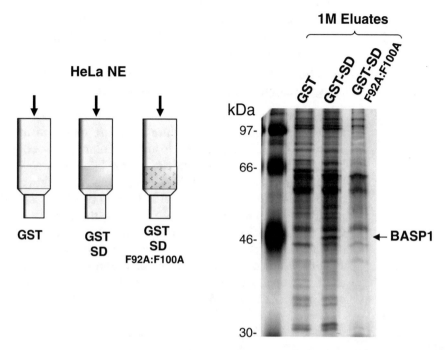

Fig. 5 Identification of WT1 cofactors by protein affinity chromatography. GST, GST-SD (containing the suppression domain of WT1, residues 71–101), and GST-SD F92A:F100A (containing residues 71–101 with F92A and F100A substitutions) were prepared from *E. coli* and retained as GST-fusion proteins bound to glutathione agarose. The glutathione agarose containing the fusion proteins was used to prepare affinity columns. 100 mg of HeLa nuclear proteins was fractionated over each column, and then the columns were washed with 20 column volumes of Buffer D. The stably bound proteins were eluted with Buffer D containing 1 M KCl. After precipitation of the proteins, they were resolved by SDS-PAGE and the gel was subjected to silver stain. The GST-SD, but not GST-SD F92A:F100A, column showed that a 50 kDa protein specifically interacted with the wild-type functional repression domain but not the F92A:F100A mutant derivative. This 50 kDa protein was subsequently identified as BASP1 [22, 26]

1. HeLa nuclear extract prepared as described in Subheading 3.1 is fractionated over the columns. The flow through is re-applied three times to allow the columns to capture as much interacting proteins as possible.

2. Wash the column with 20 column volumes of Buffer D.

3. Elute stably bound proteins with 3 ml Buffer D containing 1 M KCl.

4. The eluted proteins are then precipitated by adding 0.25 volumes of a solution containing 100% (w/v) trichloroacetic acid/0.4% (w/v) sodium deoxycholate. Briefly vortex and place on ice for 15 min.

5. Collect the precipitated proteins by microfuge at 15,000g for 15 min.

6. Add 1 ml of acetone, vortex, and microfuge at 15,000g for 5 min.

7. After removing the acetone by pipetting the pellet is then dried under vacuum for 5 min and resuspended in SDS-PAGE loading dye (*see* **Note 14**).

8. The proteins were resolved by standard SDS-PAGE and the gel was silver-stained using a commercially available kit.

Eluates from all three columns contain a number of proteins that were retained by the column and are common in all three samples (Fig. 5). The eluate from the column that contains the functional WT1 suppression domain (GST-SD) contains a specific band of approximately 50 kDa that later analysis was revealed to be brain acid-soluble protein 1 (BASP1). The band corresponding to BASP1 is not present in the eluate from the column containing GST-SD F92A:F100A, providing a functional link between the interaction of the WT1 suppression domain with BASP1. This analysis coupled with in vitro transcription methodology allowed the functional identification of BASP1 as a transcriptional corepressor of WT1 [22, 26].

4 Notes

1. It is critical that centrifugation is performed immediately after the homogenization because the nuclei will leak essential proteins.

2. Frothing will denature the nuclear proteins and reduce the activity of the nuclear extract in transcription.

3. This is important because each time the nuclear extract is thawed, precipitate will form and this will interfere with subsequent experiments.

4. A French Press can also be used to disrupt the *E. coli*.

5. It is important to leave sufficient gaps between each 30-s pulse to ensure that the sample does not become warm. This could denature the proteins.

6. We use Pierce scientific 2 ml disposable columns. The kits for these columns also provide a reservoir to facilitate the washes.

7. We find it helpful for the release of the His-tagged protein to cap the column after 1 ml has flowed through, then wait for 5 min, and continue the elution. If the column has a high flow rate, this step will help to ensure optimal elution of the His-tagged protein.

8. Ensure that the water used is ultrapure and guaranteed free of nuclease and protease activity.

9. There is usually considerable material at the interface, so be careful to avoid it.

10. These conditions facilitate priming of the RNA specifically and do not allow annealing of the primer to the DNA template.

11. Alternatively, streptavidin agarose beads can be used. If an agarose bead is used then collect the beads by allowing them to settle to the bottom of the tube.

12. The beads containing immobilized DNA can be stored at 4 °C for several days.

13. The low level of NP40 is sufficient to prevent coagulation of the beads but does not inhibit transcription.

14. Generally it is necessary to add 1–3 μl of 1 M Tris–HCl (pH 8) to neutralize the acidity of the sample.

Acknowledgements

Work in the author's laboratory is supported by the BBSRC (BB/K000446/1), and MRC (MR/K001027/1). I would like to thank Brian Carpenter, Derek Richard, and Yuming Wang for providing the data that are included in this work.

References

1. Toska E, Roberts SGE (2014) Mechanisms of transcriptional regulation by WT1 (Wilms' tumour 1). Biochem J 461:15–32

2. Nakagama H, Heinrich G, Pelletier J et al (1995) Sequence and structural requirements for high-affinity DNA binding by the WT1 gene product. Mol Cell Biol 15:1489–1498

3. Davies R, Moore A, Schedl A et al (1999) Multiple roles for the Wilms' tumor suppressor, WT1. Cancer Res 59:1747s–1750s

4. Wang ZY, Qiu QQ, Deuel TF (1993) The Wilms' tumor gene product WT1 activates or suppresses transcription through separate functional domains. J Biol Chem 268:9172–9175

5. Madden SL, Cook DM, Rauscher FJ 3rd (1993) A structure-function analysis of transcriptional repression mediated by the WT1, Wilms' tumor suppressor protein. Oncogene 8:1713–1720

6. Wang ZY, Qiu QQ, Gurrieri M et al (1995) WT1, the Wilms' tumor suppressor gene product, represses transcription through an interactive nuclear protein. Oncogene 10:1243–1247

7. McKay LM, Carpenter B, Roberts SGE (1999) Regulation of the Wilms' tumour suppressor protein transcriptional activation domain. Oncogene 18:6546–6554

8. Richard DJ, Schumacher V, Royer-Pokora B et al (2001) Par 4 is a coactivator for a splice-isoform specific transcriptional activation domain in WT1. Genes Dev 15:328–339

9. Nachtigal MW, Hirokawa Y, Enyeart-VanHouten DL et al (1998) Wilms' tumor 1 and Dax-1 modulate the orphan nuclear receptor SF-1 in sex-specific gene expression. Cell 93:445–454

10. Maheswaran S, Park S, Bernard A et al (1993) Physical and functional interaction between WT1 and p53 proteins. Proc Natl Acad Sci U S A 90:5100–5104

11. Wang W, Lee SB, Palmer R et al (2001) A functional interaction with CBP contributes to transcriptional activation by the Wilms' tumor suppressor WT1. J Biol Chem 276:16810–16816

12. Toska E, Campbell HA, Shandilya J et al (2012) Repression of transcription by WT1-BASP1 requires the myristoylation of BASP1 and the PIP2-dependent recruitment of histone deacetylase. Cell Rep 2:462–469

13. Essafi A, Webb A, Berry RL et al (2011) A Wt1-controlled chromatin switching mechanism underpins tissue-specific wnt4 activation and repression. Dev Cell 21:559–574

14. Xu B, Zeng DQ, Wu Y et al (2011) Tumor suppressor menin represses paired box gene 2 expression via Wilms' tumor suppressor protein–polycomb group complex. J Biol Chem 286:13937–13944

15. Dignam JD, Lebovitz RM, Roeder RG (1983) Accurate transcription initiation by RNA polymerase II in a soluble extract from isolated mammalian nuclei. Nucleic Acids Res 11:1475–1489

16. Lee KA, Bindereif A, Green MR (1988) A small-scale procedure for preparation of nuclear extracts that support efficient transcription and pre-mRNA splicing. Gene Anal Tech 5:22–31

17. Reece RJ, Rickles RJ, Ptashne M (1993) Overproduction and single-step purification of GAL4 fusion proteins from Escherichia coli. Gene 126:105–107

18. Lin YS, Green MR (1991) Mechanism of action of an acidic transcriptional activator in vitro. Cell 64:971–981

19. Fairley JA, Evans R, Hawkes NA et al (2002) Core promoter-dependent TFIIB conformation and a role for TFIIB conformation in transcription start site selection. Mol Cell Biol 22:6697–6705

20. Deng W, Roberts SGE (2005) A core promoter element downstream of the TATA box that is recognized by TFIIB. Genes Dev 19:2418–2423

21. Lin YS, Carey MF, Ptashne M et al (1988) GAL4 derivatives function alone and synergistically with mammalian activators in vitro. Cell 54:659–664

22. Carpenter B, Hill KJ, Charalambous M et al (2004) BASP1 is a transcriptional cosuppressor for the Wilms' tumor suppressor protein WT1. Mol Cell Biol 24:537–549

23. Choy B, Green MR (1993) Eukaryotic activators function during multiple steps of preinitiation complex assembly. Nature 366:531–536

24. Roberts SGE, Choy B, Walker SS et al (1995) A role for activator-mediated TFIIB recruitment in diverse aspects of transcriptional regulation. Curr Biol 5:508–516

25. Roberts SGE, Green MR (1996) Purification and analysis of functional preinitiation complexes. Methods Enzymol 273:110–118

26. Green LM, Wagner KJ, Campbell HA et al (2009) Dynamic interaction between WT1 and BASP1 in transcriptional regulation during differentiation. Nucleic Acids Res 37:431–440

Chapter 14

Measuring Equilibrium Binding Constants for the WT1-DNA Interaction Using a Filter Binding Assay

Paul J. Romaniuk

Abstract

Equilibrium binding of WT1 to specific sites in DNA and potentially RNA molecules is central in mediating the regulatory roles of this protein. In order to understand the functional effects of mutations in the nucleic acid-binding domain of WT1 proteins and/or mutations in the DNA- or RNA-binding sites, it is necessary to measure the equilibrium constant for formation of the protein-nucleic acid complex. This chapter describes the use of a filter binding assay to make accurate measurements of the binding of the WT1 zinc finger domain to the consensus WT1-binding site in DNA. The method described is readily adapted to the measurement of the effects of mutations in either the WT1 zinc finger domain or the putative binding sites within a promoter element or cellular RNA.

Key words WT1, Protein-nucleic acid interactions, Equilibrium binding, Filter binding assay, Zinc finger protein, DNA-protein, RNA-protein

1 Introduction

Many of the proteins that regulate gene expression at the level of transcription or pre-mRNA processing do so by forming a specific protein-nucleic acid complex *via* a bimolecular equilibrium. Being able to accurately measure the equilibrium binding constants for such interactions is key to understanding normal and disrupted functions of these proteins. For example, determining accurate equilibrium binding constants can help explain how up- and down-regulation by overlapping regulatory proteins takes place, how mutations in the nucleic acid-binding domain of these proteins increases or decreases their ability to regulate gene expression, how alternative splicing that creates isoforms of the nucleic acid-binding domain influences DNA/RNA target selection and affinities, and finally how the affinities for different targets relate to functional outcome. All of these examples are relevant to the WT1 protein: it potentially competes with EGR-1 for the same binding site within promoters [1–5]; Denys-Drash syndrome mutations map to the

Nicholas Hastie (ed.), *The Wilms' Tumor (WT1) Gene: Methods and Protocols*, Methods in Molecular Biology, vol. 1467,
DOI 10.1007/978-1-4939-4023-3_14, © Springer Science+Business Media New York 2016

zinc finger domain of WT1 as does the WILMS3 mutation [6, 7]; one alternative splicing event inserts three additional amino acids (+KTS) between zinc fingers 3 and 4 [2, 8, 9]; while the –KTS isoforms of WT1 appear to execute the major DNA binding and transcriptional activity of WT1, the +KTS isoforms associate with splicing complexes and are more implicated in posttranscriptional processes [10–14].

While there are many optical and thermal methods for determining equilibrium binding constants for protein-ligand interactions, they are unsuitable for protein-nucleic acid interactions because of their inability to measure the high association constants typical of these interactions. Traditionally, two methods that utilize isotopically labeled nucleic acids are used to determine the fraction of complex formed between the nucleic acid ligand and the interacting protein. One of these methods is the gel mobility shift assay and the other is the filter binding assay [15, 16].

Precisely measuring the equilibrium binding constants of proteins to nucleic acid ligands involves titrating a constant amount of DNA/RNA with an increasing concentration of protein in individual assay tubes (the assay can also be done by holding protein concentration constant and titrating it with increasing concentrations of ligand). The concentration-dependent fraction of ligand bound can then be used to determine the association constant (K_a) and its inverse, the dissociation constant (K_d), as illustrated in Fig. 1. Assays that use only a single protein concentration to compare DNA-protein interactions are far less precise, as indicated in Fig. 1.

Determining a K_a requires a way to separate bound and unbound DNA and quantify the amount of each. Although this separation and quantification can be readily accomplished by gel electrophoresis (gel mobility shift assay), each K_a measurement requires a gel making the process slow and tedious. The filter binding assay is in some ways more convenient and allows for higher throughput in determining K_a values compared to the gel mobility shift assay. This is helpful when comparing a number of parameters of a protein-nucleic acid interaction. The assay mixture is filtered through a stack of two filters: a nitrocellulose filter on top of either a nylon or DEAE-cellulose filter. As the assay mixture passes through the nitrocellulose filter, all of the protein, including protein that has formed complexes with the DNA/RNA, binds to the nitrocellulose. Free DNA/RNA passing through the nitrocellulose filter is then bound by the nylon filter underneath [17]. The fraction of DNA/RNA bound is the amount trapped by the nitrocellulose (bound DNA/RNA) divided by the sum of the radioactivity bound to both filters (total DNA/RNA). Certain testable assumptions must be made to use the data obtained by the filter binding assay to calculate the K_a of the protein-nucleic acid interaction [18]. In the application of the filter binding method to the study of the DNA and RNA binding properties of WT1, these assumptions have been rigorously tested and found to be sound.

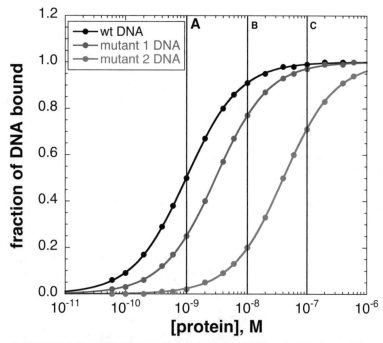

	wild type		mutant 1		mutant 2	
[protein], M	% bound	% wt	% bound	% wt	% bound	%wt
A: 10^{-9}	0.50	–	0.25	0.50	0.02	0.04
B: 10^{-8}	0.91	–	0.77	0.85	0.20	0.22
C: 10^{-7}	0.99	–	0.97	0.98	0.71	0.72

wild type		mutant 1		mutant 2	
K_a, M^{-1}	% wt	K_a, M^{-1}	% wt	K_a, M^{-1}	% wt
1.0×10^{9}	–	3.3×10^{8}	0.33	2.5×10^{7}	0.03

Fig. 1 Equilibrium protein-DNA binding curves for a wild-type DNA site and two mutant sites with reduced affinity for the protein. The *horizontal lines A*, *B*, and *C* demonstrate the fraction of DNA bound for each site at one specific protein concentration. The curves are fit to the data using the equation for a simple bimolecular equilibrium (*see* Fig. 7), generating the K_a values shown in the *bottom* table. The table immediately below the *graph* shows the data that would be obtained from single-point assays using each of the indicated protein concentrations. Comparing the data in the two tables illustrates that the relative affinities of each DNA site calculated from a single-point assay vary depending upon the concentration of protein used, and are not indicative of the actual relative affinities calculated from the true K_a values

Use of this methodology to study the nucleic acid binding properties of the WT1 protein has yielded a wealth of insight, for example, the demonstration of overlapping and unique regulatory sites for WT1 and EGR1 [3]; the contribution of individual base pairs to the binding of WT1 to DNA [5]; the identification of the effects of the +KTS splice variant on DNA and RNA binding [13]; the effects of the Denys-Drash and WILMS3 mutations on DNA and RNA binding [7, 19]; and the contributions of individual amino acids in the WT1 zinc fingers to the interaction with DNA and RNA [20].

2 Materials

2.1 Bacterial Transformation

1. One Shot® BL21 Star™ (DE3) Chemically Competent *E. coli* (Life Technologies).
2. 1× LB medium: Weigh out 20 g of LB broth into a 2 l Erlenmeyer flask. Suspend the broth in 1 l of deionized H_2O (dH_2O). Sterilize by autoclaving at 121 °C for 20 min. Cool to room temperature and store at 4 °C until required.
3. LB-ampicillin agar plates, stored at 4 °C.
4. Heat block or tempered water bath for heat shock step.
5. Shaking incubator with tube rack.

2.2 Expression of Recombinant His-Tagged WT1 Proteins

1. Ampicillin: 50 mg/ml Solution in dH_2O, filter sterilized.
2. Shaking incubator with clamps for 1 l flasks.
3. Isopropyl ß-d-1 thiogalactopyranoside (IPTG): 1 M Solution in dH_2O, filter sterilized.
4. A UV/VIS spectrophotometer.
5. A floor centrifuge with rotors that accommodate 250 ml GSA bottles and 15 ml Corex tubes.
6. A benchtop microcentrifuge.
7. 2× SDS sample buffer: 125 mM Tris–HCl pH 6.8, 4 % SDS, 10 % ß-mercaptoethanol, 0.05 % bromophenol blue, 20 % glycerol.
8. A pre-cast SDS 15 % polyacrylamide gel, or a home-poured gel.
9. Vertical gel apparatus with power supply.

2.3 Affinity Purification of His-Tagged WT1 Protein

1. Buffer A: 10 mM Tris–HCl pH 7.5 at 4 °C, 5 mM $MgCl_2$, 250 mM NaCl, 1 mM PMSF, 5 mM DTT, 5 mM imidazole.
2. His-Select® Nickel Affinity Gel (Sigma Aldrich).
3. Sonicator for cell disruption (e.g., Sonicator 3000, Qsonica LLC, USA).
4. Buffer B7: Buffer A plus 7 M urea.
5. Buffer B5: Buffer A plus 5 M urea.

6. Buffer B5-50Im: Buffer B5 plus 50 mM imidazole.

7. Buffer B5-150Im: Buffer B5 plus 150 mM imidazole.

8. Buffer B5-250Im: Buffer B5 plus 250 mM imidazole.

9. Bradford protein reagent (BioRad).

10. Bovine serum albumin (BSA): 10 mg/ml Solution in dH_2O.

11. A visible spectrophotometer or plate reader.

12. A pre-cast SDS 15 % polyacrylamide gel, or a home-poured gel.

13. Vertical gel apparatus with power supply.

2.4 Radiolabeling DNA

1. Vertical gel electrophoresis apparatus with power supply.

2. 30 % Acrylamide (29:1 bis:acrylamide) solution in dH_2O.

3. 10× TBE buffer: 0.89 M Tris base, 0.89 M boric acid, 20 mM EDTA.

4. 10 % Ammonium persulfate in dH_2O (make fresh just before use).

5. Tetramethylethylenediamine (TEMED).

6. WT1-TGT oligonucleotides:

(a) Top strand: 5′-AATTCTCTGCGTGGGCGTGTAGACG-3′

(b) Bottom strand: 5′-AATTCGTCTACACGCCCACGCAGACG-3′

7. 5× Annealing buffer: 50 mM Tris, pH 7.5, 250 mM NaCl, 5 mM EDTA.

8. dNTP mix: 0.2 mM each of dGTP, dTTP, dCTP.

9. DNA polymerase I large fragment (Klenow).

10. 10× DNA polymerase I buffer (as provided by supplier of enzyme).

11. α-^{32}P dATP within 1 half life of calibration date (Perkin Elmer).

12. Standard plexiglass safety shielding, tube racks, waste containers for working with ^{32}P radioisotope.

13. 6× Nondenaturing sample buffer: 0.1 M EDTA pH 8.0, 0.05 % bromophenol blue, 0.05 % xylene cyanol, 60 % glycerol.

14. Autoradiography Ruler (Electron Microscopy Sciences).

15. Gel elution buffer: 0.6 M Ammonium acetate, 1 mM EDTA, 0.1 % SDS.

16. 10 mg/ml Glycogen in DNase- and RNase-free H_2O.

2.5 Measuring Equilibrium Binding of WT1 to DNA with a Filter Binding Assay

1. 10× TK buffer: 200 mM Tris–HCl pH 7.5, 1 M KCl. This buffer can be stored at room temperature.

2. 1.1× TMK buffer (note: this buffer must be made fresh immediately before each assay): 1.1× TK buffer plus 0.55 mM Tris-(2-carboxyethyl) phosphine (TCEP), 0.11 mg/ml BSA, 5.5 mM $MgCl_2$, 11 µM $ZnCl_2$.

3. 96-Well NBS plates (Corning).

4. poly[dIdC] (Sigma Aldrich): To make a 1 mg/ml solution, dissolve 25 units of solid poly[dIdC] in 1 ml of 1× TK buffer. Once the solid is completely dissolved, heat the solution for 5 min at 42 °C. Store frozen at –20 °C in 100 μl aliquots.

5. Whatman Protran BA85 nitrocellulose filters, 0.45 μm.

6. Whatman Nytran N Nylon filters, 0.45 μm.

7. Blotting paper.

8. Phosphorimager.

9. Phosphorimager cassette.

10. Scientific plotting software.

3 Methods

3.1 Bacterial Transformation

1. Thaw two 50 μl aliquots of BL21(DE3)* competent cells quickly by holding them in your hands. Immediately chill on ice once the cells are thawed. If necessary, transfer each aliquot of thawed cells into a sterile 1.5 ml Eppendorf tube.

2. Add 10 ng of a pET-WT1ZFP, pET-16b plasmid containing the WT1 zinc finger domain [3] to one of the aliquots of competent cells. Add 10 μl of sterile distilled water to the other aliquot of competent cells to act as a negative control for transformation and antibiotic selection.

3. Chill on ice for 5 min.

4. Transfer the tubes to a 42 °C water or dry bath and heat shock for 2 min.

5. Transfer the tubes back to ice and chill for 5 min.

6. Add 800 μl of room temperature 1× LB medium to each tube. Mix each tube gently by inversion. Incubate the tubes at 37 °C for 1 h with shaking (250 rpm).

7. Transfer the tubes to a benchtop microcentrifuge. Pellet the cells to the bottom of the tubes by spinning at $3000 \times g$ for 5 min.

8. Remove the supernatant, taking care not to disturb the cell pellet. Resuspend the cells in 50 μl of 1× LB by gently pipetting up and down several times with a 200 μl micropipettor.

9. Spread the resuspended cells on an LB-agar plate containing 50 μg/ml ampicillin. Place the plates into a 37 °C incubator and grow overnight (no more than 16 h).

10. Take the plates out of the incubator and inspect them for colonies. The plate that received the cells transformed with the pET16b plasmid should show 100–200 single colonies. The plate that received the cells transformed with sterile water should be clear (no colonies). If this negative control plate has more than 2–3 colonies, you should make fresh LB-agar/ampicillin plates and repeat the transformation procedure (see **Note 1**).

11. Wrap the plates with parafilm and store at 4 °C. Colonies from the plates can be used for cell culture for 7–14 days before a fresh transformation needs to be done.

3.2 Expression of Recombinant His-Tagged WT1 Proteins

1. Inoculate 5 ml of 1× LB medium containing 5 µl of 50 mg/ml ampicillin (50 µg/ml final concentration) in a sterile, capped test tube with a single colony of BL21 (DE3) *E. coli* cells transformed with the pET-WT1ZFP plasmid on your LB-agar plate.

2. Incubate the culture overnight (~18 h) at 37 °C while shaking at 250 rpm.

3. Making sure that the cells are homogeneously suspended in the medium, add 2.5 ml this overnight culture to a 1 l Erlenmeyer flask containing 250 ml of sterile 1× LB medium with 50 µg/ml ampicillin.

4. Incubate the flask at 37 °C while shaking at 250 rpm.

5. After 2 h of incubation, remove 1 ml of the suspended culture and place in a disposable plastic cuvette. Read the absorbance at 595 nm.

6. If the OD_{595} is less than 0.5, continue incubation of the culture and retest every 30 min. Be sure to record the incubation time and OD_{595} value every time you do a reading during this procedure (*see* **Note 2**).

7. Once the OD_{595} is ≥0.5 the culture is ready for induction of WT1 protein expression. Remove 250 µl of culture to a 1.5 ml Eppendorf tube and store at 4 °C. This will be your $t=0$ sample for checking protein induction.

8. Induce the expression of protein by adding 250 µl of 1 M IPTG (final concentration 1 mM) and continue to grow for another 3–4 h at 37 °C with shaking.

9. At 1-h intervals after adding the IPTG, transfer a 1 ml aliquot to the plastic cuvette. Read and record the OD_{595}.

10. Transfer 250 µl of this aliquot to a 1.5 ml Eppendorf tube and store at 4 °C.

11. Three to four hours after the addition of IPTG, remove the flask from the incubator.

12. Pour the culture into a 250 ml GSA bottle and pellet the cells by centrifugation at $4000 \times g$ for 15 min at 4 °C.

13. Discard the supernatant and store the cell pellet at –80 °C until you are ready to purify the His-tagged WT1 protein.

14. Check for induction on an SDS-PAGE gel.

15. To clearly see the induction of protein, it is necessary to load an equivalent amount of bacterial cells to each well. To determine the volume needed for equal cell density at each time point, solve the equation $C_0 V_0 = C_x V_x$ for V_x, where C_0 is the

OD_{595} reading at $t=0$, $V_0=250$ μl, and C_x is the OD_{595} reading at $t=x$ (e.g., 1 h, 2 h). For example, if at $t=0$ the $OD_{595}=0.5$ and at $t=1$ the $OD_{595}=0.9$, then $(0.5)(250$ μl$)=(0.9)V_x$ and $V_x=139$ μl. Therefore, you would only use 139 μl of your $t=1$ sample for loading on the gel.

16. Transfer the tubes to a benchtop microcentrifuge. Pellet the cells to the bottom of the tubes by spinning at $3000 \times g$ for 5 min.

17. Remove all of the supernatant and resuspend the cell pellet in 20 μl of dH_2O and 20 μl of 2× SDS sample buffer.

18. Heat the samples for 30 min at 95 °C.

19. Run 10 μl of each sample on a 15 % SDS-PAGE gel with a protein size ladder. After staining the gel with Coomassie Blue, you should see a band at approximately 22 kDa that increases in intensity with each additional hour of incubation after induction (Fig. 2). *See* **Note 3**.

3.3 Affinity Purification of His-Tagged WT1 Protein

1. Resuspend the cell pellet in 10 ml of Buffer A by pipetting the solution up and down until the entire pellet is suspended in the buffer. Do not vortex!

2. Transfer the resuspended cell pellet to a 15 ml Corex glass centrifuge tube. Keep on ice.

3. Sonicate the resuspended pellet at Output 6 five times for 15 s with 1–1.5-min intervals to allow for cooling. Always keep proteins on ice (*see* **Note 4**).

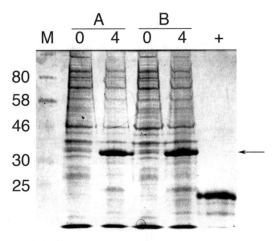

Fig. 2 Induction gel for two separate cultures of *E. coli* expressing recombinant WILMS3 zinc finger domain (A, B), which has a frameshift mutation that disrupts zinc finger 4 and lengthens the zinc finger domain [7]. The strong band at around 33 kDa indicated by the *arrow* shows the recombinant protein expression after 4 h of induction. Molecular weight markers are shown in lane M, and the positive control (lane +) is the WT1 zinc finger domain protein

4. Centrifuge the cell lysate for 15 min at $16,000 \times g$ at 4 °C.

5. Remove the supernatant (this contains soluble proteins) and store at 4 °C. The His-tagged WT1 protein is insoluble and therefore in the pellet.

6. Resuspend the pellet containing inclusion bodies in 5 ml of Buffer B7. It may be necessary to mash the pellet with a spatula in order to resuspend it. Do not use a vortex mixer for resuspending the pellet.

7. Add a small magnetic stir bar and place on stir plate for 3 h to solubilize the His-tagged WT1 protein with constant stirring (*see* **Note 5**).

8. Prepare column by spinning down 500 μl His-Select Ni resin in a 1.5 ml Eppendorf tube at $250 \times g$ for 1 min.

9. Pipette off storage buffer and resuspend in 1 ml of sterile dH_2O.

10. Using a Pasteur pipette transfer His-Select resin to a 1.4 cm diameter column with the outflow turned to the "off" position.

11. Let the resin pack by gravity for 1 h.

12. Using a Pasteur pipette, gently insert the upper frit so that it snugly packs onto the top of the settled resin.

13. Turn the outflow to the "on" position and wash the column by adding 5 ml of dH_2O.

14. Store column with both top and bottom caps on and refrigerate at 4 °C if prepared ahead.

15. Once the inclusion bodies have resolubilized, centrifuge the lysate for 15 min at $16,000 \times g$ at 4 °C. Be sure to keep the supernatant since this contains the resolubilized his-tagged WT1 protein. Store the remaining pellet at 4 °C. It can be resuspended in dH_2O to run as an extraction control on an SDS gel.

16. Equilibrate the column with 5 ml of freshly made Buffer B5.

17. Load the protein supernatant on the column. Collect the flow through in a small beaker and store at 4 °C. The loading step may be quite slow because of the high concentration of resolubilized protein in the supernatant.

18. Wash the column with 10 ml of Buffer B5. Collect the flow through in a small beaker and store at 4 °C.

19. Wash the column with 2 ml Buffer B5-50Im containing 50 mM imidazole. Collect the flow through in a small beaker and store at 4 °C.

20. Elute the protein off the column with 1 ml of Buffer B5-150Im. Collect the flow through in two 500 μl fractions in 1.5 ml Eppendorf tubes. Label these fractions E1 and E2. Keep these fractions on ice. They should contain the majority of the purified His-tagged WT1 protein.

21. Do a further elution of the column with 1 ml of Buffer B5-250Im. Collect the flow through in two 500 µl fractions in 1.5 ml Eppendorf tubes. Label these fractions E3 and E4. Keep these fractions on ice. They may contain a significant amount of purified His-tagged WT1 protein as well.

22. Wash the column with 10 ml dH$_2$O; the flow through can be discarded.

23. Add 5 ml dH$_2$O to the column and store tightly capped at top and bottom at 4 °C. Columns can be reused for the SAME protein multiple times. Alternatively, the resin can be regenerated according to the supplier's instructions.

24. Determine the protein concentration in all fractions collected by Bradford assay.

25. Dilute 3 ml of Bradford reagent with 12 ml dH$_2$O.

26. Aliquot 200 µl of diluted reagent into individual wells on a 96-well ELISA plate.

27. Set up your BSA standards: add 10 µl of dH$_2$O into a well with the Bradford reagent as a blank, and then 10 µl from each of the following solutions of BSA: 100, 200, 300, 400, and 500 µg/ml are added to separate wells containing Bradford reagent.

28. Set up your protein samples: Aliquot 10 µl of fractions E1–E4 from your column into separate wells containing Bradford reagent. Repeat with 10 µl aliquots of all other fractions collected.

29. Incubate at room temperature for a minimum of 5 min, but do not exceed 60 min.

30. Using an ELISA reader, measure the absorbance at 595 nm. The curve relating A_{595} to µg of BSA standard should be linear.

31. If the absorbance of any of your His-tagged WT1 protein fractions E1–E4 exceeds the absorbance of the 500 µg/ml BSA standard, you should take 3 µl of that fraction and dilute it with 7 µl of Buffer B5-150Im and re-do the Bradford assay (*see* **Note 6**).

32. Using the BSA standard curve, from the A_{595} values for your protein samples, determine the uncorrected concentration of E1–E4 in µg/ml. Multiply this value by 0.8 to get the correct concentration of His-tagged WT1 protein in µg/ml (this value corrects for a difference in dye binding between the BSA standard and the His-tagged WT1 protein). Using the molecular weight of the protein (20.2 kDa), convert from µg/ml to a concentration in µM.

33. Protein fractions must be aliquoted into 0.2 ml Eppendorf tubes the SAME day they are purified. Aliquots are generally 10–50 µl, depending on protein concentration (<25 µM: 20–30 µl, >25 µM: 10 µl). Store the aliquots frozen at –80 °C.

34. Purity of the His-tagged WT1 protein can be assessed by running 0.25–0.5 µg of fractions E1–E4 on a 15 % SDS-PAGE gel as described in the previous section (Fig. 3). If the yield of protein is low, troubleshooting can be accomplished by running 10 µl of the resuspended residual pellet from **step 16** and each of the flow-through fractions from the column purification on a 15 % SDS-PAGE gel (*see* **Note 6**).

3.4 Radiolabeling DNA

1. You will need to run the labeling reaction on a 20 % nondenaturing polyacrylamide gel to purify the labeled DNA.

2. Properly clean the glass plates for your gel apparatus. Assemble the gel plates using 0.75 mm spacers. Tape the sides and the bottom of the gel plate sandwich to prevent leaks.

3. Mix an appropriate amount of acrylamide solution for your gel plates. For example, 35 ml of a 20 % solution will consist of 23.3 ml of 30 % acrylamide (29:1 acrylamide:bis-acrylamide), 3.5 ml of 10× TBE, and 8.2 ml of dH_2O. Mix well.

4. Make a fresh solution of 10 % ammonium persulfate (APS). Add 350 µl (or the equivalent if your acrylamide solution is more or less than 35 ml) of the APS to the acrylamide solution and mix thoroughly.

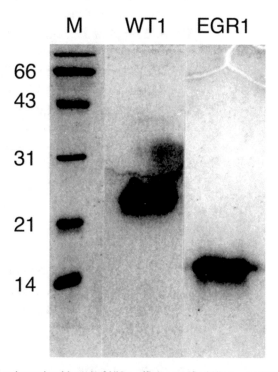

Fig. 3 SDS polyacrylamide gel of Ni2+ affinity-purified His-tagged WT1 zinc finger domain protein and EGR1 zinc finger domain protein

5. Initiate polymerization by adding 30 µl of TEMED to the acrylamide/APS solution. Mix thoroughly by swirling the flask.

6. Immediately begin pouring your gel. Once you have filled the gel plate sandwich with acrylamide solution, insert a comb with 10 deep wells into the top of the acrylamide solution.

7. Lay the assembled gel on the lab bench with the top of gel slightly elevated. Monitor for leaks until the gel has finished polymerizing.

8. Leave for a minimum of 1.5 h before use. The gel can be prepared the day before it is needed, but then must be wrapped well with plastic wrap and stored at 4 °C (*see* **Note 7**).

9. If you do not already have annealed WT1-TGT oligonucleotides in the freezer, put together the following mixture in a 0.2 ml Eppendorf tube:

    2 µl 5× Annealing buffer

    2 µl 100 µM top-strand oligonucleotide

    2 µl 100 µM bottom-strand oligonucleotide

    4 µl DNase-, RNase-free H_2O

10. Heat the tube at 94 °C in a heat block for 5 min.

11. Remove the tube from the heat block and slow cool on the lab bench for 60 min.

12. Add 90 µl of 1× annealing buffer to the tube and mix well by pipetting up and down.

13. Distribute the annealed WT1-TGT oligonucleotides into 5 µl aliquots in 0.2 ml Eppendorf tubes and store frozen at –20 °C.

14. Prepare your radioactive labeling reaction in the designated hot area, using all required safety and monitoring equipment as specified by your institutional radioisotope safety officer (*see* **Note 8**).

15. In a 0.2 ml Eppendorf tube behind shielding equipment, assemble the following reaction:

    1.0 µl 10× DNA polymerase I buffer

    1.0 µl Annealed oligonucleotides

    1.0 µl 0.2 mM dGTP, dTTP, dCTP mix

    4.5 µl DNase-, RNase-free H2O

    0.5 µl DNA pol I Large Fragment (Klenow)

    2.0 µl α-32P dATP (**RADIOACTIVITY**)

16. Incubate the reaction at room temperature for 30 min with proper safety shielding.

17. While the reaction is incubating, assemble your gel in the gel-running apparatus with 1× TBE buffer in the upper and lower buffer chambers.

18. Add 2 μl of 6× nondenaturing sample buffer to the tube, and mix by pipetting up and down.

19. Load the radioactive sample on the gel, maintaining safety shielding between you and the gel.

20. Run the gel at 300 V (constant voltage) for about 1 h at room temperature.

21. After the run is finished, turn off the power supply and disconnect the leads.

22. Carefully check the upper and lower buffer compartments with a Geiger counter for the presence of radioisotope. Carefully transfer the buffer from each compartment into an approved ^{32}P liquid waste receptacle.

23. Remove the gel from the apparatus and carefully separate the glass plates. The gel should stick to one of the plates.

24. Wrap the plate with the gel on it in saran wrap.

25. Place the wrapped gel onto absorbent bench paper in a plexiglass box.

26. Take the gel in the plexiglass box behind a shield to the darkroom. Put the box on the bench in the darkroom, with the shield between you and the radioactive gel.

27. Place the autoradiography ruler on the gel. Put a pied of X-ray film on the gel and hold it snuggly in place by putting a clean glass plate on top.

28. Expose the film to the radioactive gel for 2 min.

29. Remove the film and develop (Fig. 4) (*see* **Note 9**).

30. Take the developed film and orient it correctly on top of the gel by aligning the ruler marks on the film with those on the ruler itself. Using a permanent marker, mark the position of the bands shown on the film onto the backside of the glass that the gel is stuck to.

31. Using a clean single-edge razorblade, cut out each rectangle of the gel corresponding to a marked band. Using tweezers, place the gel slice into a 1.5 ml Eppendorf tube.

32. Add 250 μl gel elution buffer to each tube that has a gel slice.

33. Rotate the tubes slowly end over end behind a shield at room temperature for 12–16 h.

34. Transfer the buffer containing the radioactive DNA to a clean 1.5 ml Eppendorf tube for ethanol precipitation of the DNA.

35. Add 1–2 μl of 10 mg/ml glycogen to the tube, and then add 750 μl 95 % ethanol. Cap the tube tightly and mix well by inversion or using a vortex mixer.

36. Place the tube in a shielded plexiglass block in a −80 °C freezer for 30–60 min.

37. Spin for 20 min at maximum speed in a microcentrifuge.

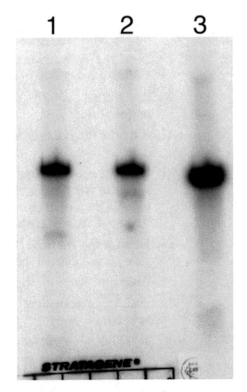

Fig. 4 Autoradiograph of a DNA-labeling gel of the wild-type and two mutant versions of the WT1 DNA-binding site. The autoradiographic ruler used to orient the film for extraction of the labeled DNA is shown at the bottom of the film

38. Carefully remove the radioactive supernatant (you may want to save it until you have confirmed successful precipitation of the labeled DNA). Take great care not to disturb the pellet of labeled DNA in the bottom of the tube.

39. Carefully wash the precipitated DNA with 200 μl of 95 % ethanol by adding the ethanol slowly to cover the pellet. It is not necessary to mix or otherwise disrupt the pellet.

40. Carefully transfer the ethanol wash, again taking care not to disturb the radioactive pellet.

41. Allow the radioactive DNA pellet to air-dry for 2 h (inverting the tube over absorbent lab bench paper helps drain residual ethanol on the sides of the tube).

42. Resuspend the radioactive DNA in 50 μl of DNase-, RNase-free H_2O.

43. Count 1 μl of the resuspended DNA in a scintillation counter.

44. Aliquot the labeled DNA by pipetting 4 μl into individual 0.2 ml Eppendorf tubes.

45. Store the labeled DNA aliquots in a shielded plexiglass box at −20 °C.

3.5 Measuring Equilibrium Binding of WT1 to DNA with a Filter Binding Assay

1. Defrost a frozen aliquot of His-tagged WT1 protein by removing it from the −80 °C freezer and placing the tube on ice.

2. Once the aliquot has thawed, dilute the protein to 10 µM concentration by adding the appropriate volume of 1.1× TMK buffer. Mix well by pipetting up and down. Store on ice.

3. Add 25 µl of the 10 µM protein stock to 225 µl of 1.1× TMK buffer to make a 1 µM solution of His-tagged WT1 protein. Mix well by pipetting up and down. Store on ice (*see* **Note 10**).

4. Align two 96-well plates as shown in Fig. 5. The top plate will hold wells 16-9, the bottom plate will hold wells 8-1 for each assay (*see* **Note 11**).

5. Aliquot the amount of 1.1× TMK buffer into each well as indicated in Table 1 for all assays. It is convenient to pour the 1.1× TMK buffer into a plastic trough and use a multichannel pipettor for this.

6. Aliquot out the volume of the 1 µM protein stock into wells 16-13 for each assay as indicated in Table 1. Each time, mix well by pipetting up and down.

7. Using a multichannel pipettor set to 10 µl, and starting with well 16, create the serial dilutions as indicated in Table 1. After adding protein to a new row of wells, mix by pipetting up and down several times.

8. Once the protein dilutions have been created, transfer the plates to your designated radioactive work area. Place the plates behind a plexiglass shield and cover the plates with parafilm.

9. Protected by the shield, thaw a frozen aliquot of your ^{32}P-labeled DNA. For each assay, dilute 200,000 cpm of the DNA into 180 µl of DNase-, RNase-free dH$_2$O containing 2 µg of poly[dIdC].

10. Protected by the shield, use a pipettor dedicated to radioactive use to aliquot 10 µl of ^{32}P-DNA into each well of the assay. It is convenient to start addition from well #1 (no protein control) and work up to well #16. Because you are moving from more dilute towards more concentrated protein dilutions, you can use the same pipet tip to aliquot all DNA for the same assay. Change tips when you start aliquoting DNA for the next assay.

11. Keep the plates covered with parafilm and incubate at room temperature for 90 min (*see* **Note 12**).

12. While the plates are incubating, prepare your nitrocellulose and nylon filters by soaking them for 10–20 min in DNase-, RNase-free dH$_2$O. It is important that you pick up the dry filters using gloves, not bare hands. You can soak the filters together in the same tray of water, but be sure to notch one or the other, so you can determine which is nylon and which is nitrocellulose. At the same time, soak a piece of blotting paper.

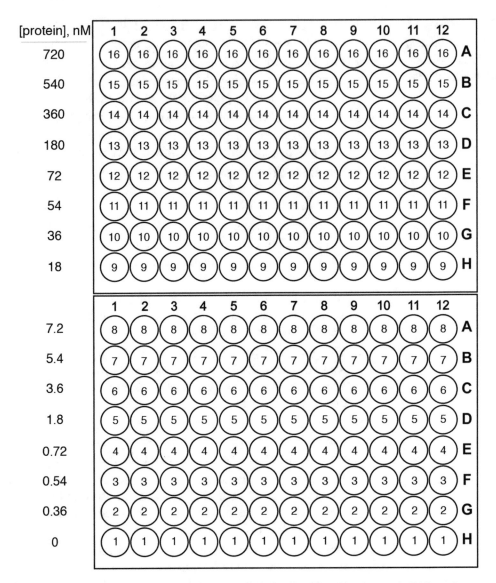

Fig. 5 Plate layout for setting up 12 filter binding assays for WT1 zinc finger domain protein. Well numbers appear within each well and the final concentration of protein in each assay well is indicated on the left-hand side

13. After preparation of the filters, assemble your 96-well dot blot apparatus. Using a flat-tongued tweezer, first transfer the blotting paper onto the base of the apparatus. Next place the nylon filter on top of the blotting paper. Then place the nitrocellulose filter on top of the nylon filter. Finally, add the top of the dot blot apparatus and clamp it closed.

14. Transfer the dot blot apparatus behind the plexiglass shield and attach the hose from a water vacuum to the outlet on the base of the apparatus.

15. When the incubation of the assay is complete, turn on the water vacuum. You will use a constant vacuum during the filtering process.

Table 1
Protocol for setting up the filter binding assay plate

Well #	1.1× TMK buffer	Protein	[protein], nM
16	20 μl	80 μl 1 μM	720
15	40 μl	60 μl 1 μM	540
14	60 μl	40 μl 1 μM	360
13	80 μl	20 μl 1 μM	180
12	90 μl	10 μl #16	72
11	90 μl	10 μl #15	54
10	90 μl	10 μl #14	36
9	90 μl	10 μl #13	18
8	90 μl	10 μl #12	7.2
7	90 μl	10 μl #11	5.4
6	90 μl	10 μl #10	3.6
5	80 μl	10 μl #9	1.8
4	80 μl	10 μl #8	0.72
3	80 μl	10 μl #7	0.54
2	80 μl	10 μl #6	0.36
1	90 μl	–	0

Note: Up to 12 assays can be done simultaneously. Start by aliquoting the 1.1× TMK buffer into the wells as indicated in column 2. Then add the specified amount of 1 μM stock protein to wells 16-13 for each assay. Then create the serial dilutions by removing 10 μl from well 16 and adding it to well 12, and so on as indicated in column 3

16. It is important that all pipetting steps, filtering, and steps handling the filters are performed behind a plexiglass safety shield.

17. Using a multichannel pipettor, remove 80 μl from each #1 well and transfer to the corresponding wells of the dot-blot apparatus. Let the vacuum pull the solution through the filters.

18. Repeat the filtering procedure for wells #2–#8.

19. Once all wells on the first plate with the lowest protein concentrations is complete, disconnect the vacuum hose from the base of the dot blot apparatus, and then turn off the vacuum.

20. Unclamp the apparatus and remove the top. Using flat-tongued tweezers, remove the nitrocellulose filter first, and place it on a piece of dry paper behind the shield. Then remove the nylon filter and place it on a second piece of dry paper behind the shield. The blotting paper can be discarded into a proper container for solid radioactive waste. Pour the liquid from the

bottom reservoir of the dot blot apparatus into a proper container for liquid radioactive waste.

21. For the second plate containing wells #9–16, repeat **steps 13–20**.

22. Allow the filters to air-dry completely.

23. Wrap the filters in saran wrap, and place into the phosphorimaging cassette. Expose overnight at room temperature. Make a note of where the filters have been placed on the screen grid.

24. The next morning, remove the filters from the phosphorimager cassette and store behind plexiglass shielding.

25. Scan the phosphor screen with the phosphorimager. You should see dots of increasing intensity moving up from well #1 to well #16 on the nitrocellulose filters, and dots of decreasing intensity moving up from well #1 to well #16 on the nylon filter (Fig. 6) (*see* **Note 13**).

26. Using the phosphorimager software, measure the intensity of each dot on the nitrocellulose and nylon filters. Save the data in a spreadsheet.

27. Calculate the raw fraction of DNA bound for each well by dividing the intensity of the dot on the nitrocellulose filter for

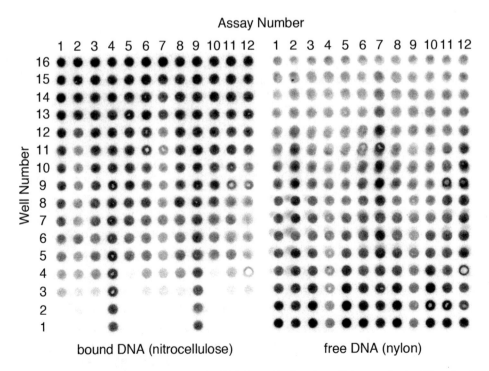

Fig. 6 Phosphorimager scan showing radioactive DNA bound to the nitrocellulose and nylon filters for 12 WT1-DNA equilibrium binding assays

that well by the sum of the intensity of the dots for that well on the nitrocellulose and nylon membranes.

28. Calculate the net fraction of DNA bound for each protein-containing well by subtracting the raw fraction of DNA-bound value for well #1 of that assay (no protein control) from the raw fraction of DNA-bound value for each protein-containing well (*see* **Note 14**).

29. Plot the results for each assay using scientific plotting software such as Kaleidagraph. Protein concentrations are plotted logarithmically on the *x*-axis, and fraction DNA bound is plotted linearly on the *y*-axis (Fig. 7) (*see* **Note 15**).

30. Calculate the association constant using the curve fitting algorithm for a simple bimolecular equilibrium (Fig. 7). Because retention of protein-DNA complexes on nitrocellulose is rarely 100% efficient, it is necessary to add a floating variable for fractional retention efficiency to the curve fitting algorithm (*see* **Notes 16** and **17**).

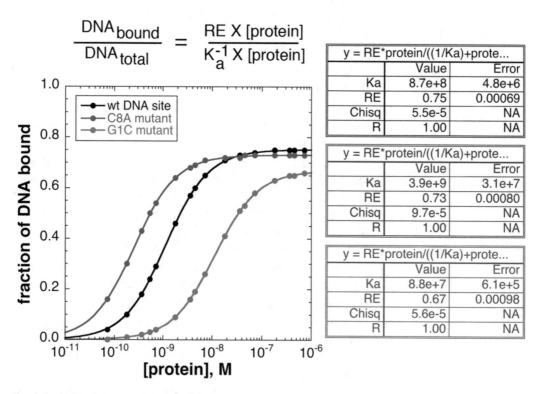

Fig. 7 Equilibrium binding of the WT1 zinc finger domain protein to the wild-type DNA site and sites mutated at base pairs 1 and 8. The equilibrium binding equation used for curve fitting in Kaleidagraph software is shown above the graph. RE refers to the retention efficiency of DNA-protein complexes trapped on the nitrocellulose filter. The tables to the right of the graph show the values for K_a and RE determined by the curve fitting function of the software

4 Notes

1. Although expiration of the ampicillin in the LB-agar plates is the most likely explanation for getting a large number of colonies on the negative control plate, there are a couple of other possibilities. The first is contamination of the sterile dH$_2$O used for the negative control transformation. The other is contamination of the competent cells. It is simple to test for these possibilities by doing three additional transformations: one with your original sterile dH$_2$O, one with freshly sterilized dH$_2$O, and one without anything added to the competent cells.

2. If the culture is very slow growing, it is unlikely that induction of expression will be successful. Slow growth is most commonly observed when the plated cells have been stored for too long. The best course of action is to do a fresh transformation of *E. coli* with the pET-WT1ZFP WT1 plasmid.

3. If there is no clear evidence of protein expression on the induction gel, either the ampicillin has expired and the culture has been overgrown with bacteria lacking the plasmid, or the IPTG solution has expired and induction of protein expression has failed. The best course of action is to make fresh solutions of IPTG and ampicillin and repeat the culture and expression steps.

4. Other methods of cell disruption can be used (e.g., French press, chemical lysis).

5. Alternatively, the pellet can be resuspended in 5 ml Buffer B containing 5 M urea and rotated overnight at 4 °C and the purification process can be continued the next day.

6. If fractions E1–E4 show little or no protein by the Bradford assay, use the diagnostic gel as outlined in **step 34** to determine at what point the purification failed. The most common problem is with binding of the protein to the Ni^{2+} resin during loading of the sample. The solution is to use the supplier's protocol for regenerating the resin, and to check the pH of the loading buffer.

7. If the gel is going to be stored longer than overnight (say for 2–3 days), first wrap the gel with two layers of wet paper towels, and then wrap with the plastic wrap.

8. Institutional approval of the use of radioisotopes is absolutely required, as is training of lab personnel by the institution's Radiation Safety Officer before any work with isotopes can be undertaken.

9. If the bands are faint or absent, the labeling reaction did not work. If you were using a frozen aliquot of previously annealed oligonucleotides, make a fresh annealing reaction. Other possible sources of problems are with the age of the DNA polymerase, and the number of freeze-thaw cycles the 10× buffer and the dNTP solution have gone through.

10. Serial dilution of zinc finger peptides to effect stepwise reduction of the urea concentration is an efficient refolding procedure. However, it is necessary to do the dilution stepwise (i.e., to 10 μM then to 1 μM) to get the most efficient refolding.

11. Having four protein concentrations per decade assures the highest accuracy in determining the K_a for the protein-nucleic acid interaction. For quick screening purposes, it is possible to use one 96-well plate oriented vertically and three protein concentrations per decade (e.g., 1.8, 3.6, 7.2).

12. Incubation must be long enough to ensure that equilibrium has been reached in all wells. The time necessary must be determined experimentally for each specific interaction; 90 min has been determined to be sufficiently long to reach equilibrium for WT1-DNA interactions [3].

13. If the spots are too faint even after adjusting the threshold value, it will be necessary to repeat the binding assay and add a higher number of cpm per well. If there are no spots on the nitrocellulose filter, and all spots on the nylon filter are uniformly dark, this indicates that the protein failed to bind the DNA. Typical reasons for this failure include expired TK buffer; reducing agent that has been freeze-thawed too many times; and errors in making the stock dilution of the protein.

14. In the absence of protein, a small amount of DNA (typically ≤10%) is held up on the wet nitrocellulose filter and that must be subtracted from all of the protein-containing wells in the same assay to accurately determine the fraction of DNA bound to the protein.

15. Strictly speaking, the plot should be fraction of DNA bound vs. [free protein]. It is possible to plot [total protein] on the x-axis in this case because the concentration of radioactive DNA in the assay is far less than even the lowest concentration of protein. Since [free protein] = [total protein] − [bound protein], when [DNA] << [total protein], [bound protein] is negligible.

16. Most protein-nucleic acid complexes are not fully retained on the nitrocellulose filter. In fact, if the nucleic acid ligand is quite large compared to the protein, the complexes can be pulled through the nitrocellulose filter. In the case of WT1-DNA complexes, the retention efficiency is typically 0.7 ± 0.5.

17. The assay as outlined in this chapter is suitable for comparing the binding of a single protein to a variety of novel DNA-binding sites or site-directed mutants of a previously characterized DNA-binding site. If the intention is to compare the DNA binding activity of a series of protein isoforms/mutants, this assay is not suitable because it would require the assumption that all isoforms/mutants refold to the same fractional activity. To compare a series of protein isoforms/mutants, the

assay can be reconfigured to titrate a constant concentration of each protein with increasing amounts of the DNA ligand. For more information about the applications of filter binding assays please see references [17, 18].

References

1. Rauscher FJ, Morris JF, Tournay OE et al (1990) Binding of the Wilms' tumor locus zinc finger protein to the Egr-1 consensus sequence. Science 250:1259–1262
2. Drummond IA, Rupprecht HD, Rohwernutter P et al (1994) DNA recognition by splicing variants of the Wilms' tumor suppressor, WT1. Mol Cell Biol 14:3800–3809
3. Hamilton T, Barilla K, Romaniuk PJ (1995) High affinity binding sites for the Wilms' tumour suppressor protein WT1. Nucleic Acids Res 23:277–284
4. Nakagama H, Heinrich G, Pelletier J et al (1995) Sequence and structural requirements for high-affinity DNA binding by the WT1 gene product. Mol Cell Biol 15:1489–1498
5. Hamilton TB, Borel F, Romaniuk PJ (1998) Comparison of the DNA binding characteristics of the related zinc finger proteins WT1 and EGR1. Biochemistry 37:2051–2058
6. Pelletier J, Bruening W, Kashtan CE et al (1991) Germline utations in the Wilms' tumor suppressor gene are associated with abnormal urogenital development in Denys-Drash syndrome. Cell 67:437–447
7. Busch M, Schwindt H, Brandt A et al (2014) Classification of a frameshift/extended and a stop mutation in WT1 as gain-of-function mutations that activate cell cycle genes and promote Wilms' tumour cell proliferation. Hum Mol Genet 23:3958–3974
8. Haber DA, Sohn RL, Buckler AJ et al (1991) Alternative splicing and genomic structure of the Wilms' tumor gene-WT1. Proc Natl Acad Sci U S A 88:9618–9622
9. Bickmore WA, Oghene K, Little MH et al (1992) Modulation of DNA binding specificity by alternative splicing of the Wilms' tumor WT1 gene transcript. Science 257:235–237
10. Caricasole A, Duarte A, Larsson SH et al (1996) RNA binding by the Wilms' tumor suppressor zinc finger proteins. Proc Natl Acad Sci U S A 93:7562–7566
11. Bardeesy N, Pelletier J (1998) Overlapping RNA and DNA binding domains of the wt1 tumor suppressor gene product. Nucleic Acids Res 26:1784–1792
12. Ladomery MR, Slight J, McGhee S et al (1999) Presence of WT1, the Wilm's tumor suppressor gene product, in nuclear Poly(A)(+) ribonucleoprotein. J Biol Chem 274:36520–36526
13. Zhai G, Iskandar M, Barilla K et al (2001) Characterization of RNA aptamer binding by the Wilms' tumor suppressor protein WT1. Biochemistry 40:2032–2040
14. Ladomery M, Sommerville J, Woolner S et al (2003) Expression in Xenopus oocytes shows that WT1 binds transcripts in vivo, with a central role for zinc finger one. J Cell Sci 116:1539–1549
15. Fried M, Crothers DM (1981) Equilibria and kinetics of lac repressor-operator interactions by polyacrylamide gel electrophoresis. Nucleic Acids Res 9:6505–6525
16. Riggs AD, Suzuki H, Bourgeois S (1970) Lac repressor-operator interaction. I. Equilibrium studies. J Mol Biol 48:67–83
17. Wong I, Lohman TM (1993) A double-filter method for nitrocellulose-filter binding: application to protein-nucleic acid interactions. Proc Natl Acad Sci U S A 90:5428–5432
18. Hall KB, Kranz JK (1999) Nitrocellulose filter binding for determination of dissociation constants. Methods Mol Biol 118:105–114
19. Borel F, Barilla KC, Hamilton TB et al (1996) Effects of Denys-Drash syndrome point mutations on the DNA binding activity of the Wilms' tumor suppressor protein WT1. Biochemistry 35:12070–12076
20. Weiss TC, Romaniuk PJ (2009) Contribution of individual amino acids to the RNA binding activity of the Wilms' tumor suppressor protein WT1. Biochemistry 48:148–155

Chapter 15

Identifying Direct Downstream Targets: WT1 ChIP-Seq Analysis

Fabio da Silva, Filippo Massa, and Andreas Schedl

Abstract

Identifying targets of transcriptional regulators such as the Wilms' tumor-suppressor protein (WT1) is an integral part of understanding the mechanisms governing the spatial and temporal activation of different genes. A commonly used strategy for studying transcription factors involves performing chromatin immunoprecipitation (ChIP) for the protein of interest with an appropriate antibody in crosslinked cells. Following ChIP, the enriched DNA is sequenced using next-generation sequencing (NGS) technologies and the transcription factor target sites are identified via bioinformatics analysis. Here we provide a detailed protocol for performing a successful ChIP-Seq experiment for WT1. We have optimized and simplified the several steps necessary for the immunoprecipitation of WT1's target-binding sites. We also suggest several strategies for validating the experiment and provide brief guidelines on how to analyze the large amounts of data generated from high-throughout sequencing. This method can be adapted for a variety of different tissues and/or cell types to help understand the role of WT1 in regulating gene expression.

Key words Wilms' tumor suppressor 1 (WT1), Next-generation sequencing (NGS), Chromatin immunoprecipitation (ChIP)

1 Introduction

Chromatin immunoprecipitation (ChIP) refers to a procedure used to identify DNA sequences bound by proteins in vivo. In ChIP assays, the protein of interest is cross-linked to its target DNA sequences and the protein-DNA complex purified by immunoprecipitation using specific antibodies. While in the past precipitated DNA was analyzed by hybridization to dedicated microarrays (ChIP-Chip analysis on tiling arrays), the rapid development of next-generation sequencing (NGS) technologies nowadays allows a comprehensive and unbiased approach. Indeed, due to its ability to effectively cover complex genomes such as that of *Mus musculus*, chromatin immunoprecipitation followed by sequencing (ChIP-Seq) has become an invaluable tool for studying genome-wide targets of transcriptional regulators.

Nicholas Hastie (ed.), *The Wilms' Tumor (WT1) Gene: Methods and Protocols*, Methods in Molecular Biology, vol. 1467,
DOI 10.1007/978-1-4939-4023-3_15, © Springer Science+Business Media New York 2016

Due to its pivotal role in developmental processes, WT1 has been one of the first proteins to be studied using ChIP experiments. Studies in the developing kidney have helped clarify its in vivo targets [1] and identified it as a modulator of the major molecular pathways involved in renal progenitor survival [2]. In addition, bioinformatic analysis confirmed its role as a key regulator of glomerular cell differentiation [3–5]. Taken together, this data demonstrates the merit of using ChiP-Seq approaches to study the function of transcription factors such as WT1 in different tissues.

1.1 ChIP-Seq Workflow

To perform a successful ChIP-Seq experiment, several steps have to be carried out sequentially and should be individually controlled (Fig. 1). Briefly, cells or tissues expected to express WT1 are treated with formaldehyde to covalently cross-link proteins to DNA. This is followed by sonication to mechanically shear the chromatin into fragments of 100–300 bp in size. Immunoprecipitation with a WT1-specific antibody is then carried out to enrich for WT1-bound DNA compared to the total chromatin. We routinely use the Santa Cruz C19 antibody, a rabbit polyclonal antibody that has been validated by several publications [1–5]. Of importance, individual batches of polyclonal antibodies are by nature unique and need to be tested for their suitability in ChIP experiments, ideally by comparing them with a previously validated batch.

After enrichment, the cross-links are reversed by heating, and the purified DNA is prepared for sequencing. Since ChIP-assays can vary between independent experiments, it is important to determine the DNA concentration and validate the enrichment of specific targets before NGS. To achieve this, semiquantitative PCR with primers specific for known or expected target-binding sites of WT1 can be employed. The enrichment must be normalized against the non-treated fragmented chromatin (input control), or to a mock ChIP in which a nonspecific antibody of the same species (IgG control) can identify unspecific binding of the chromatin to the antibody and/or magnetic beads. To ensure specificity of the enrichment, a putative negative region (randomly chosen region several kb away from the target site) should also be tested. This is especially important when the amounts of chromatin in mock controls are low. For WT1 ChIP experiments we routinely observe an enrichment of a minimum of fivefold. Not surprisingly, enrichment differs greatly for different genes and different tissues (cell types), and to date we have not been able to identify a universal target site that could serve as an internal control for each ChIP experiment.

Once validated, ChIP samples can be prepared for high-throughput sequencing. The chromatin fragments are amplified and tagged with adaptors to create a library. Library preparation can be performed in-house with specific kits or by the chosen sequencing platform. Sequencing depth will depend on the platform used, as well as the associated cost. The ENCODE Consortium suggests a minimum of 20 million reads per sample for mammalian transcription

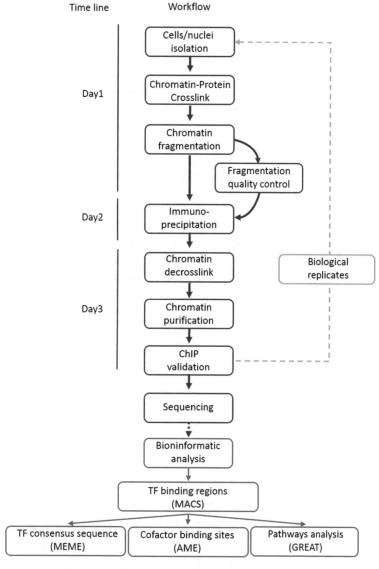

Fig. 1 ChIP-Seq workflow. Schematic representation of Chip-seq procedure

factors [6]. However, since WT1 shows a higher number of binding sites than traditional TFs, we would recommend aiming for 30–40 million reads to ensure proper coverage. Choosing an appropriate negative control is another issue that may depend on the experiment. We would recommend sequencing the mock-IgG immunoprecipitated chromatin to a similar depth as WT1, since it more closely mimics the experimental conditions than the input control. In addition, thorough coverage of the input control may require up to 3× more reads than the mock control adding to the total cost of the experiment. In some cases, however, it may prove difficult to obtain sufficient material from the mock IgG precipitated chromatin for adequate sequencing. Thus, the input should always be kept aside and, if possible, sequenced alongside the WT1 and mock IgG control.

Following sequencing a thorough bioinformatic analysis of the reads must be performed in order to correctly identify *bona fide* targets. This involves applying a quality cutoff for the sequencing data in order to filter and eliminate false-positive reads, and mapping the reads to a reference genome. An appropriate statistical analysis of the mapped data must then be undertaken and compared to the control in order to produce reliable data. To ensure reproducibility, the experiment should be repeated at least once (biological replicate).

Previous studies have revealed that WT1 occupies an unusually high number of sites throughout the genome. Canonical promoter regions lie normally within 1000 bp upstream of the transcription start site of a gene, but only a small percentage of the overall WT1-binding sites fall within these regions. This observation suggests that WT1 may have other functions unrelated to promoter activation. These may include long-distance organization of chromatin domains or the organization of the highly complex 3D architecture within the nucleus. Identifying in vivo WT1-binding sites in different tissues and integrating them with chromatin marks and bindings sites for chromatin modifiers will aid in discovering these functions.

2 Materials

2.1 Special Equipment

1. Rabbit polyclonal WT1 antibody (C19), ref no. sc-192, Santa Cruz.
2. Normal Rabbit IgG, ref no. 272295, Cell Signalling Technology.
3. 6-Tube Magnetic separation Rack ref no. S1506S New England Biolabs.
4. Minelute PCR purification kit, ref no. 28004, QIAGEN.
5. Dynabeads Protein G, ref no. 10003D, Life Technologies.
6. RNase A (stock solution 10 mg/ml), ref no. R4875, Sigma.
7. Proteinase K (stock solution 10 mg/ml), ref no. P6911, Sigma.

2.2 Buffers

1. Cell wash buffer: 20 mM HEPES pH 7.4, 150 mM NaCl, 0.125 M glycine, 1 mM PMSF.
2. Cell lysis buffer: 20 mM HEPES pH 7.4, 1 mM EDTA, 150 mM NaCl, 1% SDS, 0.125 M glycine, 1 mM PMSF.
3. Sonication buffer: 20 mM HEPES pH 7.4, 1 mM EDTA, 150 mM NaCl, 0.4% SDS, 1% Triton × 100, 1 mM PMSF.
4. SDS dilution buffer: 20 mM HEPES pH 7.4, 1 mM EDTA, 150 mM NaCl, 1% Triton X100, 1 mM PMSF.
5. Wash buffer A: 20 mM HEPES pH 7.4, 1 mM EDTA, 500 mM NaCl, 0.8% Triton X100, 0.1% SDS, 1 mM PMSF.

6. Wash buffer B: 20 mM Tris–HCl pH 8.0, 1 mM EDTA, 250 mM LiCl, 0.5 % NP40, 0.5 % sodium deoxycholate, 1 mM PMSF.

7. TE buffer: 20 mM Tris–HCl pH 8.0, 1 mM EDTA, 1 mM PMSF.

8. Elution buffer: 100 mM NaHCO₃, 1 % SDS.

3   Methods

3.1   Cell Cross-linking, Nuclear Lysis, and Chromatin Fragmentation

1. Grow cultured cells in appropriate medium to desired density. Detach them by trypsin treatment and evaluate the number of cells/ml. Usually, a final volume of 35–50 ml of confluent cells in a 175 cm² flask should be sufficient to perform a successful ChIP experiment. If working with tissue samples, dissociate until obtaining a single-cell suspension (*see* **Note 1**).

2. Replace the growth media with PBS and then cross-link the cells by adding formaldehyde to 1 % final concentration. Incubate at room temperature with gentle shaking for 10 min.

3. Add glycine to 0.125 M (final concentration) quench the formaldehyde and incubate at room temperature for 5 min.

4. Wash the cells 2×5 min in cold wash buffer with gentle shaking.

5. Resuspend cells in 6–10 ml of cell lysis buffer and then scrape off the cells with a rubber policeman. Spin cells at $2000 \times g$ for 5 min at room temperature. Remove the supernatant and resuspend in 4 ml cell lysis buffer.

6. Transfer the cells to 4×1.5 ml centrifuge tubes and run each aliquot through a 0.3 ml insulin syringe 6–7× to lyse the cells and isolate the nuclei (fixed nuclei are generally resistant to lysis in 1 % SDS). If working with low amounts of material this step can be skipped (*see* **Note 2**).

7. Spin the suspension at $2000 \times g$ 5 min room temperature for 5 min to precipitate the nuclei. Remove as much of the supernatant as possible and resuspend and combine the nuclear pellets in a total of 600 μl of sonication buffer. Split the suspension in two separate centrifuge tubes (2×300 μl). In case additional conditions or antibodies need to be tested adjust the volumes accordingly to have a total of 300 μl per condition.

8. Chromatin fragmentation: Sonicate each sample with a suitable machine (Soni probe, Diagenode Bioruptor, Covaris sonicator). This step is required to reduce the chromatin to small fragments in order to properly identify the protein-binding sites. For ChIP-seq purposes, the optimal fragment size is 150–300 bases. Different methods can be adopted, but mechanical fragmentation (sonication) is considered the most reliable, since the fragmentation of the chromatin is considered to be random. For detailed instructions on sonication procedures, please *see* **Note 3**.

9. Spin down chromatin at $16,000 \times g$ for 5 min at 4 °C to pellet insoluble material.

10. Pool supernatants to ensure that the same starting material is used for all samples. At this point, the samples can be stored at −20 °C or processed to assess the degree of fragmentation. Following this assessment it is best to continue immediately with the immunoprecipitation (*see* **Note 4**).

3.2 Fragmentation Quality Assay

1. In order to assess the quality of the fragmentation, decross-link 1/10 of the total chromatin by boiling in a water bath for 10 min (*see* **Note 5**).

2. Allow eluted chromatin and input to cool to room temperature and then treat with 30 µg/ml RNase A at 37° for 30 min

3. Add proteinase K to a final concentration of 30 µg/ml and incubate for 30 min at 55 °C.

4. Isolate the chromatin with a QIAGEN PCR purification kit and quantify it: the amount of chromatin usually obtained in this step is enough to have a correct estimation with a spectrophotometer, i.e., Nanodrop technology (Nanodrop Thermo Fischer, Wilmington, USA). In case of low amount of starting material, fluorimetric quantification might be more accurate, i.e., Qubit assay (Invitrogen).

5. Load 0.5–1 µg of purified chromatin on a 2% agarose gel to assess the quality of the DNA fragmentation (Fig. 2).

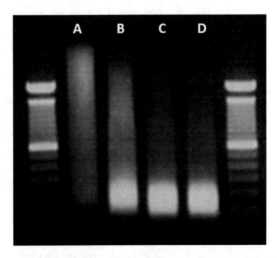

Fig. 2 Chromatin fragmentation test. Typical profile from 0.5 mg of fragmented chromatin (Bioruptor) separated on a 2% agarose gel. Line (**a**) represents very low fragmentation of the chromatin (five cycles of Bioruptor). Line (**b**) (15 cycles) shows a first enrichment of chromatin fragment of proper size, 150–300 bp. Lines (**c, d**) (25 and 30 cycles, respectively) represent ideal chromatin fragmentation, suitable for IP and sequencing

3.3 Immuno-precipitation and DNA Purification

1. Aliquot 300 µl of pooled chromatin into individual tubes. To each tube add 1.2 ml SDS dilution buffer to reduce the SDS concentration to around 0.08 % so that it does not interfere with antibody binding. If volumes used for sonication are greater than 300 µl adjust the amount of SDS dilution buffer accordingly. Remove 30 µl of the pooled chromatin as the input control and store at –20 °C.

2. *Antibody-chromatin incubation.* Add 3 µg of WT1 C19 antibody to one tube and 3 µg of rabbit IgG control to the other. Incubate O/N at 4° with gentle rotation.

3. *Magnetic bead blocking.* Aliquot 20 µl of Protein G Dynabeads per µg of antibody used and wash twice in 200 µl PBS. For each step, keep the tubes on the magnetic rack for 1 min and discard the supernatant. Resuspend beads in 200 µl PBS-BSA 1 mg/ml and incubate O/N at 4 °C with gentle rotation.

4. *Immunoprecipitation and washes.* After the O/N blocking, wash protein G beads 2× 5 min with PBS at 4 °C with gentle rotation. Resuspend the beads in SDS dilution buffer and aliquot an equal amount of beads into each WT1 and IgG chromatin tube. Incubate for 2–3 h at 4 °C with gentle rotation.

5. While waiting for the antibody to bind to the beads, prepare wash buffers A, B, and TE and keep them on ice. Washes are all performed at room temperature with chilled buffers and gentle rotation. To replace the media, use a magnetic holder to bind the beads and pipette out the supernatant.

6. Wash 3× 5 min with chilled wash buffer A at room temperature.

7. Wash 3× 5 min with chilled wash buffer B at room temperature.

8. Wash 1× 5 min with chilled TE buffer at room temperature.

9. Resuspend in 250 µl TE buffer and transfer to a new 1.5 ml centrifuge tube. Add 250 µl of TE buffer and wash for another 5 min.

10. *Chromatin elution and purification.* Remove TE wash and resuspend the beads in 300 µl elution buffer. Incubate for 1 h at room temperature with gentle rotation.

11. Transfer supernatant containing the eluted chromatin to a new centrifuge tube and remove any excess beads with magnet. Repeat transfer of the supernatant to a new centrifuge tube.

12. At this step, the input can be included in the procedure. Thaw 10 µl of the saved input chromatin from Subheading 3.3, **step 1**, and add 290 µl of elution buffer.

13. *Chromatin decross-linking.* Incubate eluted chromatin and input at 65 °C O/N with gentle shaking.

14. Allow eluted chromatin and input to cool to room temperature and then treat with 30 µg/ml RNase A at 37° for 30 min.

15. Add proteinase K to a final concentration of 30 µg/ml and incubate for 30 min at 55 °C.

16. Chromatin can be purified with QIAGEN MinElute columns according to the manufacturer's protocol. The columns increase the purity of the DNA, but generally give low overall yields. Alternatively, DNA can be purified using phenol/chloroform extraction, allowing higher yield, but lower purity.

17. *DNA quantification*. Due to the low amount of purified chromatin, it is preferable to quantify the purified chromatin by fluorimetric quantitation (i.e., Qubit assay) instead of less sensitive techniques based on absorbance (i.e., Nanodrop).

18. *ChIP validation*. Once the chromatin is quantified it must be analyzed by semiquantitative qPCR (SYBR green) with primers specific to known or expected WT1 target sites. Ideally, the target sites should be enriched 5–100× in the WT1-purified chromatin compared to the controls. For more details please *see* **Note 6**.

3.4 Analysis of Sequencing Data

Next-generation sequencing of ChIP material can be carried out on any suitable platform with Solexa machines (Illumina) being the most widely used. Primary data produced by sequencers need to be converted and aligned to allow analysis of ChIP-Seq data. A basic workflow to obtain the peak regions and visualize the results on the UCSC genome browser (https://genome.ucsc.edu/) is given below. All tools necessary for the analysis are publically available on the Galaxy website (www.usegalaxy.org).

1. *Sequence conversion* (*FASTq Groomer tool*) [7]. The first step is to convert the raw data into files that can be understood by the tools available on the Galaxy website. In this case, the raw data, which comes in the form of *fastq* files, must be converted into *fastqsanger* files. To proceed with the conversion, previously uploaded *fastq* files can be run through the tool "FASTq Groomer" that converts input sequences according to the database chosen, i.e., the latest built for the mouse genome (mm10) or human genome (hg38).

2. *Sequence alignment* (*Bowtie2 or BWA tools*) [8, 9]. The next step is to map the reads to a reference genome. For this purpose, two main tools are available on Galaxy: Bowtie2 or BWA. The two programs differ in terms of algorithms and the speed with which mapping can be performed. We routinely use Bowtie2. Sequence alignment results in output files in SAM (=uncompressed BAM file) format that can be visualized on the UCSC browser, showing the exact position of each read on the genome.

3. *Peak calling* (*MACS or MACS2 tool*) [10]. The aligned SAM files can be used to define the genomic regions that are significantly enriched. To achieve this, files obtained from ChIP samples are compared to controls (mock or input) using specific peak-calling algorithms. Model-based analysis of ChIP-Seq (MACS or the updated MACS2) is the most commonly used tool for this purpose.

Once peaks have been identified a detailed bioinformatic analysis can be performed to determine the consensus-binding sequence (position weight matrix), identify potential cofactors binding in the vicinity of target sites, and reveal major pathways regulated by WT1. A detailed description of all bioinformatic tools available would be beyond the scope of this chapter and we concentrate in the remaining text on some basic tools available on the Internet.

4. *Transcription factor consensus sequence identification* (*MEME tool*) [11]. Each transcription factor recognizes specific sequences of nucleotides in the genome and the length of this sequence can be variable from one protein to the other. The MEME suite (Multiple Expectation maximization for Motif Elicitation; http://meme.nbcr.net/meme/) provides the necessary tool to extract this sequence from the list of sequences obtained in a ChIP-Seq experiment. Normally the top 1000 peaks are used to elaborate *de novo* binding sequence for the transcription factor of interest. MEME produces a position-probability matrix (PPM) or a position weight matrix (PWM; calculated as log likelihoods) that provides for each position the statistical probability for a given nucleotide.

5. *Identification of cofactors* (*AME tool*) [12]. Transcription factors are rarely acting individually, but usually form part of multi-protein complexes with other cofactors. The analysis of sequences adjacent to binding regions obtained by ChIP-Seq analysis can offer hints of such potential cofactors. The Analysis of Motif Enrichment (AME) tool (http://meme.nbcr.net/meme/doc/ame.html) screens the supplied list of top enriched sequences for the presence of known binding sites for other transcription factors and provides a score for enriched motifs. Predicted interactions can then be verified using standard biochemical methods (e.g., CoIP).

6. *Pathways analysis* (*GREAT tool*) [13]. The last tool we present is intended to assess the functional relevance of the transcription factor-binding regions identified by ChIP-seq. The Genomic Regions Enrichment of Annotations (GREAT) tool (http://bejerano.stanford.edu/great/public/html/) takes into consideration all of the peaks, independently from their position in relation to the transcription starting points of genes. These regions are analyzed according to the annotations of 20 different gene ontology databases to evaluate the most significantly enriched pathways or biological functions (*see* also **Note 7**).

4   Notes

1. *Amount of starting material.* This protocol is designed for a total of 1×10^8 WT1-expressing cultured cells. We realize that obtaining such a high number of cells may be difficult for certain

experiments (e.g., FACS sorted) and the protocol may need to be scaled down according to the total number of cells available. When performing ChIP on freshly dissected tissues, great care should be taken to optimize tissue dissociation in order to obtain a single-cell suspension (avoid overdigestion). This protocol may also be applied to FACS-sorted cells, but further optimization steps for fixation and /or cross-linking are required.

2. *Quality of starting material.* Isolating the nuclei prevents cytoplasmic proteins from interfering with the immunoprecipitation step and normally improves overall specificity and enrichment. However, when starting with very small amounts of material, isolation of nuclei may be skipped to avoid the loss of precious material. In this case proceed to Subheading 3.1, **step 7**, once a single-cell suspension has been obtained.

3. *Choice of sonicator.* We suggest to perform the mechanical fragmentation of chromatin using ultrasound sonication: the high-frequency waves induce the formation of micro air bubbles in the sample and their explosion causes the DNA to break (event known as cavitation). Sonicators are available from different companies. We discuss here the use of two of them (one with immersion probe and one using a cooled water bath) that we have used routinely.

   Sonication with Bioruptor (Diagenode, water bath): Samples are resuspended in max 300 μl of sonication buffer for up to 10^8 cells/nuclei. The sonication program is set according to the manufacturer's manual and the number of cycles has to be defined empirically. We generally use 30 cycles of 30″on/30″off, in an ice-chilled water bath. Every five cycles, the melted ice is replaced with fresh ice.

   Sonication with a soniprobe (immersion probe): Sonicate each sample for 5 s at amplitude 10 with a Soniprep 150. For this, find an appropriate holder for the tubes and immerse the probe 2/3 of the way into the sample. Sonicate each sample a total of 6–10×. Between each sonication keep the samples on ice for at least 30 s to cool them down. Make sure not to leave them too long on ice; otherwise the SDS may precipitate. Also, be very careful to avoid foaming. If foaming is a problem try increasing the volume of sonication buffer. The amount of cycles may vary from sample to sample and will depend on the type of cells, the efficiency of the sonicator, as well as the conditions used. Usually frozen cells may require more cycles than fresh material. This sonication protocol should shear the chromatin down to an average size of 100–300 bp.

4. *Sonicated chromatin stability.* Subjecting the chromatin to freeze–thaw cycles can reduce the efficiency of antibody-chromatin immune-complex formation; therefore, we recommend performing the ChIP on fresh rather than frozen material.

5. *Decross-linking procedure.* Decross-linking by heat shock (10 min in boiling water bath) is a fast, but harsh way to check chromatin fragmentation. A milder alternative would be to decross-link O/N at 65 °C with gentle shaking. Boiling the samples is very useful to avoid freezing the rest of chromatin while waiting for the result of the standard milder decross-linking at 65 °C O/N. The chromatin resulting from this procedure is single-stranded, denatured DNA, which has to be taken into consideration during quantification.

6. *Semiquantitative qPCR analysis.* It is important to check the quality of the precipitated chromatin before proceeding with sequencing. Towards this aim, a semiquantitative or quantitative PCR analysis of possible or known binding sites of WT1 is the fastest and most reliable approach. Ensure that the same amount of chromatin is used from each condition (antibody, input, and mock controls). Empirically, we have determined that very low amounts of sample chromatin can be used for this purpose, ranging from 0.02 to 0.2 ng.

In order to validate the ChIP-seq for organs or cells other than kidney, putative binding regions can be obtained taking advantage of already published WT1-binding regions in renal samples: the coexpression of peak associated genes in the organ of interest along with WT1 may suggest a direct target of the transcription factor that can be tested for ChIP validation.

Here we propose some examples of binding sites and their respective primers that can be used in different organs (Table 1). These primers are based on our own experimental data and can

Table 1
Putative WT1-binding sites for ChIP validation

Name	Sequences	Organ/tissue of interest
Sox4_peak	CACCCCAGAGCCTTCTTTCT GAAAATCCAGCGTGCCCC	Bone marrow
Sox4_negative region	CGTTGGTAGCCGGAGTATCT TCGTGAACTGCAATCGACTG	
RSPO1_peak	TCTCACAGGCAGCTTAACCA CCCACCTGCACTGGAGATAA	Adipose tissue Developing kidney
RSPO1_negative region	AACCCTTCTCTCTCCTTGCC TGTCCTGCTTGAATCCACCT	
Gli1_peak	GGAGACCTCGTTTCAGTCCA ACGCTCTGCTCTGAAGTCTT	Hepatic stellate cells
Gli1_negative region	AGGACTCAACATACTACTCCACA TCAGGTTGTTCTCATTTCCTAGC	

be used in simple qPCR experiments with SYBR green. The concentration of the primers used must be determined empirically but generally falls within the range of normal qPCR experiments. Enrichment will depend on the target site and tissue of interest.

7. *Alternative pathway analysis tool (GOrilla)* [14]. In order to study the functional relevance of binding regions, other tools besides GREAT are available online. For example, the Gene Ontology enRIchment anaLysis and visuaLizAtion (GOrilla) can be used to visualize the molecular pathways controlled by transcription factors. However, in contrast to GREAT analysis that directly uses genomic coordinates, the GOrilla algorithm uses a ranked gene list and therefore requires manipulation of the data to sort the genes correlated to each peak and to rank them according to their significance and enrichment.

References

1. Hartwig S, Ho J, Pandey P et al (2010) Genomic characterization of Wilms' tumor suppressor 1 targets in nephron progenitor cells during kidney development. Development 137:1189–1203

2. Motamedi FJ, Badro DA, Clarkson M et al (2014) WT1 controls antagonistic FGF and BMP-pSMAD pathways in early renal progenitors. Nat Commun 5:4444

3. Lefebvre J, Clarkson M, Massa F et al (2015) Alternatively spliced isoforms of WT1 control podocyte-specific gene expression. Kidney Int 88(2):321–331

4. Kann M, Ettou S, Jung YL et al (2015) Genome-wide analysis of Wilms' tumor 1-controlled gene expression in podocytes reveals key regulatory mechanisms. J Am Soc Nephrol 26(9):2097–2104

5. Dong L, Pietsch S, Tan Z et al (2015) Integration of cistromic and transcriptomic analyses identifies Nphs2, Mafb, and Magi2 as Wilms' tumor 1 target genes in podocyte differentiation and maintenance. J Am Soc Nephrol 26(9):2118–2128

6. Landt SG, Marinov GK, Kundaje A et al (2012) ChIP-seq guidelines and practices of the ENCODE and modENCODE consortia. Genome Res 22:1813–1831

7. Blankenberg D, Gordon A, Von Kuster G et al (2010) Manipulation of FASTQ data with Galaxy. Bioinformatics 26:1783–1785

8. Langmead B, Salzberg SL (2012) Fast gapped-read alignment with Bowtie 2. Nat Methods 9:357–359

9. Li H, Durbin R (2010) Fast and accurate long-read alignment with Burrows-Wheeler transform. Bioinformatics 26:589–595

10. Zhang Y, Liu T, Meyer CA et al (2008) Model-based analysis of ChIP-Seq (MACS). Genome Biol 9:R137

11. Machanick P, Bailey TL (2011) MEME-ChIP: motif analysis of large DNA datasets. Bioinformatics 27:1696–1697

12. McLeay RC, Bailey TL (2010) Motif enrichment analysis: a unified framework and an evaluation on ChIP data. BMC Bioinformatics 11:165

13. McLean CY, Bristor D, Hiller M et al (2010) GREAT improves functional interpretation of cis-regulatory regions. Nat Biotechnol 28:495–501

14. Eden E, Navon R, Steinfeld I et al (2009) GOrilla: a tool for discovery and visualization of enriched GO terms in ranked gene lists. BMC Bioinformatics 10:48

Chapter 16

WT1-Associated Protein–Protein Interaction Networks

Ruthrothaselvi Bharathavikru and Alex von Kriegsheim

Abstract

Tumor-suppressor protein Wt1 has been shown to interact with specific proteins that influence its function. These protein interactions have been identified as direct individual interactions but with the potential to exist as a part of a multiprotein complex. In order to obtain the global proteome interaction map of Wt1, an unbiased label-free endogenous immunoprecipitation was performed followed by mass spectrometry to identify protein interactions that are Wt1 centric. This chapter details the different techniques that have been used to identify and characterize Wt1-interacting proteins.

Key words Immunoprecipitation, Proteome, Protein interaction, Mass spectrometry

1 WT1-Associated Proteome

Tumor-suppressor protein Wt1 is a transcription factor that has been shown to have both transcriptional activation and repression properties. Studies have shown that Wt1 interacts with other proteins with functional implications. Wt1-interacting proteins can be broadly classified into three functional categories, (a) transcription-related proteins, (b) cell cycle and apoptosis regulators, (c) splicing pathway components. These have been identified using several biochemical techniques such as yeast two-hybrid analysis, immuno pulldowns, and mass spectrometric analyses and validated by immunoprecipitation (IP) followed by immunoblots/western blotting approaches as well as by performing immunofluorescence to observe colocalization. A brief overview of these different functional categories of interacting proteins is followed by detailed protocols that have been used to identify and understand the significance of Wt1 interactome.

1.1 Functional Categories of Wt1-Interacting Proteins

(A) **Transcription-Related Proteins**: Tumor-suppressor protein p53 was one of the first Wt1-interacting proteins to be identified. This was later extended to include p63 and p73 as well. Several important transcription factors including STAT3, ERα, SRY, and

Nicholas Hastie (ed.), *The Wilms' Tumor (WT1) Gene: Methods and Protocols*, Methods in Molecular Biology, vol. 1467, DOI 10.1007/978-1-4939-4023-3_16, © Springer Science+Business Media New York 2016

Pax2 as well as general transcription factors such as TBP and TFIIB have been shown to physically interact with Wt1 (reviewed in ref. 1). Wt1 has also been shown to interact with transcription cofactors both coactivators and corepressors such as CBP, WTIP, and Basp1 to influence the transcriptional response.

(B) **Cell Cycle Regulators**: Wt1-interacting proteins with an implication towards cell cycle regulation such as p53 were identified initially. However, a few recent studies have identified Wt1 interaction with Htra2, a serine protease [2] with a role in apoptosis as well as interaction with a cell cycle checkpoint regulator MAD2 [3]. The heat-shock protein hsp70 which has several important regulatory roles including cell cycle is also a well-known Wt1-interacting protein [4].

(C) **Components of the Splicing Pathway**: Wt1 and its association with splicing factors and hnRNPs have been known for more than a decade. The study with U2AF65 was the outcome of a yeast two-hybrid assay, leading to the identification of a Wt1-interacting protein associated with the splicing machinery [5]. The +KTS isoform was seen to have better interaction with U2AF65. Incidentally, U2AF65 is essential for the recruitment of U2 snRNP. Yet another Wt1-interacting protein, WTAP, has also been implicated in alternative splicing events, especially the splice site selection. The Wt1 and RBM4 interaction is yet another study linking Wt1 and alternative splicing wherein minigenes were used to understand the contribution of Wt1 and RBM4 on their splicing (reviewed in ref. 6). The contribution of the isoforms as well as the actual mechanism in these processes needs further investigation.

(D) **Other Interacting Proteins**: Wt1 has also been shown to interact with structural proteins such as actin [7] and also with epigenetic factors such as DNMT1 [8] and the dioxygenase Tet2 [9] recruiting them to their target-binding sites to facilitate epigenetic modifications.

2   Materials

1. **Proteins:**

   The protein–protein interaction studies have been mostly performed with overexpression constructs wherein tagged versions of the proteins were transfected and purified from cells with the help of a tag. Thus far, only few interaction and global proteomics experiments have been performed with endogenous Wt1-expressing cell lines. All the centrifugation steps have been performed in a microfuge.

2. **Reagents:**

Agarose resins for tag purifications such as GST (Amersham), hexa-histidine (SIGMA), and anti-FLAG (SIGMA) have been used for enriching the tagged proteins as well as for interaction studies. Agarose-conjugated Wt1 antibody (sc-192) was used for the IP. Protein A/G agarose beads (sc-2003) used routinely for pre-clearing of lysates and control IPs.

2.1 Buffer Composition

1. **Gentle Lysis Buffer**: 10 mM Tris–HCl at pH 7.5, 10 mM NaCl, 10 mM EDTA, 0.5% Triton X-100, 1 mM PMSF, 1× protease inhibitor cocktail, 1 mM DTT, and 10 µg/ml of RNase A.

2. **RIPA Buffer**: 150 mM NaCl, 1% Triton X-100, 0.5% sodium deoxycholate, 0.1% SDS, 50 mM Tris–HCl, pH 8.0 with protease inhibitors (see Notes for further information)

3. **For RNA-binding proteins** (RBPs), the lysis buffer is modified to gentle lysis buffer, gentle lysis buffer: 10 mM Tris–HCl pH 7.5, 10 mM NaCl, 10 mM EDTA, 0.5% Triton X-100, 1 mM PMSF, 1× protease inhibitor cocktail, 1 mM DTT, and 10 µg/ml of RNase A. NaCl was added to the cleared lysate to a final concentration of 200 mM.

4. **Buffer 1**: 20 mM Tris–HCl (pH 7.9), 20% glycerol, 1 mM EDTA, 5 mM MgCl$_2$, 0.1% NP-40, 1 mM dithiothreitol (DTT),0.2 mM phenylmethylsulfonyl fluoride (PMSF), 0.1 M NaCl (DTT and PMSF added on the day of the experiment).

5. **Buffer 2**: 20 mM Tris–HCl (pH 7.9), 20% glycerol, 1 mM EDTA, 5 mM MgCl$_2$, 0.1% NP-40, 1 mM DTT, 0.2 mM PMSF, 1 M NaCl (add the DTT and PMSF on the day of the experiment).

6. **Buffer 3**: 20 mM Tris–HCl (pH 7.9), 20% glycerol, 5 mM MgCl$_2$, 5 mM CaCl$_2$, 0.1% NP-40, 1 mM DTT, 0.2 mM PMSF, 0.1 M NaCl (add the DTT and PMSF on the day of the experiment).

3 Methods

3.1 Yeast Two Hybrid

1. Plasmids were transformed into the respective strains using the lithium acetate method followed by analysis for interactions which was tested by growing leu–trp–his– media supplemented with 50 mM 3-amino triazole [5].

2. The β-galactosidase activity was tested by using filters from leu–trp– plates and liquid assays in leu–trp– media.

3. The activity of β-galactosidase was calculated using the following formula: $1000 \times A420 / (\text{volume} \times \text{time} \times \text{protein concentration})$.

3.2 Co-immuno-precipitation

1. To examine the interactions between Wt1 and interacting proteins, 8×10^6 cells that express Wt1 were collected by manual scraping using a scraper and pelleted by centrifugation.

2. Cell pellet was resuspended in 400 µl of gentle lysis buffer and incubated on ice for 15 min. Insoluble materials were removed by centrifugation at $13,400 \times g$ in a microcentrifuge at 4 °C for 15 min. NaCl was added to the cleared lysate to a final concentration of 200 mM.

3. Lysates are subjected to pre-clearing with 20 µl of protein A/G agarose beads at 4 °C for 1 h. Spin, at $735 \times g$ for 5 min, supernatant transferred to fresh tube.

4. 350 µl of the lysate incubated with 2 µl of Wt1-agarose-conjugated antibody, pre-immune IgG at 4 °C overnight.

5. The next day, beads were washed and bound fractions eluted by 2× SDS-sample buffer by heating at 95 °C for 5 min.

6. Proteins were resolved by SDS-PAGE, followed by western blot analysis.

3.3 Silver Staining Protocol for Mass Spec-Compatible Gel Bands

1. Gel washed in water (dH$_2$O freshly autoclaved), 2×5 min.

2. Gel fixed in 30 % ethanol: 10 % acetic acid solution, 2×15 min.

3. Gel washed in 10 % ethanol, 2×5 min, and in water, 2×5 min.

4. Gel sensitized in sensitizer working solution (50 µl sensitizer in 25 ml water), 1 min, washed in water, 2×1 min.

5. Gel stained in stain working solution (0.5 ml enhancer in 25 ml developer) for 5 min.

6. Gel developed in developer working solution (0.5 ml enhancer in 25 ml developer). Washed with water, 2×20 s. Developed for 1 min. Reaction stopped with the addition of 5 % acetic acid for 10 min. Washed with water, 2×15 min (see Notes for further information).

3.4 Label-Free Proteomics

1. $20–30 \times 10^6$ cells at confluence, monolayer washed with PBS, cells scraped in 5 ml PBS, centrifuge, pellet washed with PBS.

2. Lysed in RIPA buffer (ten times pellet cell volume (PCV)).

3. Lysate pre-cleared for 1 h using agarose slurry/beads, 4 °C on end-to-end rotor, spin, $735 \times g$ for 5 min, supernatant transferred to fresh tube (see Notes for further information).

4. IP using 1–1.5 mg of whole-cell extract (WCE) with 2–4 µg of antibody, 4 °C on end-to-end rotor, overnight.

5. Samples centrifuged at 2000 rpm for 5 min. Supernatant transferred to fresh tube and discarded after confirmation of the IP.

6. Beads washed four times with RIPA buffer at 2000 rpm for 5 min, 4 °C.

7. Beads washed twice with PBS at 2000 rpm for 5 min, 4 °C.

8. The immunoprecipitated beads subjected to snap freezing using liquid nitrogen.

3.5 Mass Spec Acquisition

The samples were digested with trypsin and then analyzed on a Q-Exactive coupled to an LC with a homemade C18 ReproSil Aq 1.8 μm column as previously described in ref. 10. Peptides were eluted using a linear gradient from 2 to 32 % acetonitrile over 40 min. Data analysis and label-free quantification were done by using MaxQuant searching against a mouse IPI database. The overall schematic of the label-free proteomic experiment is represented in Fig. 1a.

3.6 In Vitro Protein–Protein Interaction Assay

1. GST resin (10 μl packed volume so about 25 μl of resin) is taken per IP reaction.

2. Wash the resin three times with **buffer 1** (ten times volume of beads so 100 μl).

3. Protein GST and GST-Wt1 (500 ng each) mixed individually with the resin in buffer 1 and left on rotor in cold room for 1½ to 2 h.

4. Above samples centrifuged (735 × g, 4 °C, 5 min). Washed with **buffer 2**, three times, and **buffer 3**, three times (100 μl each).

5. Target protein diluted (His-tagged interacting protein X) in **buffer 3** such that there is 500 ng of protein in 5 μl volume. The washed beads from **step 4** mixed with the target protein and IP is performed in **buffer 3** in a total volume of 50 μl. In cold room, on rotor for 2 h. Samples centrifuged at 735 × g, 4 °C, 5 min. Supernatant to be used as unbound protein during western blotting.

6. Beads washed with **buffer 1,** four times (100 μl each). Sample eluted from the beads using 30 μl of SDS loading dye. Western to be probed with antibodies against the GST and His tag.

3.7 Colocalization by Immunofluorescence Analysis

1. Cells grown on cover slips, subjected to required treatment. Media aspirated. Washed with PBS (1×), three times for 2 min each.

2. Fixation with 4 % PFA (use 0.2 ml if cells on cover slips in a 24-well plate/50 μl for cells in 16-well chamber slide), 10 min at RT on shaker. PFA removed. Washed with PBS (1×), three times for 5 min each.

3. Permeabilization with 0.25 % Triton X 100 (use 0.2 ml if cells on cover slips in 24-well plate/50 μl for cells in 16-well chamber slide), 10 min RT on shaker (do not exceed the time). Triton removed, washed with PBS (1×), three times for 5 min each.

4. Blocking with 1 % BSA in 1× PBST, 30 min at RT on shaker (0.2 ml for cover slips/50 μl for 16-well chamber slide). Blocking solution discarded.

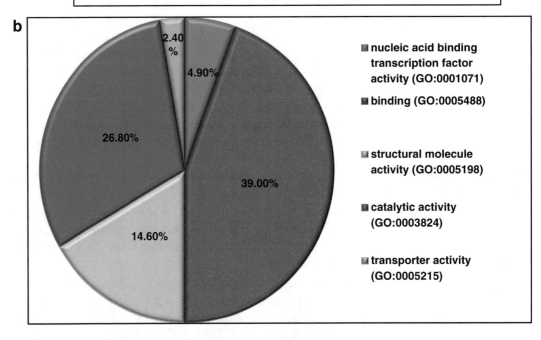

Fig. 1 An unbiased global WT1-interacting protein analysis by label-free mass spectrometry. (**a**) A brief schematic of the different steps involved in identifying Wt1-interacting proteins by label-free mass spectrometric approach. (**b**) A pie chart representation of the different gene ontology categories of Wt1-interacting proteome. The percentage in each category is also represented

5. Primary antibody to be added (if two different host antibodies are to be used, a mix of the two antibodies can also be used). 0.2 ml for cover slips/50 µl for 16-well chamber slide. Incubate at RT for 1 h. Aspirate antibody. Wash with 1× PBS (three times for 5 min each).

6. Secondary antibody or a mix added, 0.2 ml for cover slips/50 µl for 16-well chamber slide. Incubated at RT for 1 h wrapped in foil. Antibody aspirated. Washed with 1× PBS (three times for 5 min each), wrapped in foil.

7. If using chamber slide, wells and the protective seal removed. A drop of Vectashield H1200 added, cover slip placed on top. If using cover slips, on a glass slide, a drop of Vectashield H1200 added, the cover slip inverted on to the drop such that the cells are on the bottom side. Edges can be sealed with enamel for later visualization.

Antibody solutions are made in 1 % BSA in 1× PBST.

3.8 Discussion

The interactome analysis utilizes a series of different biochemical techniques to identify and characterize specific interactions. However, recent advances have allowed visualization of molecular interactions, thus providing spatial and temporal resolution to the protein interaction studies in the context of cell biology. Protein–protein interactions can now be visualized in living cells with the help of fluorescence-associated techniques such as FRET and FCS. FRET refers to the fluorescence/Förster resonance energy transfer which employs the differences in the excitation and emission energy of two fluorophores tagged to proteins as explained in ref. 11. FCS is fluorescence correlation spectroscopy which also relies on fluorophore-tagged proteins and their hydrodynamic diameter which represents changes based on interaction between the proteins [12]. These most often require additional cloning strategies to introduce the tagged version of the protein; however these techniques facilitate cellular biochemical interactions to be visualized in real time. Proximity ligation assays are yet another way of visualizing the dynamics of protein–protein interaction [13].

3.9 Protein Interaction Networks

Global protein–protein interactions can be depicted as interaction networks with the help of databases such as STRING. Alternatively, interaction data can also be analyzed for an over-representation of any particular category of proteins by using the gene ontology tools available online. An example of this is represented in Fig. 1b, where Wt1-interacting proteins identified in the epicardial cell line, enriched over a threshold of 2 in comparison to the control, were selected and submitted to the Panther database for analysis of distinct functional categories. This depicts an enrichment for Wt1-interacting proteins in the binding category, structural proteins, and catalytic activity.

4   Notes

1. Use agarose-conjugated antibodies wherever possible: If not antibodies need to be bound to the agarose slurry. (Beads equilibrated in IP buffer by washes at $326 \times g$ 3 min, twice, add antibody at required concentration in 1 ml of IP buffer, end-to-end rotor, 4 °C for 1 h, spin $326 \times g / 3$ min, remove supernatant, use these beads as the conjugated antibody for the IP.)

2. Overexpression strategies work well when matched with a good empty vector-transfected control.

3. Endogenous protein IPs are best since it does not perturb any interactions based on changes in transfection and/or expression efficiency. However, this approach requires additional controls so as to improve the efficiency of identifying true interactions.

4. Incorporation of DNase or RNase along with the lysis buffer and the IP buffer also facilitates the exclusion of nonspecific interactions.

5. PIERCE staining kit (24612) alternatively can also use the following kit (24600). Make all solutions fresh, use freshly autoclaved water (unopened before), wear gloves at all times, handle gel only with forceps if needed, and use new plates for the processing if possible.

References

1. Toska E, Roberts SG (2014) Mechanisms of transcriptional regulation by WT1 (Wilms' tumour 1). Biochem J 461(1):15–32

2. Hartkamp J, Carpenter B, Roberts SG (2010) The Wilms' tumor suppressor protein WT1 is processed by the serine protease HtrA2/Omi. Mol Cell 37(2):159–171

3. Shandilya J, Toska E, Richard DJ et al (2014) WT1 interacts with MAD2 and regulates mitotic checkpoint function. Nat Commun 5:4903

4. Maheswaran S, Englert C, Zheng G et al (1998) Inhibition of cellular proliferation by the Wilms' tumor suppressor WT1 requires association with the inducible chaperone Hsp70. Genes Dev 12(8):1108–1120

5. Davies RC, Calvio C, Bratt E et al (1998) WT1 interacts with the splicing factor U2AF65 in an isoform-dependent manner and can be incorporated into spliceosomes. Genes Dev 12(20):3217–3225

6. Morrison AA, Viney RL, Ladomery MR (2008) The post-transcriptional roles of WT1, a multifunctional zinc-finger protein. Biochim Biophys Acta 1785(1):55–62

7. Dudnakova T, Spraggon L, Slight J et al (2010) Actin: a novel interaction partner of WT1 influencing its cell dynamic properties. Oncogene 29(7):1085–1092

8. Xu B, Zeng DQ, Wu Y et al (2011) Tumor suppressor menin represses paired box gene 2 expression via Wilms' tumor suppressor protein-polycomb group complex. J Biol Chem 286(16):13937–13944

9. Wang Y, Xiao M, Chen X et al (2015) WT1 recruits TET2 to regulate its target gene expression and suppress leukemia cell proliferation. Mol Cell 57(4):662–673

10. Turriziani B, Garcia-Munoz A, Pilkington R et al (2014) On-beads digestion in conjunction with data-dependent mass spectrometry: a shortcut to quantitative and dynamic interaction proteomics. Biology (Basel) 3(2):320–332. doi:10.3390/biology3020320

11. Truong K, Ikura M (2001) The use of FRET imaging microscopy to detect protein-protein interactions and protein conformational changes in vivo. Curr Opin Struct Biol 11(5):573–578

12. Macháň R, Wohland T (2014) Recent applications of fluorescence correlation spectroscopy in live systems. FEBS Lett 588(19):3571–3584

13. Söderberg O, Leuchowius KJ, Gullberg M et al (2008) Characterizing proteins and their interactions in cells and tissues using the in situ proximity ligation assay. Methods 45(3):227–232

Chapter 17

Methods to Identify and Validate WT1–RNA Interaction

Ruthrothaselvi Bharathavikru and Tatiana Dudnakova

Abstract

Tumor suppressor protein, Wt1 is a transcription factor that binds to DNA sequence similar to the Early Growth Response gene, EGR1 consensus binding sequence. Biophysical and biochemical validations have shown that the zinc fingers of Wt1 are capable of binding to both DNA and RNA albeit with different binding affinities which potentially is also isoform specific. SELEX based identification of the RNA binding motifs led to the identification of motifs which could not be translated into the in vivo context. With the advent of recent technologies that allow cross-linking of RNA and protein and high throughput sequencing techniques, it is now possible to analyze the in vivo RNA binding interactome of Wt1. This chapter outlines the initial studies that were aimed at addressing the Wt1 RNA interactome and also provides a detailed overview of some of the recent techniques used.

Key words RNA, NGS, IP, CLIP

1 Introduction

1.1 Wt1 Binds to DNA and RNA

Wilms' tumor suppressor protein, Wt1 is a transcription factor with four zinc fingers in the C-terminus. Several isoforms of this protein exist because of features like alternative start sites, RNA editing, and splicing. Of these different isoforms, the evolutionarily conserved isoforms are two, that differ from each other by the presence of absence of three amino acids KTS. An alternative splice site results in the insertion of these three amino acids between exon 9 and 10, referred to as the +KTS isoform (reviewed in ref. 1). The –KTS isoform binds to DNA sequences similar to the EGR1 consensus site. Due to the insertion of the amino acids, the +KTS isoform is structurally impeded in its DNA binding and hence has less affinity towards DNA. However, colocalization studies have shown the predominant +KTS isoform to be present in spliceosomes implicating an association with RNA. Biochemical validations have indeed shown that the +KTS isoform binds to RNA with greater affinity than the –KTS isoform which are summarized below.

Nicholas Hastie (ed.), *The Wilms' Tumor (WT1) Gene: Methods and Protocols*, Methods in Molecular Biology, vol. 1467, DOI 10.1007/978-1-4939-4023-3_17, © Springer Science+Business Media New York 2016

1.2 In Vitro and In Vivo RNA Interaction

One of the compelling pieces of evidence of Wt1 and RNA interaction was the observation wherein the mouse +KTS of Wt1 in *Xenopus* oocytes was shown to be preferentially enriched on nascent transcripts [2]. It also led to the identification that zinc finger 1 is more important for the RNA binding ability because the absence led to the failure to sediment with the RNP components. Subsequent experiments also revealed that Wt1 associates with mRNP particles both in fetal as well as cancer cell lines [3]. There have also been data to show the localization of the Wt1 isoforms with snRNPs. It is also of interest to mention that it has been observed that the Wt1 consensus sequence is present in the 5′ UTR of several candidate genes. A putative RNA recognition motif (RRM) was identified by structural modeling at the N-terminus but no functional study has shown its importance. There have been attempts to study this interaction using SELEX based approaches using the zinc fingers of Wt1. Biophysical binding studies have shown that the zinc fingers have RNA binding ability [4]. Some structural investigations have been done with the RNA aptamers, however their functional validation has not been done yet. Other experiments using IP followed by enrichment for RNAs has led to the identification of a structural protein associated network [5]. Based on all the above findings, it is clear that Wt1 and RNA interplay is involved in several steps of RNA metabolism with functional implications in different cellular events.

2 Materials

2.1 Cell Lines

Mesonephric cell line M15 and epicardial cell line, CoMEEC were used for the experiments.

2.2 Reagents

3′ linkermiRCat-33 linker (IDT) AppTGGAATTCTCGGG TGCCAAG/ddC/5′ linkers (barcode marked red)L5Aa invddT-ACACrGrArCrGrCrUrCrUrUrCrCrGrArUrCrUrNrNrNrUrArA rGrC-OH L5Ab invddT-ACACrGrArCrGrCrUrCrUrUrCrCrGr ArUrCrUrNrNrNrArUrUrArGrC-OHL5Ac invddT-ACACrGrA rCrGrCrUrCrUrUrCrCrGrArUrCrUrNrNrNrGrCrGrCrArGrC-OHL5Bb invddT-ACACrGrArCrGrCrUrCrUrUrCrCrGrArUrCr UrNrNrNrGrUrGrArGrC-OHL5Bc invddT-ACACrGrArCrGrCr UrCrUrUrCrCrGrArUrCrUrNrNrNrCrArCrUrArGrC-OHL5Bd invddT-ACACrGrArCrGrCrUrCrUrUrCrCrGrArUrC rUrNrNrNrUrCrUrCrUrArGrC-OHL5Ca invddT-ACACrGrAr CrGrCrUrCrUrUrCrCrGrArUrCrUrNrNrNrCrUrArGrC-L5Cb invddT-ACACrGrArCrGrCrUrCrUrUrCrCrGrArUrCrUr NrNrNrGrGrArGrC-OHL5Cc invddT-ACACrGrArCrGrCrUrCr UrUrCrCrGrArUrCrUrNrNrNrArCrTrCrArGrC-OHL5Cd invddT-ACACrGrArCrGrCrUrCrUrUrCrCrGrArUrCrUrNrN rNrGrArCrTrTrArGrC-Barcode sequence together with short experiment title in each case is used in the sample name for the ease of data processingNNNTAAGC for L5AaNNNATTAGC for L5AbNNNGCGCAGC for L5AcNNNCGCTTAGC for L5AdNNNGTGAGC for L5BbNNNCACTAGC for L5Bc NNNTCTCTAGC for L5BdNNNCTAGC for L5CaNNNTGGA GCforL5CbNNNACTCAGCforL5CcNNNGACTTAGCforL5Cd PCR primersmiRCat-33 primer (IDT) CCTTGGCACCCGA GAATT primer for RLibrary Amplification Primers:PE_miRCat_ PCR CAAGCAGAAGACGGCATACGAGATCGGTCTCGGCAT TCCTGGCCTTGGCACCCGAGAATTCCP5 AATGATACGGC GACCACCGAGATCTACACTCTTTCCCTAC ACGACGCTCTTCCGATCTOligos for EMSAs are ordered from SIGMA

2.3 Equipment

1. UV cross-linking is done in a Stratagene cross-linker.
2. Centrifugation is performed in an Eppendorf microfuge.

2.4 Buffer Composition

1. Binding buffer 10×: 100 mM Tris–HCl pH 7.9, 500 mM KCl, 10 mM DTT, 10 mM EDTA.
2. Lysis buffer: 50 mM HEPES, 140 mM NaCl, 1 mM EDTA, 1% (v/v) Triton X-100, 0.1% (w/v) sodium deoxycholate (before use add protease inhibitors and 40 U RNasin).
3. Wash buffer: 50 mM HEPES, pH 7.5, 500 mM NaCl, 1 mM EDTA, 1% (v/v) Triton X-100, 0.1% (w/v) sodium deoxycholate (before use add 40 U RNasin per ml buffer).
4. CLASH buffers:
   (a) Lysis buffer: (20 mM Tris-HCl pH 7.4, 150 mM NaCl, 0.4% NP-40, 2 mM MgCl$_2$, 1 mM DTT, protease inhibitors (Roche, cOmplete, EDTA-free), RNAse Inhibitor (Promega)).
   (b) PBS-WB buffer: (PBS, +150 mM NaCl, 2 mM MgCl$_2$, 0.4% NP-40).
   (c) EB (elution buffer: NuPAGE protein sample buffer plus 20 mM Tris–HCl, 1% SDS, 100 mM ME (β-mercaptoethanol)).
   (d) HS-PBS-WB: (PBS, 0.3 M NaCl, 2 mM MgCl2, 0.4% NP-40).
   (e) UB: (20 mM Tris–HCl pH 7.4, 2 M UREA, 0.15 M NaCl, 0.4% NP-40).
   (f) PNK buffer: (50 mM Tris–HCl pH 7.5, 10 mM MgCl2, 0.5% NP-40, 50 mM NaCl).
   (g) Proteinase K buffer: (50 mM Tris–HCl pH 7.8, 50 mM NaCl, 0.4% NP-40, 0.5% SDS, 5 mM EDTA).
5. RNP Lysis buffer: (20 mM Tris–HCl, pH 8, 140 mM KCl, 1.5 mM MgCl$_2$, 0.5% NP-40, 0.5 mM DTT).
6. Interaction buffer: 20 mM Tris–HCl, pH 8.0, 140 mM KCl, 4 mM MgCl$_2$, 0.75 mM DTT, 0.1% NP-40, 0.1 u/µl *E. coli* tRNA.

3   Methods

3.1   RNA Immunoprecipitation (RIP)

This protocol involves three distinct stages: (1) cross-linking, (2) immunoprecipitation, and (3) recovery of RNA.

3.1.1   Cross-Linking

This is variable based on the experimental strategy and can either be native when there is no cross-linking involved or formaldehyde cross-linking which leads to more general cross-linking or UV cross-linking which involves capturing interactions at distinct sites [6]. The UV cross-linking strategy can be further modified such that individual nucleotides can be cross-linked and identified. A representation of these different strategies is represented in Fig. 1.

(a) Formaldehyde Cross-Linking:

1. Confluent cells are washed with PBS (10 ml per 15 cm dish) after aspirating media.

2. The cells are cross-linked using 0.25 ml of 38% formaldehyde directly on the cells and incubated on shaker platform for 10 min at room temperature.

3. The cross-linking is neutralized by the addition of 1 ml of 2 M glycine and incubated on shaker platform for 10 min at room temperature.

4. The above solution is removed and the cells are scraped in 10 ml of ice-cold PBS, and centrifuged at $76 \times g$ for 10 min.

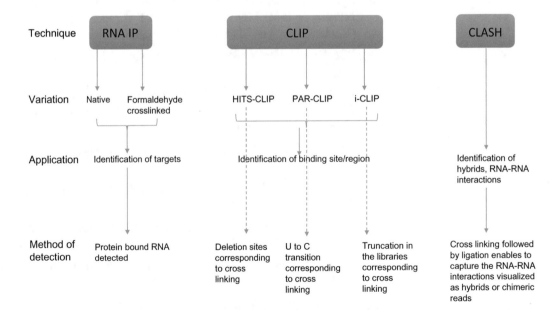

Different Approaches to Study RNA interactome

Fig. 1 Different approaches to study RNA interactome

5. The supernatant is discarded and the pellet is transferred to a 1.5 ml microfuge tube using 1 ml PBS.

(b) UV Cross-Linking:

1. Confluent cells are washed with PBS (10 ml per 15 cm dish) after aspirating media.

2. Cells are cross-linked using the cross-linker at (1200 μjoules/s) using the optimal cross-link function. (see Notes for further information)

3. The cells are scraped in minimal volume of PBS (1–2 ml) and centrifuged at $81.6 \times g$ for 10 min.

4. The pellet is washed with 5 ml PBS and processed as in (a), **step 5**.

(c) Native Cross-Linking:

1. Confluent cells are washed with PBS (10 ml per 15 cm dish) after aspirating media.

2. Cells are scraped in minimal volume of PBS (1–2 ml) and centrifuged at $81.6 \times g$ for 10 min.

3. The pellet is washed with 5 ml PBS and processed as in (a), **step 5**.

3.1.2   RIP

1. Cell pellet is resuspended in ice-cold PBS, and centrifuged at $117.5 \times g$ for 5 min at 4 °C.

2. Cell pellet is resuspended in lysis buffer (0.4 ml), and kept on ice for 5 min.

3. Sonicated at 5 sec on and 5 sec off pulse, six times.

4. To the sonicated extract, the following components are added, 25 mM $MgCl_2$, 5 mM $CaCl_2$, RNasin (3 μl of 40u/μl stock), RNase free DNaseI (6 μl of 1500 k Ustock), and incubated at 37 °C for 15 min.

5. The above reaction stopped by the addition of 20 mM EDTA and samples are centrifuged at $11752 \times g$ for 5 min.

Bead Preparation

1. Magnetic beads (Pierce A/G) resuspended by gentle shaking and pipetting.

2. Tubes labeled as per the IP conditions.

3. 25 μl of the magnetic beads is added to each of the tubes, 0.25 ml of the RIP wash buffer is added to each tube and vortexed. Tubes placed on the magnetic rack. After solution has separated, the supernatant is removed.

4. The above step repeated once again to wash the beads.

IP

1. Tubes are removed from the magnetic stand; 0.1 ml of RIP lysis buffer added to the tube, 2 μg of WT1 antibody added to the tube and incubated at RT for 30 min on end to end rotor.

2. After incubation with the antibody, tubes are centrifuged at $734 \times g$ for 2 min, placed on magnetic stand and supernatant discarded.

3. 0.5 ml of RIP lysis buffer is added to the beads, and vortexed. Placed on magnetic stand and supernatant discarded. The above step repeated twice.

4. IP done with RIP lysis buffer: 860 μl + 0.5 M EDTA (35 μl) and RNase inhibitor (5 μl).

5. 0.6 ml of above RIP buffer added to each tube and 0.4 ml of lysate added to each tube (adjusted according to the lysate volume).

6. 10% of the above lysates is stored to be included as input sample in the Subheading 3.1.3.

7. IP was done overnight on end to end rotor at 4 °C.

Washes

1. Post IP the tubes are placed on the magnetic stand to facilitate separation.

2. 0.5 ml of RIP lysis buffer is used for wash, six times (each time, buffer added, vortexed and placed on magnetic stand for aiding in separation), followed by washes with wash buffer for three times.

3.1.3 RNA Precipitation

1. To the magnetic beads, the following is added, 150 μl of proteinase K buffer, 117 μl of RIP wash buffer +15 μl of 10 % SDS +18 μl of 10 mg/ml proteinase K.

2. Input samples from **step 6**, Subheading 3.1.2.2 (10 μl) + 107 μl of RIP wash buffer +15 μl of 10 % SDS +18 μl of proteinase K and incubated at 55 °C for 30 min, on thermomixer.

3. Reverse cross-linking is performed at 65 °C for 1 h, on a thermomixer.

4. Samples are centrifuged briefly to collect all the contents and placed on magnetic rack for separation. Supernatant transferred to fresh tube.

5. 0.25 ml of RIP wash buffer is added to each tube, and 0.4 ml of acidified phenol–chloroform is added, then vortexed for 15 s, centrifuged at $13792 \times g$ for 10 min.

6. Supernatant transferred to fresh tube, and to each of the tubes, the following is added, 40 μl of sodium acetate +1 μl of glycogen +850 μl of absolute ethanol. Mixed well and left at −80 for minimum 1 h.

7. Samples centrifuged at $13792 \times g$ for 30 min at 4 °C. Pellet washed with 70 % ethanol and air-dried.

8. Sample resuspended in 20 μl of nuclease free water. Vortexed mildly and concentration estimated by bioanalyzer.

3.1.4 cDNA Library Preparation

Double stranded cDNA synthesis of RNA-IP samples.

First Strand cDNA Synthesis (Done in a Thermal Cycler)

1. IP RNA—9.5 µl.
2. Random Primers—1 µl (200 pmol in total).
3. Water—to a total volume of 10.5 µl.

   Incubate at 70 °C for 10 min, followed by incubation on ice.

   To the above reaction, the following components are added.

1. RT buffer 5X—4 µl.
2. DTT—2 µl.
3. AMV 25u/µl—1 µl.
4. Protector RNase inhibitor—0.5 µl.
5. dNTP mix—2 µl.

   Incubate at 42 °C for 60 min, followed by incubation on ice to terminate the reaction.

Second Strand Synthesis (Done in a Thermal Cycler)

1. cDNA from above step—20 µl.
2. Second strand buffer—15 µl.
3. dNTP mix—0.75 µl.
4. Second strand enzyme mix—3.25 µl.
5. Water—36 µl.

   (a) Total reaction volume of 75 µl.
   (b) Incubate at 16 °C for 2 h, followed by addition of 10 µl of T4 DNA polymerase.
   (c) Incubate at 16 °C for 5 min.
   (d) Terminate reaction by addition of 8.5 µl of 0.2 M EDTA, pH 8.0.

Digestion of RNA

1. 0.75 µl of RNase I is added to the above reaction mix.
2. Incubate at 37 °C for 30 min.
3. 2.5 µl of proteinase K is added to the reaction.
4. Incubate at 37 °C for 30 min.

Cleaning of dsDNA

1. Double stranded cDNA samples are subjected to phenol–chloroform extraction.
2. Supernatant is precipitated using 0.6 volume of 5 M ammonium acetate and 2.5 volumes of absolute ethanol.
3. Incubate at –80 for minimum 1 h
4. Centrifuge at $13792 \times g$ for 20 min in a mini centrifuge.
5. Pellet is washed with ethanol.
6. Pellet is air-dried and resuspended in 13 µl of water; 2 µl is used for bioanalyzer.

3.2 CLASH

CLASH refers to the Cross-linking and Association of Hybrids [7], a modified version of CLASH has been carried out to obtain endogenous interactions.

3.2.1 UV Cross-Linking

Mouse kidney mesonephric M15 cells are grown to 90% confluency and are UV cross-linked on ice with $\lambda = 254$ nm in Stratalinker 1800, at 400 mJ/cm^2.

3.2.2 Cell Lysis and Wt1 Bound Complexes Purification

1. M15 cells are lysed by addition of ice-cold CLASH lysis buffer. 10 µl of RQ1DNAse is added and the samples are mixed by pipetting and incubated for 10 min at room temperature.

2. Lysates are centrifuged in Eppendorf mini centrifuge at 14,000 rpm and 4 °C for 10 min and supernatant is collected.

3. Protein A beads conjugated with IgG and anti-WT1 C19 antibody are washed with PBS/0.4% NP40.

4. Cell lysates are incubated with IgG- or C19-beads for 60 min at 4 °C. Supernatant is discarded and the recovered beads are washed twice with PBS-WB buffer and once in 1× PBS with 2 mM MgCl$_2$.

5. RNAse treatment: RNP complexes bound to the beads are treated with 0.5 unit RNaseA + T1 mix (RNace-IT, Stratagene) in 100 µl PBS, 2 mM MgCl$_2$ buffer for 10 min at 20 °C. To remove indirect RNA and protein binding from WT1–RNA complexes the beads are washed again twice with PBS-WB buffer.

6. Beads were re-suspended in 100 µL of PBS, followed by 100 µl of 1% formalin in PBS and complexes cross linked for 1 min at room temperature. 50 µl of 1M Tris-HCl pH 7.4 and 50 µL of 2M Glycine (neutral pH) is added and incubated 5 min on ice, then washed twice with 4M UREA/PBS/0.4% NP40 buffer, twice with PBS-NP40 buffer, thrice with 1x PNK buffer.

3.2.3 Linkers' Ligation and RNA–Protein Complexes Recovery

1. To remove unwanted 3′ phosphate groups from bound RNA fragments the complexes are treated with TSAP phosphatase in the phosphatase buffer for 40 min at room temperature.

2. To inactivate the enzyme, the beads are washed once with UB and 3 times with PNK buffer.

3. The complexes on the beads are incubated with 40 units T4 Polynucleotide kinase, first with P32 labeled ATP for 45 min, then for 20 min with 1 mM cold ATP, in PNK buffer with RNase inhibitors at room temperature. The beads are then washed as before once with UB and 4 times with PNK buffer.

4. WT1-bound RNA molecules are ligated together and with 3′ linker (1 µM miRCat-33), overnight using 40 units of T4 RNA ligase 1 in PNK buffer with RNase inhibitors at 16 °C. The next day, the beads are washed as before once with UB and four times with PNK buffer.

5. 40 units of RNA ligase 1, barcoded 5′ linkers (final conc. 5 μM; one for each sample) are ligated in RNA ligase 1 buffer with 1 mM ATP for 3–6 h at 20 °C. The beads are washed as before, once with UB and four times with PNK buffer.

6. The samples are eluted in NuPAGE protein sample buffer plus 20 mM Tris–HCl, 1 % SDS, 100 mM ME (β -mercaptoethanol). Boiled for 2 minutes at 98°C. The samples are centrifuged for a minute to recover the supernatant with RNA–protein complexes.

3.2.4 SDS-PAGE and Transfer

1. Protein–RNA complexes in NuPAGE SB plus SDS, ME are resolved on a 4–12 % bis-tris NuPAGE gel in NuPAGE SDS MOPS running buffer followed by transfer to nitrocellulose membrane in NuPage transfer buffer with 10 % methanol for 1 h at 100 V.

2. Depending on the strength of the signal the membrane is exposed on film for 1 h or overnight at –70 °C.

3. The developed film is aligned with the membrane and the radioactive bands corresponding to the WT1–RNA complexes are excised.

3.2.5 Proteinase K Treatment and RNA Isolation

1. The excised bands are incubated with 150 μg of Proteinase K (Roche) and proteinase K buffer for 2 h at 55 °C.

2. The RNA is extracted with phenol–chloroform–isoamyl alcohol (PCI) mixture and ethanol-precipitated overnight with 10 μg of glycogen.

3.2.6 cDNA Library Preparation

1. The isolated RNA is dissolved in 12 μl of distilled RNAse-free water and reverse-transcribed using miRCat-33 primer with Superscript III Reverse Transcriptase in its buffer for 1 h at 50 °C.

2. RNA is then degraded by addition of RNase H for 30 min at 37 °C. cDNA is amplified using primers P5 and primer PE_miRCat_PCR and TaKaRa LA Taq polymerase.

3. PCR products are separated on a 2 % MetaPhor agarose gel with SYBRSafe in 1× TBE at 4 °C. The gel band corresponding to 150–200 bp is excised.

4. cDNA is purified with MinElute Gel Extraction Kit and the purified cDNA libraries are sent for high-throughput sequencing.

3.3 Electrophoretic Mobility Shift Assays (EMSA)

1. Nuclear extract aliquots are prepared using cytoplasmic nuclear fractionation kit as per manufacturer's protocols. The nuclear extracts are verified by western blotting to confirm Wt1 expression. The nuclear extracts (NE) are quantified for their protein content and stored as aliquots in –80 °C.

2. Competitor oligos and labeled oligos also referred to as the "hot" oligo is 3′ boitin tagged are reconstituted to 100 μM

concentration. Also needed are the complementary oligo and a non-tagged version.

3. 6% acrylamide gel is prepared with 0.5% TBE.

4. 100 μM oligos are diluted 1:1000 with water and the following annealing reaction is carried out.

F oligo	10 μl
R oligo*	10 μl
H restriction buffer	10 μl
Water	70 μl
The above components heated to 95 °C for 5 min, and allowed to cool to room temperature	

5. Competitor oligos are processed as follows:

F oligo	10 μl
R oligo	10 μl
H restriction buffer	10 μl
Water	70 μl
Heated to 95 °C for 5 min, and allowed to cool to room temperature	
The competition oligos are diluted 1:10 to give 50× excess	

6. Binding reaction is prepared as follows:

– NE	2 μl (4 μg of protein)
– dI/dC	1 μl (1 mg/ml solution)
– Binding buffer	1.5 μl
– Competitor if required	2 μl (50× excess, 1 pmol)
– Water	
– Oligo*	2 μl (20 fmols)
– Total	15 μl
All reagents except the hot* oligo are added together and incubated for 10 min on ice	

7. Hot oligo* is added and incubated at room temperature for 20 min.

8. The samples are mixed with 4 μl of 30% sucrose/BPB loading dye and loaded on to the 6% gel from **step 3**.

9. The samples are electrophoresed in 0.5% TBE until dye front reaches the bottom of the gel and transferred in 0.5% TBE on nitrocellulose (in the cold room).

10. Filters are subjected to UV cross-linking using the optimal cross-link option.

11. The filters are developed with Chemiluminescent Nucleic Acid Detection Kit as per the manufacturers' instructions.

3.4 RNA–Protein Cross-Linking Experiment

1. Cells (2×10^7) are pelleted and resuspended in 1 ml of RNP lysis buffer and centrifuged at $14,000 \times g$ for 10 min at 4 °C.

2. Glycerol is added to the supernatant at a final concentration of 5%.

3. Cytoplasmic extract is stored in –80 °C freezer, in aliquots at a concentration of 5–7 μg/μl.

4. Radiolabeled (RNA regions such as 5′ UTR, fragments of coding regions, 3′ UTR) fragments are synthesized at a 30 Ci uridine/mmol concentration.

5. Oligo template hybridized to T7 promoter primer.

T7 promoter primer	2 μl
DNA hyb buffer	6 μl
Oligo template (100 μM)	2 μl

6. Samples are heated to 70 °C for 5 min, left at room temperature for 5 min to hybridize.

7. Klenow filling

To the above reaction, the following components are added.	
10X Klenow reaction buffer	2 μl
10X dNTP mix	2 μl
Nuclease free water	4 μl
Exo-klenow	2 μl
Components are mixed well, centrifuged briefly, and incubated at 37 °C for 30 min.	

8. Transcription of probe:

10X transcription buffer	2 μl
dsDNA template	5 μl
A/C/G 10 mM	1 μl
Alpha-UTP*	5 μl
T7 RNA pol	2 μl
Water	5 μl
Incubated for 30 min at 37 °C.	
To the above, 1 μl of DNase I is added and further incubated for 10 min at 37 °C.	
Samples are heated for 1 min at 95 °C, placed on ice followed by addition of 10 ml of hybridization buffer added.	

9. Approximately, 15 μg of protein (lysate) is incubated with 100 nCi of labeled RNA fragments for 25 min at room temperature in 10 μl of the interaction buffer.

10. The above samples are irradiated with 254 nm wavelength UV for 30 min at 5.4 J/cm^2 on ice.

11. Excess probe is removed by digestion with 0.5 μg of RNase A at 37 °C for 25 min.

12. The samples are electrophoresed on 10 % SDS-PAGE and subjected to autoradiography.

3.5 Discussion

Recent techniques coupled with next generation sequencing technologies have hugely impacted the field of RNA protein interactions. The earlier approaches such as SELEX identified a few potential RNA binding motifs; however, when these were used as baits, no physiological targets were identified except α-actinin. This was an indication towards the possibility that the endogenous interactions are likely to be tissue specific and also transient or dynamic thus necessitating approaches that can exploit endogenous interactions. The RNA IP approach and the CLASH approaches are precisely engineered towards these needs since RIP can provide information about Wt1 interacting RNA targets (an example depicted in Fig. 2), whereas the latter can provide information about binding sites as well as provide insights about the potential Wt1 RNA complex. Although CLASH relies on tagged proteins, it should be possible to adopt this to endogenous proteins using modifications to the cross-linking approaches.

3.6 Future Perspectives

The identification and elucidation of the Wt1 RNA interactome has only been possible by employing a variety of techniques including biochemical and sequencing approaches. This is very similar to the early advances in the field of protein–protein interactions which have now moved on to visualization of these interactions within the cell. There have been a few studies recently wherein the RNA–protein interaction have been attempted to be visualized in the

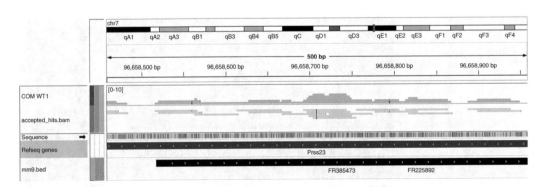

Fig. 2 CoMEEC cells that express endogenous Wt1 are subjected to RNA IP, followed by sequencing of the libraries. Represented above is an example of an alignment of the sequencing reads obtained to the noncoding regions within the Prss23 coding region

in vivo context. Although this involves fluorescent tagging of the molecules involved, thus not exactly a correlation of what is relevant in the physiological scenario, it is possible that with the CRISPR strategy, endogenous molecules can be visualized interacting in real time.

4   Notes

1. The cross-linking approaches can be varied depending on the need of the experiment. If the overall experimental strategy is towards identifying RNA targets of a particular protein, native or formaldehyde cross-linking suffice. However, UV cross-linking can provide more information on the binding sites.

2. Cells that are being processed for cross-linking should be always kept on ice so as to preserve any transient interactions. For cells that are to be subjected to UV cross-linking, it is advised to grow them on dishes rather than flasks, to maximize the cross-linking. The cells should be covered with minimal volume of PBS (about 1–2 ml) during the UV cross-linking procedure.

3. The samples during the processing for RNA interactions can be frozen at various time points such as after cross-linking in Subheading 3.1.1. The pellets can be subjected to flash freezing.

4. The fragmentation of RNA either before the IP or during the input sample preparation also influences the outcome of the experiment. Generally, if no fragmentation step has been included, the entire molecule is purified and thus impedes any binding motif identification. However, if sonicated fragments are used, or RNase digestion is performed, the overall enrichment of smaller fragments can lead to identification of potential binding motifs.

References

1. Hohenstein P, Hastie ND (2006) The many facets of the Wilms' tumour gene, WT1. Hum Mol Genet 15(Spec No 2):R196–R201

2. Ladomery M, Sommerville J, Woolner S et al (2003) Expression in Xenopus oocytes shows that WT1 binds transcripts in vivo, with a central role for zinc finger one. J Cell Sci 116(Pt 8):1539–1549

3. Niksic M, Slight J, Sanford JR et al (2004) The Wilms' tumour protein (WT1) shuttles between nucleus and cytoplasm and is present in functional polysomes. Hum Mol Genet 13(4):463–471

4. Zhai G, Iskandar M, Barilla K et al (2001) Characterization of RNA aptamer binding by the Wilms' tumor suppressor protein WT1. Biochemistry 40(7):2032–2040

5. Morrison AA, Venables JP, Dellaire G et al (2006) The Wilms' tumour suppressor protein WT1 (+KTS isoform) binds alpha-actinin 1 mRNA via its zinc-finger domain. Biochem Cell Biol 84(5):789–798

6. König J, Zarnack K, Luscombe NM et al (2012) Protein-RNA interactions: new genomic technologies and perspectives. Nat Rev Genet 13(2):77–83

7. Helwak A, Tollervey D (2014) Mapping the miRNA interactome by cross-linking ligation and sequencing of hybrids (CLASH). Nat Protoc 9(3):711–728

Chapter 18

Bioinformatic Analysis of Next-Generation Sequencing Data to Identify WT1-Associated Differential Gene and Isoform Expression

Stuart Aitken and Ruthrothaselvi Bharathavikru

Abstract

Differential gene expression analysis has been conventionally performed by microarray techniques; however with the recent advent of next-generation sequencing (NGS) approaches, it has become easier to analyze the coding as well as the noncoding components. Additionally, NGS data analysis also provides information regarding the expression changes of specific isoforms. There are several bioinformatics tools available to analyze NGS data but with different parameters. This chapter provides a comparative insight into these tools by utilizing NGS datasets available from Wt1 knockout and embryonic stem cell line model.

Key words Next-generation sequencing (NGS), Cuffdiff2, DESeq2, edgeR

1 Next-Generation Sequencing Data Analysis: Current Challenges

High-throughput sequencing is a rapidly developing technology with diverse applications including de novo DNA sequence assembly, SNP detection, and the detection of differentially expressed genes. In contrast with earlier techniques, there is no need to specify probe sequences or any restriction to a reference genome assembly [1]. Sequencing costs are reducing and this is another factor contributing to the increased use of this technique.

However, estimating the abundance of RNA transcripts from sequencing data is not without difficulty. Early approaches treated the read data simply as count data—read counts per transcript have been shown to be linearly related to transcript abundance—and used the Poisson distribution as the underlying statistical model [2]. Problems have subsequently been identified with this assumption as counts typically show a variance that is greater than the mean (mean and variance are the same in the Poisson distribution, which has a single parameter λ) [2]. The assumed distribution plays a role in testing for differential expression, hence impacts on the assignment of differential expression.

Nicholas Hastie (ed.), *The Wilms' Tumor (WT1) Gene: Methods and Protocols*, Methods in Molecular Biology, vol. 1467,
DOI 10.1007/978-1-4939-4023-3_18, © Springer Science+Business Media New York 2016

It has been noted that the variance in sequencing read counts varies with the mean; hence many attempts have been made to estimate dispersion (the disparity between the variance and the mean) from the available data, usually as a function of the mean, and use the negative binomial distribution (which has two parameters, the mean and variance) when testing for differential expression.

The state-of-the-art tools for differential expression testing include DESeq2 [3], Cuffdiff2 [4], and edgeR [5]. DESeq2 adopts the negative binomial distribution and applies sophisticated techniques to estimate dispersion on a per-gene basis, detect outliers, and prevent type I errors (false positives). DESeq2 calculates an estimate of the fold change that is moderated, that is, reduced in absolute value in comparison with a simple estimate from raw read counts. Cuffdiff2 estimates the read counts for each isoform of each gene, rather than treating each gene as a single entity, adopting the beta-negative binomial distribution for testing differential expression. Trapnell et al. note that for genes with multiple isoforms, a change in fragment count for a gene does not necessarily mean a change in expression but may indicate a change in isoform abundance [4]. Distinguishing the expression of alternative isoforms is of interest in many situations, for example, to distinguish isoforms of Wt1 with and without the KTS sequence as described below.

A recent comparison of differential expression tools [1] concluded that the number of biological replicates was a major factor: where two or more replicates were available the tools made similarly good predictions. In the absence of replicates, differences in calls of significant genes were more notable.

In this chapter, we present protocols for running Cuffdiff2 and DESeq2. Following is the protocol for generating expression data from cell line models.

2 Materials

2.1 Cell Lines

Mouse ES cell line E14 and the Wt1 knockout ES line (KO1A) were cultured as a monolayer with retinoic acid (1 μM) for 5 days in ES cell media without LIF [6].

2.2 RNA Isolation

These cell lines were processed for RNA isolation using the Qiagen RNAeasy mini columns as per the manufacturer's protocol.

2.3 Library Preparation

The isolated total RNA was subjected to Poly A selection and subjected to library preparation with the NEBnext Ultra RNA library kit for Illumina for performing NGS.

3   Methods

3.1   RNA Isolation

1. Cells were harvested by trypsinization and collected in PBS followed by lysis in RLT buffer + β-mercaptoethanol as recommended. Centrifuged at 8049 × g for 3 min in a microfuge.

2. The supernatant was mixed with equal volume of absolute ethanol and added to the RNeasy Qiagen columns (700 μl at a time). Centrifuged at 13792 × g for 1 min in a microfuge.

3. The columns were washed with RW1 buffer (700 μl). Centrifuged at 13792 × g for 1 min in a microfuge.

4. The columns were washed with RPE buffer with ethanol (500 μl), twice. Centrifuge at 13792 × g for 1 min. Centrifuge again at 13792 g for 2 min in a microfuge.

5. To the columns, 30 μl of RNase-free water was added to elute RNA. The columns were centrifuged at 13792 × g for 1 min to collect the RNA sample in a microfuge tube.

6. RNA concentration was estimated by nanodrop and stored in –80 °C till further use.

3.2   Samples for RNA Sequencing

1. mRNA was polyA+ enriched from the total RNA sample of 1 μg.

2. cDNA synthesis was performed by random hexamer priming and subjected to enrichment.

3. The above samples were barcoded and multiplexed, and subjected to sequencing on the Illumina platform to obtain 50 bp single reads.

3.3   Data Analysis Protocols

Here we present the essential steps in the computational analysis of the unpaired 50 bp reads generated by Illumina sequencing described above. The following protocols are easily adapted to the situation where sequencing data for multiple biological replicates is available.

3.3.1   Cuffdiff2 Protocol

The Cuffdiff2 analysis requires the following tools to be installed and run at the command line: bowtie2 (v2.2.3), tophat2 (v2.0.13), cufflinks (v2.2.0), and samtools (0.1.18). Files from the Ensembl mouse genome assembly mm9/mm10 must also be installed (available from http://support.illumina.com/sequencing/sequencing_software/igenome.html). The following protocol is based on [7]. The steps in the protocol are organized into bash shell scripts that specify the resource files and command arguments needed. These scripts are designed to be run at the command line (full paths to files are omitted for brevity, they should be substituted for <path>).

Each replicate sequencing data set for each condition should first be aligned to the genome (**step 1**). Note that the label "X" should be replaced by a meaningful term such as wild type (WT) or knockout (KO) (which could be read from the command line). When using a gtf annotation file (tophat2 -G option), the chromosome names, i.e., 1, 2, 3 or chr1, chr2 chr3, in the gtf file must match those in the bowtie2 index (use bowtie2-inspect –names <index-file> to check). Cufflinks can also be run with a gtf file as input when attempting to identify novel transcripts in the context of an established reference [8] but this option is not essential [7].

Cuffdiff2 Step 1. Script to run tophat2 and cufflinks on sequencing data X (bowtie2 is used for alignment). Note that the results of the alignment and cufflinks results are written to the directories tophat_X and cufflinks_X, respectively. The samtools commands sort and index the bam file for use in genome browsers such as IGV.

```
#!/bin/sh
bowtie2index="<path>/Mus_musculus/Ensembl/NCBIM37/
Sequence/Bowtie2Index/genome"
gtffile="<path>/Mus_musculus/Ensembl/NCBIM37/
Annotation/Genes/genes.gtf"

tophat2 -p 4 -o tophat_X -G $gtffile $bowtie2index
sequencing_data_X.fastq
cd tophat_X
if test -f accepted_hits.bam
then {
        samtools  sort  accepted_hits.bam  accepted_
        hitsSorted;
        samtools index  accepted_hitsSorted.bam;
        mv accepted_hitsSorted.bam accepted_hits.bam;
        mv accepted_hitsSorted.bam.bai accepted_hits.
        bam.bai; }
fi
cd ..
cufflinks -p 4 -o cufflinks_X ./tophat_X/accepted_hits.bam
```

Once all data has been aligned (X and Y in the present example), a merged assembly of transcripts found in all conditions can be created by listing the cufflinks transcript outputs in a file called assemblies.txt (**step 2**), and running cuffmerge (**step 3**).

Cuffdiff2 Step 2. Create the assemblies.txt file that identifies the cufflinks transcripts to be merged in **step 3**.

```
<path>/cufflinks_X/transcripts.gtf
<path>/cufflinks_Y/transcripts.gtf
```

Cuffdiff2 Step 3. Script to run cuffmerge on the set of transcripts in the file assemblies.txt created in **step 2**. Note that the results are written to the directory merged_XY.

```
#!/bin/sh
gtffile="<path>/Mus_musculus/Ensembl/NCBIM37/Annotation/
Genes/genes.gtf"
```

```
fastafile="<path>/Mus_musculus/Ensembl/NCBIM37/Sequence/
WholeGenomeFasta/genome.fa"

cuffmerge -o merged_XY -g $gtffile -s $fastafile -p 4
assemblies.txt
```

The merged X–Y assembly and the aligned reads in X and Y are inputs to cuffdiff which performs the differential expression analysis (**step 4**). This step is very computationally intensive, and can be time consuming even when using 4 cores (-p 4 option).

Cuffdiff2 Step 4. Script to run cuffdiff on the mapped reads in data sets X and Y using the merged transcript file created in **step 3**. Note that the labels X and Y in –L X,Y should be replaced by something more meaningful such as wild type and knockout (–L WT,KO), and that the results are written to the directory cuffdiff_XY.

```
#!/bin/sh
fastafile="<path>/Mus_musculus/Ensembl/NCBIM37/Sequence/
WholeGenomeFasta/genome.fa"

cuffdiff -o cuffdiff_XY -b $fastafile -p 4 -L X,Y -u
merged_XY/merged.gtf \          ./tophat_X/accepted_hits.bam
./tophat_Y/accepted_hits.bam
```

The final step of the Cuffdiff analysis is performed in R using the Cummerbund library. **Step 5** shows the creation of the cuffdiff database object and the extraction of significant genes and isoforms from it. R version 3.2.1 was used here; note that earlier versions of R will not load Cummerbund v2.8.2. Additional details can be found in [7].

Cuffdiff2 Step 5. R code calling methods in Cummerbund to create the cuffmerge database and to extract significant genes and isoforms.

```
cuffData      <-      readCufflinks(dir="<path>/cuffdiff_XY",
gtfFile="<path>/merged_XY/merged.gtf",
genome="mm9", rebuild=TRUE);

sigGenes              <- getSig(cuffData,level='genes',al
pha=0.05);
sigIsoforms    <- getSig(cuffData,level='isoforms',al
pha=0.05);
```

3.3.2 DESeq2 Protocol

The DESeq2 [3] analysis also requires the reads in each dataset to be aligned to the genome. The alignment performed in **step 1** of the Cuffdiff protocol can be used. It is necessary to count the reads assigned to each gene to generate a table of raw counts, and this can be performed with htseq-count (v0.6.1p1) as shown in **step 1**.

DESeq2 Step 1. Command to generate counts per gene using htseq-count using the reads mapped by bowtie2 in **step 1** of the

Cuffdiff2 protocol. Note that the final lines in X_counts.tsv contain run information.

```
$htseq-count -s no -f bam ./tophat_X/accepted_hits.bam     \
<path>/Mus_musculus/Ensembl/NCBIM37/Annotation/Genes/
genes.gtf > X_counts.tsv
```

DESeq2 Step 2. R code calling methods in DESeq2 to create a data table from the htseq-count output files, run the DESeq analysis, and order the results by p value.

```
sampleTable <- data.frame(sampleName = c("WT","KO"),
                          fileName = c("X_counts.tsv",
                          "Y_counts.tsv"),
                          condition =  c("untreated",
                          "treated"));
htseq <- DESeqDataSetFromHTSeqCount(sampleTable = sampleTable,
                          directory = <path>,
                          design= ~ condition);
colData(htseq)$condition <- factor(colData(htseq)$condition,
                          levels=c("untreated","treated"));
htseq <- DESeq(htseq);
result <- results(htseq);
result <- result[order(result$pvalue),];
```

The remainder of the analysis is performed in R using the DESeq2 library. **Step 2** shows the creation of the count object

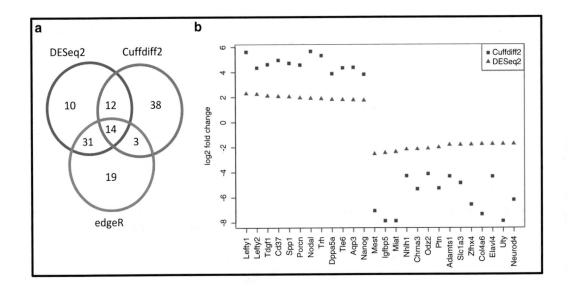

Fig. 1 Transcriptome changes in ES cells upon Wt1 knockout: (**a**) Venn diagram representation of the number of differentially regulated genes identified by the three different tools used for analysis, DESeq2, Cuffdiff2, and EdgeR. (**b**) Differential regulation of gene expression in Wt1 knockout cells compared to the ES cells represented as log2 fold change. Data points represent analysis by DESeq2 (*red triangles*) and Cuffdiff2 (*blue squares*)

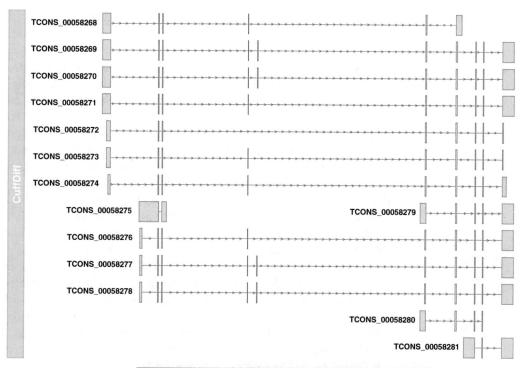

No.	Isoform Id	KTS
1	TCONS_00058269	Present
2	TCONS_00058270	Present
3	TCONS_00058272	Present
4	TCONS_00058273	Present
5	TCONS_00058276	Present
6	TCONS_00058278	Present
7	TCONS_00058279	Present
8	TCONS_00058271	Not present
9	TCONS_00058274	Not present
10	TCONS_00058277	Not present
11	TCONS_00058281	Not present
12	TCONS_00058268	No exon 9
13	TCONS_00058275	No exon 9
14	TCONS_00058280	No exon 9

Fig. 2 RNA sequencing approach identifies Wt1 isoforms in ES cells: Different isoforms of Wt1 identified in the ES cells are represented with their identification numbers. The table represents information of the presence or absence of KTS in the above isoforms

from the output files of htseq-count, running the analysis, and extracting the results.

3.4 Results

Cuffdiff2 identified 67 regulated genes, including 24 upregulated and 43 downregulated genes (using a generous alpha value of 0.2). DESeq2 did not identify any significantly changed genes (all adjusted p values were >0.9) and Cuffdiff2 did not identify any isoforms with significant changes in the E14 data. To compare DESeq2 with Cuffdiff2, a set of the highest confidence genes (those with the highest regularized log 2 fold change calculated by DESeq2) of the same size as the set calculated by Cuffdiff2 was created. As a further comparison, edgeR [5] was run using a single value for dispersion estimated from the two samples available. The results of edgeR were filtered by p value to create a gene set of size 67: the intersection of the three sets of results is shown in Fig. 1a.

The differences in estimates of fold change calculated by DESeq2 and Cuffdiff2 are illustrated in Fig. 1b, where it can be seen that DESeq2 has reduced the fold changes to moderated values of approximately +2 or −2 from the greater estimates that follow from the read counts more directly. The alternative isoforms of Wt1 identified by Cuffdiff2 are shown in Fig. 2. There is sufficient information in the isoform annotation to identify those isoforms that contain the KTS sequence, those that do not, and those that lack exon 9. Wt1 isoforms are typically reduced in expression in the KO condition, some considerably; however, the Cuffdiff2 statistical model does not assign a significant adjusted p value.

4   Notes

1. Good-quality RNA is absolutely essential for an informative sequencing experiment. Although most sequencing experiments have now been modified so as to use starting material of very low nanogram concentration as well as to include formalin-fixed, paraffin-embedded (FFPE) samples, a good coverage can be guaranteed only from reasonably well-concentrated samples with a good RNA integrity number (RIN) value.

2. The agreement between DESeq2 and Cuffdiff2 is 34% for the data set analysed. Given the small number of genes identified, a practical strategy would be to consider the union of genes called as having (more) significant changes, and to consider the wider set called by edgeR. Considering the analysis in [1] we can conclude that the discrepancy (and lack of significant genes called by DESeq2) is most likely due to the lack of biological replicates, a common situation in exploratory studies. Hence, if possible, it is always advised to sequence replicates.

References

1. Zhang ZH, Jhaveri DJ, Marshall VM et al (2014) A comparative study of techniques for differential expression analysis on RNA-Seq data. PLoS One. doi:10.1371/journal.pone.0103207

2. Anders S, Huber W (2010) Differential expression analysis for sequence count data. Genome Biol 11:R106

3. Love IM, Anders S, Huber W (2014) Moderated estimation of fold change and dispersion for RNA-seq data with DESeq2. Genome Biol 15:550

4. Trapnell C, Hendrickson DG, Sauvageau M et al (2013) Differential analysis of gene regulation at transcript resolution with RNA-seq. Nat Biotechnol 31(1):46–54

5. Robinson MD, McCarthy DJ, Smyth GK (2010) edgeR: a Bioconductor package for differential expression analysis of digital gene expression data. Bioinformatics 26:139–140

6. Spraggon L, Dudnakova T, Slight J et al (2007) hnRNP-U directly interacts with WT1 and modulates WT1 transcriptional activation. Oncogene 26(10):1484–1491

7. Trapnell C, Roberts A, Goff L et al (2012) Differential gene expression and transcript expression analysis of RNA-seq experiments with TopHat and Cufflinks. Nat Protoc 7(3):562–578

8. Roberts A, Pimentel H, Trapnell C et al (2011) Identification of novel transcripts in annotated genomes using RNA-Seq. Bioinformatics 27(17):2325–2329

Chapter 19

Immunotherapy Targeting WT1: Designing a Protocol for WT1 Peptide-Based Cancer Vaccine

Sumiyuki Nishida and Haruo Sugiyama

Abstract

There is much current excitement about the potential of cancer immunotherapy. WT1 is high on the National Cancer Institute's list of priority antigens for immune therapy. In this chapter we describe a protocol for a clinical trial using a WT1 peptide-based cancer vaccine.

Key words Cancer immunotherapy, Peptide-based vaccines, Dendritic cells, Cytotoxic T-lymphocytes, Clinical trials

1 Introduction

The immune system evolved to distinguish self and nonself and to effectively protect the individual from microorganisms, many of which cause diseases, and the resulting damage; the immune system also protects us against cancers and toxins, in order to help maintain our normal activities [1]. Cancer cells are self-cells with aberrant growth potential, acquired as a result of several gene abnormalities [2]. The idea that the immune system could control cancer growth has been discussed for over a century. "Evading immune destruction" has been recently added in the hallmarks of cancer, proposed by Hanahan and Weinberg in 2011 [2]. We clinically encounter cancer cells that have escaped from immune surveillance. Recent progress in cancer immunity has been answering questions about how the immune system is involved in the process of cancer formation [3], and whether immunotherapy eliminates cancer cells that have undergone immune escape.

The identification of MAGE-A1 in melanoma patients, described as the first cancer antigen by Boon et al. in 1991 [4], opened the door to antigen-specific cancer immunotherapies from nonspecific ones such as immune-adjuvants [5, 6] and cytokines [7]. During the next two decades, many cancer antigens have been identified, including

Nicholas Hastie (ed.), *The Wilms' Tumor (WT1) Gene: Methods and Protocols*, Methods in Molecular Biology, vol. 1467,
DOI 10.1007/978-1-4939-4023-3_19, © Springer Science+Business Media New York 2016

WT1, leading to the development of more effective cancer immunotherapies [8–10]. Currently, cancer immunotherapy is expected for the fourth most common cancer therapy, behind surgical resection, radiotherapy, and chemotherapies (including molecular target agents).

There are several methods for cancer immunotherapy targeting WT1, including peptide-based and dendritic cell (DC)-based cancer vaccines [11, 12]. In this chapter, we present the protocol of clinical trial using a WT1 peptide-based cancer vaccine.

2 Principle of Peptide-Based Cancer Vaccine

In most of cancer immunotherapy, the key process involves exploiting the intrinsic capacity of dendritic cells (DCs) in vivo or ex vivo in order to induce antigen-specific T-cell responses [13–15]. Peptide-based cancer vaccines, which are simple and easily adapted to a variety of cancer patients, are widely used in clinical trials. The principles of peptide-based cancer vaccines, which consist of HLA class I-restricted peptide and immune adjuvant, are as follows (Fig. 1) [16, 17].

1. HLA class I-restricted peptides are injected intradermally or subcutaneously along with some immune adjuvant. Peptides bind to the HLA class I molecules on the surface of DCs, or are taken up and presented on the cell surface along with HLA class I molecules by immature DCs. Immune adjuvant injected at the same time stimulates immature DCs in peripheral tissues.

2. These activated DCs migrate via lymphatics to regional lymph nodes, where they arrive as fully mature DCs that express both antigen/HLA-molecule complexes and costimulatory molecules necessary to stimulate antigen-specific T-lymphocytes.

3. Antigen-specific T-lymphocytes, especially CD8+ cytotoxic T-lymphocytes (CTLs), are stimulated to proliferate and differentiate by mature DCs and form a clone of effecter cells.

4. Ultimately, antigen-specific CTLs enter the tumor bed, and kill the targeted cancer cells by inducing apoptosis and releasing specialized cytotoxic granules, such as perforin and granzymes, upon recognition of the antigen on the surfaces of tumor cells.

3 Indications for WT1 Peptide-Based Cancer Vaccine: Essential Eligibility Criteria

Two criteria are particularly important for the clinical trial of the WT1 peptide-based cancer vaccine. The first is "whether cancer cells express the *WT1* gene". Peptide-based cancer vaccines are theoretically adapted to cancers expressing these antigens. In this

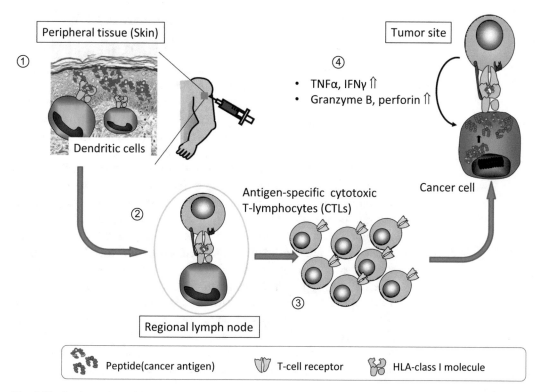

Fig. 1 Mechanism of peptide-based cancer vaccines. Cancer cells express some antigens recognized by the host immune system, and present the peptide derived from this antigen/HLA class I complex on the cell surface. Antigen-specific cytotoxic lymphocytes that are elicited by peptide-based cancer vaccines recognize peptide/HLA class I complexes via the T-cell receptor (TCR)

1. Injection of cancer antigen and immune adjuvant
2. Migration to lymph node and presentation of cancer antigen to T-cells; antigen-specific cytotoxic T-lymphocytes (CTLs)
3. Proliferation and differentiation of T-lymphocytes
4. Cytotoxicity mediated by antigen-specific CTLs

regard, WT1 peptide-based cancer vaccine is a high priority; because most malignancies express the *WT1* gene at high level, as described elsewhere in this book, such a vaccine could be adapted to a wide range of cancers [11, 18–21]. The second consideration is "which type of HLA molecules the patient has". A particular peptide may not bind to all HLA molecules. The WT1 gene products (peptides) are presented by HLA class I molecules on the surface of DCs and cancer cells; CTLs recognize this peptide/HLA class I molecule complex through the antigen-specific T-cell receptor (TCR), which activates T-lymphocytes in cooperation with costimulatory molecules. The peptides that can be used as CTL epitopes are therefore restricted by their binding to specific HLA molecules. For example, 9-mer $WT1_{126}$ peptide (RMFPNAPYL) [22, 23] and 9-mer $WT1_{235}$ peptide (CMTWNQMNL) [24] are restricted to bind HLA-A*02:01, and HLA-A*24:02, respectively.

WT1$_{126}$ peptide and modified WT1$_{235}$ peptide (CYTWNQMNL) [25] have been widely used in clinical trials and analysis of WT1-specific CTL responses, because about 50% of Caucasians and 20% of Japanese possess HLA-A*02:01, and about 60% of Japanese and 20% of Caucasians have HLA-A*24:02.

Other important considerations in planning peptide-based cancer vaccine regimens include the extent of disease and the immune condition of the patient. It seems obvious that as cancer burden grows larger, immunity will grow weaker, leading to a smaller clinical effect. Thus, better physical and immunologic conditions are required in order to obtain better clinical outcomes. The number of absolute lymphocytes, or the ratio of neutrophils and lymphocytes in the peripheral blood [26], and the density and location of immune cells infiltrated within the cancer, called the "immune score" [27] are candidate biomarkers associated with better clinical outcome. The number and phenotype of WT1-specific CTLs and the delayed-type hypersensitivity (DTH) to WT1 peptides are, of course, the most important biomarkers following vaccinations with WT1 peptides, although these factors are not prospective [17, 28, 29]. Further studies are necessary to validate them as important and useful biomarkers in clinical studies of cancer immunotherapies, including WT1 peptide-based cancer vaccine.

4 Preparation of WT1 Peptide-Based Cancer Vaccine

Peptide-based vaccines generally consist of peptides and immune adjuvants. Peptides can be further divided into two groups: HLA-restricted short peptides, and non-HLA-restricted long peptides [30]. A majority of clinical studies of cancer immunotherapies targeting WT1 have used HLA-restricted short peptide-based vaccines. In this section, we describe how to prepare the WT1 peptide-based cancer vaccines in our clinical setting.

1. Peptides: HLA-restricted short peptides are used; specifically, HLA-A*24:02-restricted modified 9-mer WT1$_{235}$ peptide and/or HLA-A*02:01-restricted 9-mer WT1$_{126}$ peptide. The doses of peptide are usually 3 mg/body, although the recommended doses (RD) of the peptides have not been determined in dose-escalation studies [28, 31]. In our recent studies, HLA class II-restricted peptides (WT1$_{332}$ peptide: KRYFKLSHLQMHSRKH [32]), which are designed to stimulate CD4$^+$ helper T-lymphocytes, are also used alone or in combination with HLA class I-restricted peptides.

2. Adjuvants: Immune adjuvants are materials that enhance the immune response. Their functions can be broadly divided into two categories: (1) transport medium, by which antigen presenting cells (APCs), including DCs, engulf vaccine antigens

effectively; and (2) immune modulator. The latter role is the more important of the two. The activation of DCs through the pattern recognition receptors (PRRs), such as Toll-like receptors (TLRs), is the most important process and is crucial for initiating the innate immunity response: such signaling makes immature DCs, whose sole function is to capture microbes and the dead cells, differentiate into mature DCs, which can process and present their antigens to T-lymphocytes in regional lymph nodes [33–35]. Immune adjuvants work like pathogen-associated molecular patterns (PAMPs) and damage-associated molecular pattern (DAMPs) to activate DCs. Different adjuvants are currently used in therapeutic vaccines [35]. Montanide ISA51, called incomplete Freund's adjuvant, is one of the most frequently used immune adjuvants for peptide-based cancer vaccines [28]. Keyhole limpet hemocyanin (KLH) [36–39], GM-CSF [30, 36, 37, 40], BCG-CWS [41], imiquimod [42], and CpG-oligodendronucleotide (CpG-ODN) [43, 44], which stimulate tissue-resident DCs to induce stronger immune response, are also often used in clinical studies of WT1 peptide-based cancer vaccine.

3. Products: We describe the vaccine product frequently used in our clinical setting as follows: 3 mg of WT1 peptide is dissolved in a small volume of dimethyl sulfoxide (DMSO), and then the peptide solution is diluted to 400 μl with 5 % glucose. Ultimately, the mixture is emulsified with an equal weight of Montanide ISA51 adjuvant [28].

5 Treatment Schedule for WT1 Peptide-Based Cancer Vaccine Alone

A standardized treatment schedule has not been ascertained in terms of number and frequency of vaccinations. Vaccination frequently ranges from weekly to monthly administration [12]. However, no controlled study has investigated which schedule is better for inducing the immune response and exerting clinical effects. In our original study, which was reported in 2004 [28], WT1 peptide-based cancer vaccines were administrated biweekly over a 2-months protocol, followed by administration every 1–2 months. Next, we investigated the safety of weekly vaccination for 3 months, followed by biweekly or monthly vaccinations. It remains unknown which schedule is better, although no grade 3 or higher treatment-related toxicity was observed during weekly administration [31, 45, 46].

In our recent study, the WT1 peptide-based cancer vaccine contains both HLA class I and class II short peptides; for each, the dose is 2 mg/body. Vaccines are administered biweekly to boost the immune response for the first 3 months, and then monthly to maintain the immune response induced by the first vaccinations.

6   Combination Therapies with WT1 Peptide-Based Cancer Vaccine

Cancer immunotherapies targeting WT1 are expected to be used in combination with generally used cancer therapies, such as surgery, radiotherapy, and chemotherapy, because there is no cross-reaction between these modalities in terms of toxicity. However, it may be difficult to decide a suitable treatment schedule for the combination therapies, because each conventional therapy differs in terms of immunogenic or immunosuppressive aspects. Here, we describe some treatment schedules used in our studies.

1. Combination therapy with gemcitabine for advanced pancreatic cancer [29, 47, 48]

   Gemcitabine, a nucleotide analogue and the key cytotoxic agent for the treatment of the pancreatic cancer, has been recently evaluated for its immunogenic functions in the combination with cancer immunotherapies. The immunogenic effects of gemcitabine at clinical doses are follows: (1) elevation of the expression of HLA class I molecules on the surface of cancer cells; (2) enhancement of cross-presentation of cancer antigens to CD8+ cytotoxic T-lymphocytes; and (3) selective killing of myeloid-derived suppressor cells (MDSCs) [49, 50]. These effects are expected to facilitate T-cell-dependent anticancer immunity, although the detailed molecular mechanisms of immunomodulation by gemcitabine remain unknown. In our clinical study, WT1 peptide-based cancer vaccine, which consists of 3 mg of peptide and the immune adjuvant Montanide, is administered on day 1 and 15 of a 28 days schedule in combination with the standard gemcitabine (1000 mg/m², day 1, 8, and 15 every 28 days) for advanced pancreatic cancer [29].

2. Combination therapy with imatinib for chronic myeloid leukemia (CML) [51, 52]

   Imatinib mesylate inhibits tyrosine kinase encoded by the *bcr-abl* oncogene, resulting in decreased proliferation and enhanced apoptosis in the cells of Philadelphia-positive (Ph+) hematological malignancies such as CML and acute lymphoblastic leukemia (ALL).

   The immunogenic or immunosuppressive functions of imatinib remain unclear. However, WT1 peptide-based cancer vaccine, which consists of 3 mg of peptide and the immune adjuvant Montanide, has been combined with imatinib (400–600 mg/day) for the treatment of CML in the chronic phase [51].

3. Maintenance therapy to preserve complete remission after complete surgical resection or chemotherapy

At lower tumor load, cancer immunotherapy is predicted to be more effective [53]. Moreover, because peptide-based cancer vaccine seems less toxic than other modalities, it may be acceptable to use them as the maintenance therapies after complete remission. However, it remains unclear how many times the vaccinations should be performed, and how long they should be continued, in these situations. For some cancers with higher relapse rates, the maintenance should be continued at least until the patient has surpassed the progression-free survival time reported elsewhere, even if tumor has been resected completely.

7 Maintenance Therapies with WT1 Peptide-Based Cancer Vaccine After Allogeneic Hematopoietic Stem Cell Transplantation

When designing therapy that combines allogeneic hematopoietic stem cell transplantation (allo-HSCT) with WT1 peptide-based cancer vaccine, it is necessary to consider the unique immunological conditions following allo-HSCT. In order to engraft the hematopoietic cells without rejection, lymphocytes derived from the recipients are completely ablated by conditioning therapies. This lymphoablation leads to lymphopenia-induced proliferation of lymphocytes derived from the donor grafts, which is called "homeostatic proliferation" [54–56]. Homeostatic proliferation facilitates and enhances the proliferation not only of T-lymphocytes that respond to nonself-antigens but also of those that respond to low-affinity self-antigens expressed in cancer cells; this process is called "GVL-oligoclonal expansion" (GVL: graft-versus-leukemia) [57]. In this immunologic environment, we can expect that the vaccinations against cancer antigens induce stronger antigen-specific CTL responses and generate long-lived memory T-lymphocytes. Several preclinical murine models have evaluated the effect of lymphoablation in combination with cancer antigen-specific vaccinations, which allow for rapid expansion of antigen-specific CTLs [58, 59]. These findings allow us to carry out maintenance therapies with WT1 peptide-based cancer vaccine after allo-HSCT, especially for patients who are still at high risk of relapse [60, 61].

Our group and others recently reported promising results in maintenance therapies with WT1 peptide-based vaccines, albeit in small early-phase studies [62–64]. Both basic and clinical investigations are also necessary to establish the post-HSCT therapeutic strategies, which provide the maximum immunological anti-cancer effect induced by WT1 peptide-based cancer vaccine.

8   Observed or Expected Adverse Events Related to WT1 Peptide-Based Cancer Vaccine

Adverse events related to cancer immunotherapies targeting WT1 have been reported in several clinical studies [28–31, 36–48, 51–53, 62–76]. The most frequent is skin toxicity, such as redness, erythema, and induration, at vaccine injection sites. Although these reactions are, in general, well-tolerated, local inflammatory reactions occasionally form ulcers, which are sometimes difficult to treat locally with steroid ointment [48].

Systemic adverse events which are related to autoimmunity elicited by immunotherapy targeting WT1 occasionally occur, because WT1 is also expressed in normal tissues, such as kidney and hematopoietic cells [11]. We observed some severe adverse events, including hematologic toxicities (such as neutropenia and thrombocytopenia) [28] and interstitial pneumonitis, in patients treated with WT1 vaccine. The main treatment for these adverse events is immunosuppressive therapy with a steroid (e.g. prednisone 0.5–1.0 mg/kg), for which the appropriate dose should be determined by the degree or extent of adverse events.

Although immunotherapy targeting WT1 could cause more severe hematologic adverse events in combination with chemotherapies, because of the high expression of WT1 in hematopoietic progenitor cells, these adverse events have not been reported to be more frequent and serious than those of monotherapies with cytotoxic agents such as gemcitabine [29, 47, 48].

9   Future Perspectives

Elicited immune responses are theoretically expected to eradicate cancer cells; however, the clinical effects of cancer vaccines, including objective response and survival, have been disappointing in most clinical studies [77]. The clinical effects of WT1 peptide-based cancer vaccines are also still limited, although they could induce the immune response in cancer patients. We must overcome at least two hurdles inhibiting these immune responses to improve their clinical effects: one is the escape from immunity by cancer cells (e.g., antigen loss, insensitivity to immune effector mechanisms, or an immunosuppressive state within the cancer microenvironment), especially in the patients with advanced cancer [3, 78, 79], and the other is the normal expression of inhibitory molecules (called the "immune checkpoint") on effector T-lymphocytes which act as a brake on the immune system by preventing T-cell activation [80]. To overcome these hurdles and to enhance the immune response elicited by vaccination, several tools have been proposed and tested in basic and clinical studies [81].

1. Multiple peptides, both HLA class I and class II peptides as well as long-peptides, both of which are expected to elicit stronger and more durable WT1-specific CTL response [30, 32, 82–85].

2. Clinical application of new immune adjuvants based on the molecular biosciences, e.g., poly I:C (TLR2 stimulator), CpG-ODN (TLR9 stimulator), and so on [33, 35, 43, 44].

3. Clinical use of the new technique for adoptive T-cell transfer (ACT), in which a gene encoding WT1-specific TCR is transduced into T-lymphocytes isolated from the patient [86, 87].

4. Combination therapy with the immune checkpoint inhibitors such as ipilimumab (anti-CTLA-4 antibody) and nivolumab (anti-PD-1 antibody) [80, 88].

WT1 peptide-based cancer vaccines have been demonstrated to be feasible in patients with several kinds of cancers. These vaccines elicited WT1-specific CTLs and exhibited promising clinical effects, such as improvement of survival time. These clinical results, however, are from small early-phase clinical trials. In the near future, we should see verification of the clinical effects of cancer immunotherapy targeting WT1 in late-phase randomized clinical trials. Furthermore, combination immunotherapy using several tools, including cancer vaccines, antibodies that inhibit immune checkpoints, immune adjuvants, and molecular target agents to modify immunity, is expected to become a central player in the cancer treatment.

References

1. Kenneth Murphy et al (2011) Janeway's immunobiology, 8th edn. Grand Science.

2. Hanahan D, Weinberg RA (2011) Hallmarks of cancer: the next generation. Cell 144:646–674

3. Schreiber RD, Old LJ, Smyth MJ (2011) Cancer immunoediting: integrating immunity's roles in cancer suppression and promotion. Science 331:1565–1570

4. Van der Bruggen P, Traversari C, Boon T et al (1991) A gene encoding an antigen recognized by cytotoxic T lymphocytes on a human melanoma. Science 254:1643–1647

5. Reed SG, Bertholet S, Coler RN et al (2009) New horizons in adjuvants for vaccine development. Trends Immunol 30:23–32

6. Mbow ML, De Gregorio E, Valiante NM et al (2010) New adjuvants for human vaccines. Curr Opin Immunol 22:411–416

7. Banchereau J, Pascual V, O'Garra A et al (2012) From IL-2 to IL-37: the expanding spectrum of anti-inflammatory cytokines. Nat Immunol 13:925–931

8. Vigneron N, Stroobant V, Van den Eynde BJ et al (2013) Database of T cell-defined human tumor antigens: the 2013 update. Cancer Immun 13:15

9. Coulie PG, Van den Eynde BJ, van der Bruggen P et al (2014) Tumour antigens recognized by T lymphocytes: at the core of cancer immunotherapy. Nat Rev Cancer 14:135–146

10. Cheever MA, Allison JP, Ferris AS et al (2009) The prioritization of cancer antigens: a national cancer institute pilot project for the acceleration of translational research. Clin Cancer Res 15:5323–5337

11. Sugiyama H (2010) WT1 (Wilms' tumor gene 1): biology and cancer immunotherapy. Jpn J Clin Oncol 40:377–387

12. Van Driessche A, Berneman ZN, Van Tendeloo VF (2012) Active specific immunotherapy targeting the Wilms' tumor protein 1 (WT1) for patients with hematological malignancies and solid tumors: lessons from early clinical trials. Oncologist 17:250–259

13. Rosenberg SA (2001) Progress in human tumour immunology and immunotherapy. Nature 411:380–384

14. Paulucka H, Banchereau J (2012) Cancer immunotherapy via dendritic cells. Nat Rev Cancer 12:265–277

15. Alatrash G, Jakher H, Stafford PD et al (2013) Cancer immunotherapies, their safety and toxicity. Expert Opin Drug Saf 12:631–645

16. Melief CJ, Kast WM (1995) T-cell immunotherapy of tumors by adoptive transfer of cytotoxic T lymphocytes and by vaccination with minimal essential epitopes. Immunol Rev 145:167–177

17. Oka Y, Tsuboi A, Oji Y et al (2008) WT1 peptide vaccine for the treatment of cancer. Curr Opin Immunol 20:211–220

18. Miwa H, Beran M, Aunders GF (1992) Expression of the Wilms' tumor gene (WT1) in human leukemias. Leukemia 6:405–409

19. Inoue K, Sugiyama H, Ogawa H et al (1994) WT1 as new prognostic factor a new marker for the detection of minimal residual disease in acute leukemia. Blood 84:3071–3079

20. Oji Y, Ogawa H, Tamaki H, Oka Y, Tsuboi A, Sugiyama H et al (1999) Expression of the Wilms' tumor gene WT1 in solod tumors and its involvement in tumor cell growth. Jpn J Cancer Res 90:194–204

21. Nakatsuka S, Oji Y, Sugiyama H et al (2006) Immunohistochemical detection of WT1 protein in a variety of cancer cells. Mod Pathol 19:804–814

22. Oka Y, Elisseeva OA, Tsuboi A, Sugiyama H et al (2000) Human cytotoxic T-lymphocyte responses specific for peptides of the wild-type Wilms' tumor gene (WT1) product. Immunogenetics 51:99–107

23. Gao L, Bellantuono I, Elsasser A et al (2000) Selective elimination of leukemic CD34 (+) progenitor cells by cytotoxic T lymphocytes specific for WT1. Blood 95:2198–2203

24. Ohminami H, Yasukawa M, Fujita S (2000) HLA class I-restricted lysis of leukemia cells by a CD8 (+) cytotoxic T-lymphocyte clone specific for WT1 peptide. Blood 95:286–293

25. Tsuboi A, Oka Y, Udaka K, Sugiyama H et al (2002) Enhanced induction of human WT1-specific cytotoxic T lymphocytes with a 9-mer WT1 peptide modified at HLA-A*2402-binding residues. Cancer Immunol Immunother 51:614–620

26. Takakura K, Koido S, Kan S, Sugiyama H et al (2015) Prognostic markers for patient outcome following vaccination with multiple MHC Class I/II-restricted WT1 peptide-pulsed dendritic cells plus chemotherapy for pancreatic cancer. Anticancer Res 35:556–562

27. Galon J, Mlecnik B, Bindea G et al (2014) Towards the induction of the 'Immunoscore' in the classification of malignant tumours. J Pathol 232:199–209

28. Oka Y, Tsuboi A, Taguchi T et al (2004) Induction of WT1 (Wilms' tumor gene)-specific cytotoxic T lymphocytes by WT1 peptide vaccine and the resultant cancer regression. Proc Natl Acad Sci U S A 101:13885–13890

29. Nishida S, Koido S, Takeda Y et al (2014) Wilms' tumor gene (WT1) peptide-based cancer vaccine combined with gemcitabine for patients with advanced pancreatic cancer. J Immunother 37:105–114

30. Maslak PG, Dao T, Krug LM et al (2010) Vaccination with synthetic analog peptides derived from WT1 oncoprotein induces T-cell responses in patients with complete remission from acute myeloid leukemia. Blood 116:171–179

31. Morita S, Oka Y, Tsuboi A et al (2006) A phase I/II trial of a WT1 (Wilms' tumor gene) peptide vaccine in patients with solid malignancy: safety assessment based on the phase I data. Jpn J Clin Oncol 36:231–236

32. Fujiki F, Oka Y, Kawakatsu M et al (2008) A WT1 protein-derived, naturally processed 16-mer peptide, $WT1_{332}$, is a promiscuous helper peptide for induction of WT1-specific Th1-type CD4[+] T cells. Microbiol Immunol 52:591–600

33. Ishii KJ, Akira S (2007) Toll or toll-free adjuvant path toward the optimal vaccine development. J Clin Immunol 27:363–371

34. Palm NW, Medzhitov R (2009) Pattern recognition receptors and control of adaptive immunity. Immunol Rev 227:221–233

35. Kawai T, Akira S (2010) The role of pattern-recognition receptors in innate immunity: update on Toll-like receptors. Nat Immunol 11:373–384

36. Keilholz U, Letsch A, Busse A et al (2009) A clinical and immunologic phase 2 trial of Wilms' tumor gene product 1 (WT1) peptide vaccination in patients with AML and MDS. Blood 113:6541–6548

37. Rezvani K, Yong AS, Mielke S et al (2008) Leukemia-associated antigen-specific T-cell responses following combined PR1 and WT1 peptide vaccination in patients with myeloid malignancies. Blood 111:236–242

38. Kitawaki T, Kadowaki N, Kondo T et al (2008) Potential of dendritic cell immunotherapy for relapse after allogenic hematopoietic stem cell transplantation, shown by WT1 peptide-and keyhole limpet hemocyanin-pulsed, donor-derived dendritic-cell vaccine for acute myeloid leukemia. Am J Hematol 83:315–317

39. Van Tendeloo VF, van de Velde A, van Driessche A et al (2010) Induction of complete and molecular remissions in acute myeloid leukemia by Wilms' tumor 1 antigen-targeted dendritic cell vaccination. Proc Natl Acad Sci U S A 107:13824–13829

40. Krug LM, Dao T, Brown AB et al (2010) WT1 peptide vaccinations induce CD4 and CD8 T cell immune responses in patients with mesothelioma and non-small cell lung cancer. Cancer Immunol Immunother 59:1467–1479

41. Nishioka M, Tanemura A, Nishida S et al (2012) Vaccination with WT-1 (Wilms' tumor gene-1) peptide and BCG-CWS in melanoma. Eur J Dermatol 22:258–259

42. Coosemans A, Wölfl M, Berneman ZN et al (2010) Immunological response after therapeutic vaccination with WT1 mRNA-loaded dendritic cells in end-stage endometrial carcinoma. Anticancer Res 30:3709–3714

43. Kuball J, de Boer K, Wagner E et al (2011) Pitfalls of vaccinations with WT1-, Proteinase3- and MUC1-derived peptides in combination with MontanideISA51 and CpG7909. Cancer Immunol Immunother 60:161–171

44. Ohno S, Okuyama R, Aruga A et al (2012) Phase I trial of Wilms' Tumor 1 (WT1) peptide vaccine with GM-CSF or CpG in patients with solid malignancy. Anticancer Res 32:2263–2269

45. Izumoto S, Tsuboi A, Oka Y et al (2008) Phase II clinical trial of Wilms' tumor 1 peptide vaccination for patients with recurrent glioblastoma multiforme. J Neurosurg 108:963–971

46. Miyatake T, Ueda Y, Morimoto A et al (2013) WT1 peptide immunotherapy for gynecologic malignancies resistant to conventional therapies: a phase II trial. J Cancer Res Clin Oncol 139:457–463

47. Koido S, Homma S, Okamoto M et al (2014) Treatment with chemotherapy and dendritic cells pulsed with multiple Wilms' tumor 1 (WT1)-specific MHC class I/II-restricted epitopes for pancreatic cancer. Clin Cancer Res 20:4228–4239

48. Kaida M, Morita-Hoshi Y, Soeda A et al (2011) Phase 1 trial of Wilms' tumor 1 (WT1) peptide vaccine and gemcitabine combination therapy in patients with advanced pancreatic or biliary tract cancer. J Immunother 34:92–99

49. Nowak AK, Lake RA, Robinson BWS (2006) Combined chemoimmunotherapy of solid tumours: improving vaccines? Adv Drug Deliv Rev 58:975–990

50. Zitvogel L, Apetoh L, Ghiringhelli F et al (2008) Immunological aspects of cancer chemotherapy. Nat Rev Immunol 8:59–73

51. Oji Y, Oka Y, Nishida S et al (2010) WT1 peptide vaccine induces reduction in minimal residual disease in an Imatinib-treated CML patient. Eur J Haematol 85:358–360

52. Narita M, Masuko M, Kurasaki T et al (2010) WT1 peptide vaccination in combination with imatinib therapy for a patient with CML in the chronic phase. Int J Med Sci 7:72–81

53. Tsuboi A, Oka Y, Kyo T et al (2012) Long-term WT1 peptide vaccination for patients with acute myeloid leukemia with minimal residual disease. Leukemia 26:1410–1413

54. Baccala R, Gonzalez-Quintial R, Dummer W et al (2005) Tumor immunity via homeostatic T cell proliferation: mechanistic aspects and clinical perspectives. Springer Semin Immunopathol 27:75–85

55. Williams KM, Hakim FT, Gress RE et al (2008) T cell immune reconstitution following lymphodepletion. Semin Immunol 19:318–330

56. Boyman O, Letourneau S, Krieg C et al (2009) Homeostatic proliferation and survival naïve and memory T cells. Eur J Immunol 39:2088–2094

57. Goldrath AW, Bevan MJ (1999) Low-affinity ligands for the TCR drive proliferation of mature CD8+ T cells in lymphopenic hosts. Immunity 11:183–190

58. Gattinoni L, Finkelstein SE, Klebanoff CA et al (2005) Removal of homeostatic cytokine sinks by lymphodepletion enhances the efficacy of adoptively transferred tumor-specific CD8+ T cells. J Exp Med 202:907–912

59. Borrello I, Sotomayor EM, Rattis FM et al (2000) Sustaining the graft-versus-tumor effect through posttransplant immunization with granulocyte-macrophage colony-stimulating factor (GM-CSF)-producing tumor vaccines. Blood 95:3011–3019

60. Rezvani K (2011) Posttransplantation vaccination: concepts today and on the horizon. Hematology Am Soc Hematol Educ Program 2011:299–304

61. Hosen N, Maeda T, Hashii Y et al (2014) Vaccination strategies to improve outcome of hematopoietic stem cell transplant in leukemia patients: early evidence and future prospects. Expert Rev Hematol 7:671–781

62. Rezvani K, Grube M, Brenchley JM et al (2003) Functional leukemia-associated antigen-specific memory CD8+ T cells exist in healthy individuals and in patients with chronic myelogenous leukemia before and after stem cell transplantation. Blood 102:2892–2900

63. Hashii Y, Sato-Miyashita E, Matsumura R et al (2012) WT1 peptide vaccination following allogeneic stem cell transplantation in pediatric leukemic patients with high risk for relapse: successful maintenance of durable remission. Leukemia 26:530–532

64. Maeda T, Hosen N, Fukushima K et al (2013) Maintenance of complete remission after allogeneic stem cell transplantation in leukemia

patients treated with Wilms' tumor 1 peptide vaccine. Blood Cancer J 3:e130

65. Iiyama T, Udaka K, Takeda S et al (2007) WT1 (Wilms' tumor 1) peptide immunotherapy for renalcell carcinoma. Microbiol Immunol 51:519–530

66. Kawakami M, Oka Y, Tsuboi A et al (2007) Clinical and immunologic response to very low-dose vaccination with WT1 peptide (5 microg/body) in a patients with chronic myelomonocytic leukemia. Int J Hematol 85:426–429

67. Tsuboi A, Oka Y, Nakajima H et al (2007) Wilms' tumor gene WT1 peptide-based immunotherapy induced a minimal response in a patient with advanced therapy-resistant multiple myeloma. Int J Hematol 86:414–417

68. Ohno S, Kyo S, Myojo S et al (2009) Wilms' tumor 1 (WT1) peptide immunotherapy for gynecological malignancy. Anticancer Res 29:4779–4784

69. Ohta H, Hashii Y, Yoneda A et al (2009) WT1 (Wilms' tumor 1) peptide immunotherapy for child hood rhabdomyosarcoma: a case report. Pediatr Hematol Oncol 26:74–83

70. Yasukawa M, Fujiwara H, Ochi T et al (2009) Clinical efficacy of WT1 peptide vaccination in patients with acute myelogenous leukemia and myelodysplastic syndrome. Am J Hematol 84:314–315

71. Hashii Y, Sato E, Ohta H et al (2010) WT1 peptide immunotherapy for cancer in children and young adults. Pediatr Blood Cancer 55:352–355

72. Rezvani K, Yong AS, Mielke S et al (2011) Repeated PR1 and WT1 peptide vaccination in Montanide-adjuvant fails to induce sustained high-avidity, epitope-specific CD8+ T cells in myeloid malignancies. Haematologica 96:432–440

73. Shirakata T, Oka Y, Nishida S et al (2012) WT1 peptide therapy for a patient with chemotherapy-resistant salivary gland cancer. Anticancer Res 32:1081–1085

74. Rezvani K, Yong AS, Mielke S et al (2012) Lymphodepletion is permissive to the development of spontaneous T-cell responses to the self-antigen PR1 early after allogeneic stem cell transplantation and in patients with acute myeloid leukemia undergoing WT1 peptide vaccination following chemotherapy. Cancer Immunol Immunother 61:1125–1136

75. Coosemans A, Vanderstraeten A, Tuyaerts S et al (2013) Immunological response after WT1 mRNA-loaded dendritic cell immunotherapy in ovarian carcinoma and carcinosarcoma. Anticancer Res 33:3855–3859

76. Coosemans A, Vanderstraeten A, Tuyaerts S et al (2013) Wilms' Tumor Gene 1 (WT1)-loaded dendritic cell immunotherapy in patients with uterine tumors: a phase I/II clinical trial. Anticancer Res 33:5495–5500

77. Rosenberg SA, Yang JC, Restifo NP (2004) Cancer immunotherapy: moving beyond current vaccines. Nat Med 10:909–915

78. Zou W (2005) Immunosuppressive networks in the tumour environment and their therapeutic relevance. Nat Rev Cancer 5:263–274

79. Nishikawa H, Sakaguchi S (2014) Regulatory T cells in cancer immunotherapy. Curr Opin Immunol 27:1–7

80. Pardoll DM (2012) The blockade of immune checkpoints in cancer immunotherapy. Nat Rev Cancer 12:252–264

81. Makkouk A, Weiner GJ (2015) Cancer immunotherapy and breaking immune tolerance: new approaches to an old challenge. Cancer Res 75:5–10

82. Janssen E, Lemmens E (2003) CD4+ T cells are required for secondary expansion and memory in CD8+ T lymphocytes. Nature 421:852–856

83. May RJ, Dao T, Pinilla-Ibarz J et al (2007) Peptide epitopes from the Wilms' tumor 1 oncoprotein stimulate CD4+ and CD8+ T cells that recognize and kill human malignant mesothelioma tumor cells. Clin Cancer Res 13:4547–4555

84. Lehe C, Ghebeh H, Al-Sulaiman A et al (2008) The Wilms' tumor antigen is a novel target for human CD4+ regulatory T cells: implications for immunotherapy. Cancer Res 68:6350–6359

85. Anguille S, Fujiki F, Smits EL et al (2013) Identification of a Wilms' tumor 1-derived immunogenic CD4+ T-cell epitope that is recognized in the context of common Caucasian HLA-DR haplotypes. Leukemia 27:748–750

86. Restifo NP, Dudley ME, Rosenberg SA (2012) Adoptive immunotherapy for cancer: harnesting the T cell response. Nat Rev Immunol 12:269–281

87. Ochi T, Fujiwara H, Okamoto S et al (2011) Novel adoptive T-cell immunotherapy using a WT1-specific TCR vector encoding silencers for endogenous TCRs shows marked antileukemia reactivity and safety. Blood 118:1495–1503

88. Gibney GT, Kudchadkar RR, DeConti RC et al (2015) Safety, correlative markers and clinical results of adjuvant nivolumab in combination with vaccine in resected high-risk metastatic melanoma. Clin Cancer Res 21:712–720

INDEX

Nicholas Hastie (ed.), *The Wilms' Tumor (WT1) Gene: Methods and Protocols*, Methods in Molecular Biology, vol. 1467,
DOI 10.1007/978-1-4939-4023-3, © Springer Science+Business Media New York 2016

233

Printed in the United States
By Bookmasters